# CRASH COURSE
# Psychiatry
## SECOND EDITION

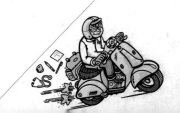

sect² 136 ⟶ public place appearing to display symptoms of / mental disorder.     POLICE

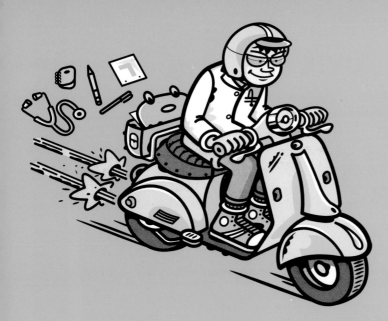

Series editor
**Daniel Horton-Szar**
BSc (Hons), MB BS (Hons)
GP Registrar
Northgate Medical Practice
Canterbury
Kent

Faculty advisor
**MJ Akhtar**
MSc, MBBS, DPM, FRCPsych
Honorary Lecturer
Newcastle University
Consultant Psychiatrist
University Hospital
Hartlepool

# Psychiatry

## SECOND EDITION

## Alasdair D Cameron

MB ChB, MRCPsych
Senior House Officer in Psychiatry
West Hampshire NHS Trust

First Edition Authors
**Darran Bloye, Simon Davies**

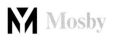 Mosby

Edinburgh • London • New York • Oxford • Philadelphia • St Louis • Sydney • Toronto 2004

MOSBY
An imprint of Elsevier Limited

Commissioning Editors          Alex Stibbe, Fiona Conn
Project Development Manager     Fiona Conn
Project Manager                Frances Affleck
Designer                       Andy Chapman
Illustration Manager           Bruce Hogarth

First edition 1999
Second edition 2004
    Reprinted 2004, 2005, 2006

ISBN 0 7234 3340 2

British Library Cataloguing in Publication Data
A catalogue record for this book is available from the British Library

Library of Congress Cataloguing in Publication Data
A catalogue record for this book is available from the Library of Congress

**Notice**
Medical knowledge is constantly changing. Standard safety precautions must be followed, but
as new research and clinical experience broaden our knowledge, changes in treatment and
drug therapy may become necessary or appropriate. Readers are advised to check the most
current product information provided by the manufacturer of each drug to be administered to
verify the recommended dose, the method and duration of administration, and
contraindications. It is the responsibility of the practitioner, relying on experience and
knowledge of the patient, to determine dosages and the best treatment for each individual
patient. Neither the Publisher nor the author assumes any liability for any injury and/or
damage to persons or property arising from this publication.

*The Publisher*

**ELSEVIER**  your source for books,
journals and multimedia
in the health sciences
**www.elsevierhealth.com**

Working together to grow
libraries in developing countries

www.elsevier.com | www.bookaid.org | www.sabre.org

ELSEVIER   BOOK AID International   Sabre Foundation

The
publisher's
policy is to use
**paper manufactured
from sustainable forests**

Typeset by Kolam, Pondicherry, India
Printed in China

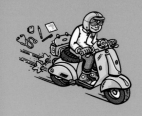

# Preface

After hearing many strong opinions expressed by students new to psychiatry, both positive and negative, I am convinced that the most common stumbling block to attaining a real understanding of the subject is difficulty in grasping some of the basic concepts that underpin it. With that in mind, I set out to write this new edition of Crash Course Psychiatry in a straightforward, unambiguous way, without sacrificing the subtleties that make psychiatry so interesting.

The book is divided into four parts. Part I, 'The Patient Presents With', and Part II, 'Diseases and Disorders', go hand-in-hand, and have been cross-referenced so that you can read them as a complete unit if this is how you prefer to study. An outline of the ICD–10 (*Tenth Revision of the International Classification of Diseases and Related Health Problems*) diagnostic criteria has been provided for many of the important disorders described, as this is the most widely used diagnostic system in Europe. However, I also refer to the DSM-IV (*Fourth Edition of the Diagnostic and Statistical Manual of Mental Disorders*), used predominantly in North America, because in some cases (for example Sleep and Psychosexual Disorders), I found the DSM-IV's criteria more useful to present a broad but brief overview to readers with little background knowledge of the topic. Part III, 'Assessment, Therapy and Service Delivery', deals with psychiatric assessment, pharmacological and psychological therapy, mental health legislation and service delivery. Part IV, 'Self-assessment', includes questions in a variety of formats for exam practice and detailed answers refer back to the original text if you find you need to go over something again.

Wherever possible I have highlighted controversies surrounding definitions and current thinking and have tried to present concisely a common sense approach to these more complicated issues. I hope that this book helps you to get to grips with this fascinating subject.

**Alasdair D Cameron**

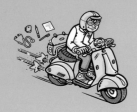

# Preface

Over the last six years since the first editions were published, there have been many changes in medicine, and in the way it is taught. These second editions have been largely rewritten to take these changes into account, and keep *Crash Course* up to date for the twenty-first century. New material has been added to include recent research and all pharmacological and disease management information has been updated in line with current best practice. We've listened to feedback from hundreds of medical students who have been using *Crash Course* and have improved the structure and layout of the books accordingly: pathology and disease management material has been moved closer to the diagnostic skills chapters; there are more MCQs and now we have Extended Matching Questions as well, with explanations of each answer. We have also include 'Further Reading' sections where appropriate to highlight important papers and studies that you should be aware of, and the clarity of text and figures is better than ever.

The principles on which we developed the series remain the same, however. Clinical medicine is a huge subject, and teaching on the wards can sometimes be sporadic because of the competing demands of patient care. The last thing a student needs when finals are approaching is to waste time assembling information from different sources, or wading through pages of irrelevant detail. As before, *Crash Course* brings you all the information you need in compact, manageable volumes that integrate an approach to common patient presentations with clinical skills, pathology and management of the relevant diseases. We still tread the fine line between producing clear, concise text and providing enough detail for those aiming at distinction. The series is still written by junior doctors with recent exam experience, in partnership with senior faculty members from across the UK.

I wish you the best of luck in your future careers!

**Dan Horton-Szar**
**Series Editor**

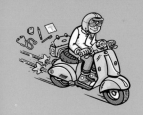

# Acknowledgements

Many people at Elsevier deserve recognition for bringing this book to print and I cannot mention all of them, but I would like to convey my special thanks to: Alex Stibbe, whose personable style and energy sold the 'Crash Course' idea to me and got me up and running; Fiona Conn, who managed to coordinate and synchronize the whole process with remarkable insight and unqualified professionalism; Stephanie Pickering, for her meticulous copy editing; and all those involved with the layout and illustrations. Thanks too to Dan Horton-Szar the Crash Course series editor. It was a joy working with him. His intelligence and application, at such short notice, was a godsend.

From the Department of Health, I would like to acknowledge Neil McIvor, Assistant Statistician, for his help in ensuring that I had the most up-to-date statistics for Chapter 17.

It also gives me great pleasure to thank the consultant psychiatrists in Winchester and Eastleigh who read sections of the book and made invaluable suggestions. These include Dr Eric Chan-Pensley (Chapters 10, 17 and 29), Dr Clio Bellenis (Chapter 23), and Dr Stefano Olivieri (Chapters 9, 16, 24), who, as college tutor, never gave a second thought to restructuring my 'day job' programme so that I could finish this book on time. I would also like to thank the Faculty Advisor, Dr MJ Akthar, and Dr Trevor Turner, for their reviews of the complete manuscript.

Although not directly involved with the writing of this book, I would like to express my appreciation to all my colleagues and friends associated with Melbury Lodge in Winchester and the associated community mental health teams in Winchester, Andover, Eastleigh and Romsey. They have helped shape my thinking, both as a psychiatrist and as a person.

All of the above helped to make this book better than it would otherwise have been. They are not responsible, however, for any of its deficiencies. That responsibility rests with me.

Finally, my deepest appreciation and gratitude to my partner Lizzy de la Porte, to whom this book is dedicated – because of her fierce emotional support during the writing process, because of the countless style and content suggestions she offered, because she spent so many hours reading, checking, correcting and formatting, and most of all because, in her work as a mental health nurse and in the way she lives her life, she exemplifies so many of the values I hold dear.

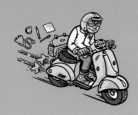

# Dedication

To Lizzy de la Porte

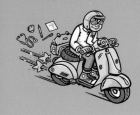

# Contents

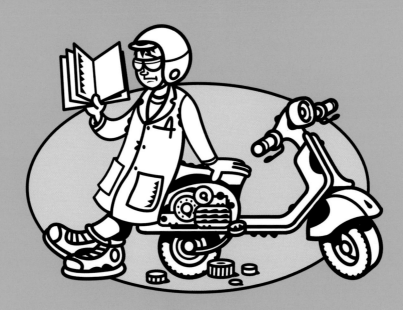

# THE PATIENT PRESENTS WITH

15-20% old people ⟶ depressive symptoms.

* Predisposing / Precepitating
   - loss events
   - change events

maternal death at young age
death of cat + dog ⟶ flake on cake.

moving house
chronic illness

pt. w/ depression
   · 20% suicide risk
   · 30% if EtOH too.

older people > likely to have comorbid anxiety
   ↳ protective factors < attendance at religious venue
                          confidant.

* Causes of organic depression
   · Hyper / hypo thyroid
   · Parkinson's ⟶ 40% present w/ depression before motor signs.
   · Dementia
   · Carcinoma
   · Stroke ⟶ close relat^ship between vascular disorders + depression.
              N.B. depression ↑ cardiovascular morbidity.

* Clinically
   · Open questions
   · Get up ok?                           objective signs ⟶ omega's sign?
     Concentrate on things?
     Psychotic features?
     Suicide? ⟶        RISKS FOR SUICIDE

Tx
   Mild ⟶ psychological > effective than drug Tx.

sect^n 12 approved

[ elderly ⟶ often don't respond to antidepressants
            ∴ ECT ¾or antipsychotic.

to be sect^ed, must suffer from;       2x doctor fills in form
mental illness under the terms of the act   social worker +
   + be a danger to yourself or others      Mx of hosp make decision.
   * Tx only possible v/in hospital.

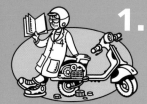

# 1. The Patient with Low Mood

*WHO → Mental illness = n° 1 cause of disability worldwide.*
*Depression = n°1 of the mental illnesses*

Mrs LM, a 32-year-old married housewife with two children aged 4 and 6 years, presented to her family doctor stating that she was persistently unhappy and had been crying repeatedly over the past few weeks. She had no previous psychiatric history or significant medical history and her only regular medication was oral contraception. She had moved to the area 3 years earlier when her husband was promoted and, at first, appeared to have integrated well into the neighbourhood by involving herself in the organization of a toddlers' group. Unfortunately, the group had dissolved a few months ago when her co-organizer and only close confidante had moved away. Deprived of her most important social outlet, Mrs LM found herself increasingly dominated by her young children. Although usually an outgoing person, she noticed that her motivation to keep in touch with other mothers from the group had started to dwindle. At the same time, she started feeling persistently weary even though her work schedule had not increased and often awakened 2–3 hours earlier in the morning. Although her appetite had not increased, she had turned to food for 'comfort' and had gained over 14 lb in weight. Mrs LM also candidly admitted that she was drinking more alcohol than usual. She described feeling incompetent because she was always miserable and had become too tired to look after the children. She felt guilty for burdening her husband and started crying when talking about her loss of interest in sex and her feelings of unattractiveness. Mrs LM maintained that no aspect of her life gave her pleasure and when asked specifically by her doctor, admitted that she had started to wonder whether her children and husband would be better off without her.

*(For a discussion of the case study see the end of the chapter)*

Feeling sad or upset is a normal part of the human condition; thus, a patient presenting with emotional suffering does not necessarily warrant a psychiatric diagnosis or require treatment. However, most psychiatrists agree that when patients present with a certain number of key *depressive features*, they are probably suffering from some form of psychopathology that will require, and usually respond to, specific kinds of treatment.

## Definitions and clinical features

Whereas *feelings* describe a short-lived emotional experience, *mood* refers to a patient's sustained, subjectively experienced emotional state over a period of time. Patients are described as having *a depressed mood* when they report feeling: depressed, sad, dejected, despondent, 'down in the dumps', miserable, 'low in spirits' or

'heavy-hearted'. They are unable to just lift themselves out of this mood and its severity is often out of proportion to the stressors in their surrounding social environment.

The term 'affect' can be used synonymously with mood or emotion, as in the *affective (mood) disorders*. This is confusing because psychiatrists most often use it in the context of a mental state examination to mean the *observed, external expression of emotion* – as perceived by another person. In this sense, the affect may be incongruous with the patient's subjectively reported mood, for example: the grinning patient who reports feeling miserable. Additionally, the range of affect (i.e. range of emotional expressivity) can be described; for example: a *blunted affect* indicates a reduction in the normal intensity of emotional expression as evidenced by a monotonous voice and minimal facial expression (see Ch. 26: Psychiatric Assessment and Diagnosis).

3

The ICD-10 classification system has identified two further important depressive features that are most commonly associated with depressed mood:

- Markedly reduced interest in almost all activities, associated with the loss of ability to derive pleasure from activities that were formerly enjoyed (anhedonia).
- Lack of energy or increased fatiguability on minimal exertion leading to diminished activity (anergia).

It is useful to consider the other depressive features associated with depressed mood under the subheadings: cognitive, biological, suicidal, psychotic and severe motor symptoms.

Remember the distinction between the terms 'mood' and 'affect'; they are not the same.

## Cognitive symptoms

In this context, cognition refers to *thoughts* patients have about themselves and the world as well as global brain functioning (thinking, concentrating, making decisions).

**Reduced concentration and attention**   Depressed patients report difficulty in sustaining attention while doing previously manageable tasks. They often appear easily distracted and may complain of memory difficulties.

**Poor self-esteem**   Self-esteem includes the interrelated concepts of personal efficacy and personal worth. Depressed patients may have thoughts that they are no longer competent to meet life's challenges and that they are no longer worthy of happiness and the healthy assertion of their needs.

**Guilt**   Depressed patients often have guilty preoccupations about minor past failings. This guilt is often inappropriate and out of proportion to the original 'offence'. Patients often have guilty thoughts about the very act of developing the depressed mood itself.

**Hopelessness**   Depressed patients can have bleak and pessimistic views of the future, believing that there is no way out of their current situation.

Know the biological symptoms of depression; they are often asked for in exams.

## Biological (somatic) symptoms

Some psychiatrists believe that there is a subgroup of depressed patients who have a 'biological' depression (also called somatic, melancholic, vital or endogenous depression). The essence of this type of depression is that there is an absence of an external environmental cause and that there is a 'biological' clinical picture. This is opposed to the so-called 'reactive' or 'neurotic' depression where it is assumed that the patient is, to some degree, understandably depressed, reacting to adverse psychosocial circumstances. Although the scientific validity of this classification is questionable, if a patient has four or more of the eight symptoms of the *somatic syndrome*, it can be coded for in the ICD-10:

1. **Loss of interest or pleasure in activities that are normally enjoyable**   Anhedonia means an inability to derive pleasure or excitement from any activities. This key symptom in depression is also associated with the related concept of having a markedly reduced interest in engaging in any of one's usual concerns.
2. **Reduced emotional reactivity**   This means an impaired emotional response to pleasurable surroundings. Patients can describe this as 'numbness', 'living in thick fog', 'or as being 'disconnected'.
3. **Early morning awakening**   Although patients may get to off to sleep at their normal time, they wake at least 2 hours earlier than they would usually, and then find it impossible to get back to sleep again. Further disturbances of sleep in depression include: difficulty falling asleep (initial insomnia), frequent awakening during the night and excessive sleeping (hypersomnia). Although all of these contribute to the diagnosis of depression, only early morning awakening is part of the *somatic syndrome*.
4. **Depression worse in the morning**   Diurnal variation of mood means that a patient's mood is more pronounced at a specific time of day. A depressive mood consistently and specifically worse in the morning is regarded as an important feature of the somatic syndrome.

5. **Psychomotor retardation or agitation** The term 'psychomotor' is used to describe a patient's motor activity as a consequence of their concurrent mental processes. Psychomotor changes in depression include *retardation* (slow, monotonous speech; long pauses before answering questions or muteness; leaden body movements and limited facial expression i.e. blunted affect) and *agitation* (inability to sit still; fidgeting, pacing or hand-wringing; rubbing or scratching skin or clothes). Note that psychomotor changes must be severe enough to be observable by others, not just the subjective experience of the patient.

6. **Marked loss of appetite** Although some depressed patients have an increased appetite and turn to 'comfort eating', only a dramatic reduction in appetite is regarded as somatic. Note that the reversed biological features overeating and oversleeping are sometimes referred to as *atypical depressive symptoms*.

7. **Weight loss** In addition to loss of appetite, a loss of 5% body weight in the past month is an important biological symptom.

8. **Loss of libido** Sensitive questioning will often reveal a reduction in sex drive that may lead to guilt when the sufferer feels unable to satisfy their partner.

Low mood, loss of interest or pleasure and fatiguability are the three core symptoms of depression.

## Suicide or self-harm

Depressed patients frequently have thoughts of death and harming themselves. In severe cases suicidal ideation may lead to an actual suicide attempt. At these times, patients may believe that they are faced with insurmountable difficulties or are trying to escape a relentlessly painful emotional state. Self-harm is discussed fully in Chapter 3.

It is crucial to always assess the risk of suicide in patients who present with low mood. Chapter 3 will help you in this regard.

> MOOD CONGRUENT
> MOOD INCONGRUENT } *describes consistency (of psych. symptoms) w/mood.*

## Psychotic and severe motor symptoms

In severe depressive episodes, patients may suffer from delusions, hallucinations or a depressive stupor; these are termed psychotic symptoms (see Ch. 4). Delusions and hallucinations can be further classified as 'mood congruent' or 'mood incongruent', which indicate whether the content of the psychotic symptoms is *consistent* with the patient's mood. Delusions and hallucinations in depression are most often mood congruent and so may involve an irrational conviction of guilt or sin or the belief that parts of the body are dead or wasting away. Hallucinations may take the form of accusatory or defamatory voices criticizing the patient in the second person (auditory hallucination) or the smell of rotting flesh (olfactory hallucination). Severe psychomotor retardation may progress to *stupor* and involves extreme unresponsiveness, lack of voluntary movement (akinesis) and near or total mutism. Severe motor symptoms are probably more common in schizophrenia and bipolar affective disorder, but they can and do occur in unipolar depression (see Ch. 4). *Nehilism* *Dellusion of enormity.*

## Differential diagnosis of low mood

*? PRIMARY OR SECONDARY*

Careful history taking and examination should reveal whether the patient presenting with low mood is suffering from a primary mood disorder, or whether their depression is secondary to a medical condition, psychoactive substance or other psychiatric condition – Figure 1.1 presents the differential diagnosis. An algorithm for the diagnosis of mood disorders is presented on page 14.

## Mood (affective) disorders
### Depressive episode

The ICD-10 has set out certain diagnostic guidelines for diagnosing a depressive episode (Fig. 1.2). The minimum duration of the episode is 2 weeks and at least two of the three symptoms of depressed mood, loss of interest or pleasure and increased fatiguability should be present. A depressive episode can be graded mild, moderate or severe depending on the number and severity of symptoms. A depressive episode occurring with hallucinations, delusions or a depressive stupor is always coded as *severe with psychotic features*.

## Differential diagnosis of low mood

Mood disorders
• Depressive episode
• Recurrent depressive disorder
• Dysthymia
• Bipolar affective disorder
• Cyclothymia

Schizoaffective disorder

Secondary to a general medical condition

Secondary to psychoactive substance use (including alcohol)

Secondary to other psychiatric disorders

• Psychotic disorders
• Anxiety disorders
• Adjustment disorder (including bereavement)
• Eating disorders
• Personality disorders
• Dementia

**Fig. 1.1** Differential diagnosis for patient presenting with low mood.

## Depressive episode

**Symptoms should be present for at least 2 weeks**
*At least two of the following core symptoms:*
• Depressed mood
• Loss of interest and enjoyment
• Reduced energy or increased fatiguability

AND...
*At least two of the following:*
• Reduced concentration and attention
• Reduced self-esteem and self-confidence
• Ideas of guilt and unworthiness
• Bleak and pessimistic views of the future
• Ideas or acts of self-harm or suicide
• Disturbed sleep
• Diminished appetite

**Severity**
*Mild*: Total of 4 or more symptoms
*Moderate*: Total of 5 (preferably 6) or more symptoms
*Severe*: Total of 7 or more symptoms including all 3 core symptoms.
*Severe with psychotic symptoms*: In cases with delusions, hallucinations or stupor
*With somatic syndrome*: If 4 or more of 8 biological symptoms present

**Fig. 1.2** ICD-10 criteria for depressive episode.

## Recurrent depressive disorder

Many patients will have a few depressive episodes in their lifetime. Recurrent depressive disorder is diagnosed when a patient has another depressive episode after their first.

## Dysthymia

This is a chronically depressed mood that usually has its onset in early adulthood and usually remains so throughout the patient's life with variable periods of wellness in between. The patient's mood is seldom severe enough to satisfy the formal criteria for a depressive episode and does not present with discrete episodes as in genuine *recurrent depressive disorder*. Sometimes dysthymia has its onset in later adult life, often after a discrete depressive episode, and is usually associated with bereavement or some other serious stress. Note that patients may develop a depressive episode on a baseline mood of dysthymia (so called *double depression*).

## Bipolar affective disorder/cyclothymia

Unipolar depression means that the patient's mood is either depressed or normal. When patients suffer from episodes of either depressed or elevated mood, the disorder is termed *bipolar*, as the mood is considered to deviate from normal to either a depressed or elated (manic) pole. When this instability of mood involves only mild elation and depression it is termed *cyclothymia*. Bipolar illness and cyclothymia are presented in Chapter 2.

## Schizoaffective disorder

A diagnosis of schizoaffective disorder can be made when patients present with both mood (depression or mania) symptoms and schizophrenic symptoms within the same episode of illness. It is important that these symptoms occur simultaneously or at least within a few days of each other. As you can imagine, this is a difficult diagnosis to establish, as it is not uncommon to have psychotic symptoms in a severe episode of depression (*depressive episode with psychotic features*); likewise, depressive symptoms often occur in patients with schizophrenia. Schizoaffective disorder is discussed in more detail in Chapter 4.

## Depression secondary to psychiatric or general medical disorders, or to psychoactive substances

The mood disorders as described above are considered primary; however, depressive symptoms are non-specific and can occur secondary to a range of other conditions. For example, a patient who has schizophrenia, an anxiety disorder, a personality disorder, an eating disorder or dementia may experience depression as a consequence. These depressive symptoms may even meet the criteria for a depressive episode.

General medical conditions that may produce depression through a presumed direct depressant effect are listed in Figure 1.3. Note that any medical condition that causes a significant degree of suffering may cause secondary depression indirectly for 'psychological reasons'.

Both prescribed (Fig. 1.4) and illicit drugs can be aetiologically responsible for symptoms of depression. For example, reserpine, an antihypertensive agent, is thought to produce depression through depletion of presynaptic catecholamine stores. Remember that alcohol is the psychoactive substance that is probably most associated with substance-induced depression.

Low mood may be one of several symptoms that appear when a patient has had to adapt to a significant change in life (e.g. divorce, retirement). When it can be confidently assumed that the symptoms would not have arisen without the stress due to the life event, the diagnosis of *adjustment disorder* is made. Bereavement is a form of adjustment reaction and is discussed in more detail in Chapter 7.

## Assessment

### Clinical

The following questions might be helpful in eliciting the key symptoms of depression:

- Have you been cheerful or quite low in mood or spirits lately?
- Do you find that you no longer enjoy things the way you used to?
- Do you find yourself often feeling very tired or worn out?
- How do you see things turning out in the future?
- Sometimes when people are depressed they have a poor sex drive. Has this happened to you?

A basic physical examination, including a thorough <u>neurological and endocrine system examination,</u> should be performed on all patients with depression.

### Special investigations

**Social**

- Collateral information from GP, community mental health team, family.
- Consider home visit to assess self-care, ability to care for family, home structure.

| General medical conditions causing low mood | | | |
| --- | --- | --- | --- |
| **Neurological** | **Endocrine** | **Infections** | **Others** |
| Multiple sclerosis | Cushing's disease | Hepatitis | Malignancies (especially |
| Parkinson's disease | Addison's disease | Infectious mononucleosis | pancreatic cancer) |
| Huntington's disease | Thyroid disorders (especially | Herpes simplex | Systemic lupus erythematosus |
| Spinal cord injury | hypothyroidism) | Brucellosis | Rheumatoid arthritis |
| Stroke (especially left | Parathyroid disorders | Typhoid | Renal failure |
| anterior infarcts) | Menstrual cycle-related | HIV/AIDS | Porphyria |
| Head injury | | Syphilis | Vitamin deficiencies (e.g. niacin) |
| Cerebral tumours | | | Chronic pain states |

**Fig. 1.3** General medical conditions causing low mood.

| Prescribed drugs causing low mood | | | | |
| --- | --- | --- | --- | --- |
| **Antihypertensives** | **Steroids** | **Neurological drugs** | **Analgesics** | **Psychiatric** |
| Beta-blockers | Corticosteroids | L-dopa | Opiates | Antipsychotics (phenothiazines, |
| Methyldopa | Oral contraceptives | Carbamazepine | Ibuprofen | butyrophenones) |
| Reserpine (no longer | | Phenytoin | Indometacin | |
| used in UK) | | Benzodiazepines | | |

**Fig. 1.4** Prescribed drugs causing low mood.

- Consider interviewing immediate family if disturbed inter-personal family dynamics are suspected.

## Psychological

- Patient may be asked to keep a mood diary.
- Self-report inventories for quantitative ratings of mood, e.g. Beck Depression Inventory (BDI), Hospital Anxiety and Depression Scale (HADS).

## Physical

*[handwritten annotations: → exclude poss Medical of substance related causes; → establish baseline values before Tx; → assess renal + Liver funct?]*

Physical investigations are performed to (1) exclude possible medical or substance-related causes of depression; (2) establish baseline values before administering treatment that may alter blood chemistry (e.g. antidepressants may cause hyponatraemia, lithium may cause hypothyroidism); and (3) assess renal and liver functioning, which may affect the elimination of medication.

- Full blood count: check for anaemia (low haemoglobin), infection (raised white count), and a high mean cell volume (MCV; a marker of high alcohol intake).
- Urea and electrolytes (renal function).
- Liver function tests and gamma glutamyl transpeptidase (γGT) (also a marker for high alcohol intake).
- Thyroid function tests and calcium.
- Erythrocyte sedimentation rate (ESR).

If indicated:

- Vitamin $B_{12}$ and folate (if deficiencies suspected).
- Urine drug screen (if drug use is suspected).
- An ECG should be done in patients with cardiac problems as tricyclic antidepressants and lithium may prolong the QT interval and have the potential to cause lethal ventricular arrhythmia.
- Serological tests for syphilis if indicated (e.g. TPHA).
- EEG (if epileptic focus or other intracranial pathology is suspected).

Despite much research on the dexamethasone suppression test (DST), there is no reliable blood test to indicate the presence of depression. However, one biological finding that is strongly associated with depression is a reduction in the latency (time to onset after falling asleep) of rapid eye movement (REM) sleep.

## Discussion of case study

Mrs LM meets the criteria for a depressive episode, at least moderate in severity. She has had all three core symptoms of depression for longer than 2 weeks: depressed mood, loss of interest or pleasure and fatiguability. The GP has also elicited associated depressive symptoms of disturbed sleep, feelings of incompetence (reduced self-esteem) and guilt and possible thoughts of self-harm. Mrs LM also has somatic symptoms of loss of interest or pleasure, early morning awakening and loss of libido. As this is a first episode, the diagnosis of recurrent depressive disorder is not appropriate. Dysthymia is not a suitable diagnosis as the period of low mood is far too short, the severity of the present episode too great and the deterioration in functioning too marked. There appear to be no instances of elated mood or increased energy, militating against a diagnosis of bipolar affective disorder or cyclothymia.

In order to grade the severity of the depression (and possibly the presence of a somatic syndrome) it would be useful to enquire about all the cognitive, biological, suicidal and psychotic components of depression. In all cases of suspected depression it is imperative to enquire about thoughts and or plans of suicide or self-harm (see Ch. 3 for a full discussion). It is also important to rule out secondary causes of depression; these include general medical conditions (Fig. 1.3), psychoactive substance use (Fig. 1.4) and other psychiatric conditions. Mrs LM admitted to using increased quantities of alcohol. Patients often use alcohol as a form of self-medication to alleviate feelings of dysphoria; however, alcohol can aggravate and in some cases even cause depressive symptoms. Mrs LM's use of oral contraception long before the onset of her depressive symptoms suggests that it is unlikely that this prescribed drug is causing her depression.

## Now go on to Chapter 13 to read about the mood disorders and their management.

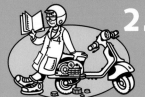

# 2. The Patient with Elevated or Irritable Mood

Feeling that she was no longer able to cope, Mrs EM consulted her GP about a Mental Health Act assessment for her husband, Mr EM, a 37-year-old freelance writer. He had no psychiatric history other than a period of depression 2 years ago. He had progressively needed less sleep over the past 2 weeks and had not slept at all for 48 hours. Recently, he had started taking on increasing amounts of work and seemed to thrive on this due to an 'inexhaustible source of boundless energy'. He told his wife and all his friends that he had a new lease of life, as he was 'happier than ever'. Mrs EM became concerned when he developed lofty ideas that he was a world expert in his field and would talk incessantly for hours about elaborate and complicated writing schemes. Mr EM's behaviour had become markedly uncharacteristic over the past day or two, when he started making sexually inappropriate comments to his neighbour's wife, and presented her with reams of poetry which he had spent the night writing. When Mrs EM suggested that he visit the GP, Mr EM became verbally aggressive saying that she was trying to bring him down because she was threatened by his 'irresistible sex appeal and wit'. Mrs EM was unable to reason with him and noticed that he struggled to keep to the point of the conversation, often bringing up issues that seemed completely irrelevant. The GP noted that, other than a recent bout of flu, Mr EM had no medical problems and was not using any prescribed medication.

*(For a discussion of the case study see the end of the chapter)*

Just as spells of feeling sad and miserable are quite normal to the human experience, so too are periods where we feel elated, excited and full of energy. Although an irritable or elevated mood is not in itself pathological, it can be when grossly and persistently so, and when associated with other manic psychopathology.

## Definitions and clinical features

In Chapter 1 we observed how a disturbance in mood in addition to various other cognitive, biological and psychotic symptoms all contribute to the recognition of a *depressive episode*. A similar approach is taken to *hypomanic* and *manic episodes*; these occur on the opposite pole of the mood disorder spectrum to depression.

### Mood

The hallmark of a manic episode is an elevated or irritable mood. When their mood is elevated, manic patients most often enjoy the experience and might describe themselves as feeling: 'high', 'on top of the world', 'fantastic' or 'euphoric'. This mood has an infectious quality, although those who know the patient well clearly see it as deviation from normal. Some patients tend to become extremely irritable or suspicious when manic and do not enjoy the experience at all. They have a low frustration tolerance and any thwarting of their plans can lead to a rapid escalation in anger or even delusions of persecution. Some patients alternate rapidly between manic and depressive symptoms from day to day or even hour to hour; this is termed a *mixed affective episode*.

Most patients with mania experience irritability (80%), depressed mood (72%), and labile or fluctuating mood (69%) just as often as euphoria (71%) – *prevalence in parentheses.*

*manifestat⁵ of flight of ideas*

# Biological symptoms

***Decreased need for sleep*** This is a very important early warning sign of mania or hypomania. Sleep disturbance can range from only needing a few hours sleep a night to a manic patient going for days on end with no sleep at all.

***Increased energy*** This initially results in an increase in goal-directed activity and, when coupled with impaired judgement, can have disastrous consequences, e.g. patients may instigate numerous risky business ventures; go on excessive spending sprees; or engage in reckless promiscuity that is unusual for them. However, in severe episodes actions can become repetitive, stereotyped and apparently purposeless even progressing to a _manic stupor in the extreme case_. If left untreated, excessive overactivity can lead to physical exhaustion and sometimes even death. On mental state examination, increased energy can be seen as _psychomotor agitation_: the patient is unable to sit still, frequently standing up, pacing around the room and gesticulating expansively.

*98% pressured speech*
*87% psychomotor agitat⁺ⁿ*

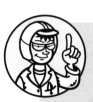 In patients with mania 98% have pressured speech 87% have psychomotor agitation; 81% have decreased need for sleep and 57% have sexual disinhibition.

# Cognitive symptoms

### Elevated sense of self-esteem or grandiosity
Hypomanic patients may overestimate their abilities and social or financial status. In severe cases, manic patients may have delusions of grandeur (see later).

***Poor concentration*** Manic patients may find it difficult to maintain their focus on any one thing as they struggle to filter out irrelevant external stimuli (background noise, other objects or people in the room), consequently, making them highly distractible.

***Accelerated thinking*** A manic patient may subjectively experience their thoughts or ideas racing even faster than they can articulate them. When thoughts are rapidly associating in this way in a stream of connected concepts it is termed *flight of ideas*. When patients have an irrepressible need to

express these thoughts verbally, making them difficult to interrupt, it is termed *pressure of speech*. Some hypomanic patients express themselves by incessant letter writing, poetry, doodling or artwork.

 Grandiosity (78%), racing thoughts (71%) and distractibility (68%) are the most common non-psychotic cognitive disturbances in patients with mania – *prevalence in parentheses*.

***Impaired judgement and insight*** This is typical of manic illness and sometimes results in costly indiscretions that patients may later regret. Lack of insight into their illness can be a difficult barrier to overcome when trying to engage patients in essential treatment.

*MANIC > DEPRESSIVE*

# Psychotic symptoms
Psychotic symptoms are far more common in manic than depressive episodes and include disorders of *thought form* and *perception*.

## Disordered thought form
Disordered thought form (see Ch. 4) commonly occurs in schizophrenia, but is regularly seen in manic episodes with psychotic features and to lesser degree in psychotic forms of unipolar depression. The most common thought form disorders in mania are probably circumstantiality, tangentiality, flight of ideas and secondary delusional thinking. However, signs of thought disorder most typical to schizophrenia can also be seen in manic episodes, e.g. loosening of association, neologisms and thought blocking.

***Circumstantiality and tangentiality*** Circumstantial (over-inclusive) speech means speech that is delayed in reaching its final goal because of the over-inclusion of details and unnecessary asides and diversions; however, the speaker, if allowed to finish, does eventually connect the original starting point to the desired destination. Circumstantiality can also be found in normal people – most families have at least one person who takes forever to finish a story! Tangential speech, on the other hand, is more indicative of psychopathology and sees the speaker diverting from the initial train of thought but never

returning to the original point, jumping tangentially from one topic to the next.

**Flight of ideas**  As described above, this occurs when thinking is markedly accelerated resulting in a stream of connected concepts. The link between concepts can be as in normal communication where one idea follows directly on from the next; through a pun or clang association; or through some vague idea which is not part of the original goal of speech, e.g. 'I need to go to bed now. Have you ever smelt my bed of roses? Ah, but a rose by any other name would smell just as sweet!' Even though manic patients may appear to be talking absolute gibberish, a written transcript of their speech will usually reveal that their ideas are related in some, albeit obscure, way.

As patients become increasingly manic, their associations tend to loosen as they find it increasingly difficult to link their thoughts. Eventually they start approaching the incoherent thought disorder of the schizophrenic patient who exhibits *loosening of association* (*derailment or knight's move thinking*), *word salad* and *neologisms* where ideas are very loosely or not at all related (see Ch. 4). Flight of ideas is regarded as a psychotic phenomenon when speech is practically incomprehensible.

**Secondary delusions**  Secondary delusions are those that develop *in response* to another psychopathological state – in this case, abnormal mood. Inherent in this definition is the implication that it is *understandable* how the delusion originated when one examines the patient's mental state. This is in contrast to primary delusions, which develop spontaneously from no pre-existing pathological mental state, thus making their genesis completely *beyond understanding*. These are almost exclusively seen in patients with schizophrenia (see Ch. 4). Patients with elated mood therefore, will typically present with *grandiose delusions* in which they believe they have special importance or unusual powers. *Persecutory delusions* are also common, especially in patients with an irritable mood, and often feature them believing that others are trying to take advantage of their exalted status. When the content of delusions matches the mood of the patient, the delusions are termed *mood-congruent*. Very often, patients with elevated mood may have overvalued ideas as opposed to true delusions, which are important to distinguish, as the former are not regarded as psychotic in nature (see p. 26).

**Perceptual disturbance**  Some hypomanic patients may describe subtle distortions of perception. These are not psychotic symptoms and mainly include altered intensity of perception such that sounds seem louder (hyperacusis) or colours seem brighter and more vivid (visual hyperaesthesia). Psychotic perceptual features develop when manic patients experience hallucinations. This is usually in the form of voices encouraging or exciting them.

Phenomenological studies have shown that in patients with bipolar affective disorder, at least two-thirds reported experiencing psychotic symptoms during a manic episode and up to one-third reported experiencing psychotic symptoms during a depressive episode.

## Differential diagnosis of elevated or irritable mood

Like depression, an elevated or irritable mood can be secondary to a medical condition, psychoactive substance use or other psychiatric disorder. These will have to be excluded before a primary mood disorder can be diagnosed. Figure 2.1 shows the differential diagnosis for patients presenting with elevated or irritable mood.

**Differential diagnosis for patient presenting with elevated or irritable mood**

Mood disorders
- Hypomania, mania, mixed affective episode
- Bipolar affective disorder
- Cyclothymia
- Depression (may present with irritable mood)

Secondary to a general medical condition

Secondary to psychoactive substance use

Psychotic disorders
- Schizoaffective disorder (may be similar to mania with psychotic features)
- Schizophrenia

Personality disorders

Delirium/dementia

**Fig. 2.1** Differential diagnosis for patient presenting with elevated or irritable mood.

# Mood (affective) disorders
## Hypomanic, manic and mixed affective episodes

The ICD-10 specifies three degrees of severity of a manic episode: *hypomania, mania without psychotic symptoms* and *mania with psychotic symptoms*. All of these share the above-mentioned general characteristics, most notably: an elevated or irritable mood and an increase in the quantity and speed of mental and physical activity. Unlike for depressive episodes, the ICD-10 does not specify a certain number of symptoms to establish the diagnosis. It does, however, require the clinician to determine the degree of psychosocial impairment, as well as to code for the presence of psychotic symptoms (Fig. 2.2 – note that the degree of impairment of social functioning is the crucial distinguishing factor between hypomania and mania). As mentioned above, episodes where patients present with rapidly alternating manic and depressive symptoms are termed *mixed affective episodes.*

## Bipolar affective disorder

A patient presenting with a second episode of a major mood disturbance (depression or mania) should be diagnosed as having *recurrent depressive disorder* or *bipolar affective disorder*. If a patient has had at least one hypomanic, manic or mixed affective episode in association with any kind of past mood episode (hypomanic, manic, depressive, mixed), then bipolar affective disorder is the correct diagnosis. Most patients who experience hypomanic or manic episodes also experience depressive episodes, hence, the commonly used term: 'manic-depression'. However, patients who only suffer from manic or hypomanic episodes with no intervening depressive episodes are also classified as having bipolar affective disorder, even though their mood does not swing to the depressive pole. It is good practice to record the nature of the current episode in a patient with longstanding bipolar affective disorder (e.g. '*bipolar affective disorder, current episode manic without psychotic features*').

## Cyclothymia

Cyclothymia is analogous to dysthymia (see p. 6) in that it usually begins in early adulthood and follows a chronic course with intermittent periods of wellness in between. It is characterized by an instability of mood resulting in alternating periods of mild elation and mild depression, none of which are sufficiently severe or long enough to meet the criteria for either a hypomanic or a depressive episode.

## Depression

There are two scenarios where a patient with a primary depressive disorder may present with an elevated or irritable mood. An 'agitated depression' can present with a prominent irritable mood, which, when coupled with psychomotor agitation, can be difficult to distinguish from a manic episode. Secondly, depressed patients who are responding to antidepressants or electroconvulsive therapy (ECT) may experience a transient period of elevated mood.

# Manic episodes secondary to a general medical condition or psychoactive substance use

A medical or psychoactive substance cause of mania should always be sought for and ruled out. Figure 2.3 lists the medical and substance-related causes of mania. The medical condition or substance use

| ICD-10 distinguishing features of hypomania and mania | | | |
|---|---|---|---|
| Features | Hypomania | Mania without psychotic features | Mania with psychotic features |
| Mood | Mildly elevated or irritable mood – greater than cyclothymia | Greatly elevated or irritable mood | Severely elevated or suspicious mood accompanied by delusions, hallucinations, incomprehensible pressure of speech or manic stupor |
| Duration | Several days | 1 week | 1 week |
| Psychosocial functioning | Considerable interference with work or social activity but disruption is not complete or severe | Disrupts work and social activities completely | Disrupts work and social activities completely. Associated with violent excitement, dehydration and self-neglect |

Fig. 2.2 ICD-10 distinguishing features of hypomania and mania.

| Medical and substance causes of mania | |
|---|---|
| **Medical conditions** | **Substances** |
| Cerebral neoplasms, infarcts, trauma, infection (including HIV) | Amfetamines |
| Cushing's disease | Anticholinergics |
| Huntington's disease | Antidepressants |
| Hyperthyroidism | Antiviral drugs |
| Multiple sclerosis | Antimalarials |
| Renal failure | Captopril |
| Systemic lupus erythematosus | Cimetidine |
| Temporal lobe epilepsy | Cocaine |
| Vitamin $B_{12}$ and niacin (pellagra) deficiency | Corticosteroids |
| | Hallucinogens |
| | L-dopa |

**Fig. 2.3** Medical and substance causes of mania.

should predate the development of the mood disorder and symptoms should resolve with treatment of the condition or abstinence from the offending substance. Absence of previous manic episodes or a family history of bipolar affective disorder also supports this diagnosis.

## Psychotic disorders

### Schizoaffective disorder
See pages 6 and 29. This can be very difficult to distinguish from a manic episode with psychotic features.

### Schizophrenia
Patients with schizophrenia can present with an excited, suspicious or agitated mood and therefore can be difficult to distinguish from manic patients with psychotic symptoms. Figure 2.4 compares relevant features that might act as clues to the correct diagnosis.

## Personality disorders
Psychiatrists often see patients with disorders of personality who present with features in common with hypomania, e.g. impulsivity, displays of temper and lability of mood in borderline personality disorder. However, personality disorders involve stable and enduring behaviour patterns unlike the more discrete episodes of bipolar affective disorder, which are characterized by a distinct, demarcated deterioration in psychosocial functioning.

## Delirium/dementia
See Chapter 9.

## Assessment

### Clinical
The following questions might be helpful in eliciting the key symptoms of mania/hypomania:
- Have you been feeling particularly happy or on top of the world lately?
- Do you sometimes feel as though you have too much energy compared to people around you?
- Do you find yourself needing less sleep but not getting tired?
- Have you had any new interests or exciting ideas lately?
- Have you noticed your thoughts racing in your head?
- Do you have any special abilities or powers?

| Schizophrenia | | |
|---|---|---|
| **Psychopathology** | **Mania** | **Schizophrenia** |
| Thought form | Circumstantiality, tangentiality, flight of ideas | Loosening of association, neologisms, thought blocking |
| Delusions | Most often mood-congruent (grandiose delusions or persecutory delusions) | Delusions unrelated to mood, bizarre delusions, delusions of passivity (e.g. thought insertion, withdrawal, broadcast) |
| Speech | Pressured speech, difficult to interrupt | Speech is often hesitant or halting |
| Biological symptoms | Significantly reduced need for sleep, increased physical and mental energy | Sleep less disturbed, less hyperactive |
| Psychomotor function | Agitation | Agitation, catatonic symptoms or negative symptoms |

**Fig. 2.4** Psychopathological distinctions between mania and schizophrenia (these are guidelines only; typically schizophrenic symptoms can occur in mania and vice-versa).

A basic physical examination, including a thorough neurological and endocrine system examination, should be performed on all patients with elevated mood.

## Special investigations

As for the depressive disorders, social, psychological and physical investigations are normally performed on manic patients mainly to establish the diagnosis and to rule out an organic or substance-related cause (see Fig 2.3). The Mood Disorders Questionnaire (MDQ), a self-report inventory, is a useful screening tool for bipolar affective disorder.

## Algorithm for the diagnosis of mood disorders

See Figure 2.5.

## Discussion of case study

Mr EM appears to be suffering from a *manic episode with psychotic features*. He has an elated mood and has developed the grandiose delusion that he is a world expert secondary to this mood (mood-congruent

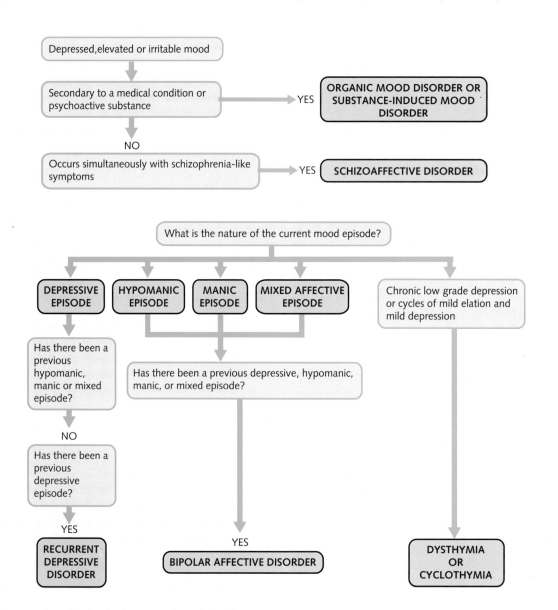

**Fig. 2.5** Algorithm for the diagnosis of mood disorders.

psychotic symptom); note also the rapid switch to irritable mood when confronted. Biological symptoms include the reduced need for sleep and increased mental and physical energy with overactivity. Cognitive symptoms include elevated sense of self-importance, poor concentration, accelerated thinking with pressure of speech and impaired judgement and insight. The episode is classified as manic because of the severe impairment in social and probably work functioning.

The past psychiatric history is extremely important in this case. A previous mood episode (hypomanic, manic, depressive, mixed) is required in order to make the diagnosis of bipolar affective disorder. Mr EM had a period of depression 2 years prior to developing this manic episode. If this was a genuine depressive episode then the correct diagnosis would be: *bipolar affective disorder, current episode manic with psychotic features*. Previous psychotic episodes should add schizoaffective disorder and schizophrenia to the differential diagnosis.

## Now go on to Chapter 13 to read about the mood disorders and their management.

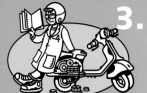

# 3. The Patient with Suicide or Self-harm Intent

At 1:30 a.m., the psychiatry senior house officer receives a call from the casualty department of an inner city hospital. He is asked for his opinion on Mr SA, a 28-year-old unemployed, recently divorced man, who was brought in by his landlord. The landlord had called round on the off-chance to discuss payment arrears, only to find the door unlocked and Mr SA asleep on his bed with an empty bottle of paracetamol tablets and several empty cans of lager littered around the bedroom floor. He also found a hastily scribbled suicide note addressed to Mr SA's children on the bedside table. Mr SA was easily roused but was upset to have been found and initially refused the landlord's persistent pleas that they should go along to the hospital. Only when he was violently sick did he finally agree. The casualty officer reports that other than the smell of alcohol on his breath, Mr SA's medical examination was normal. Special investigations revealed paracetamol in his blood, but not at a sufficiently high level to require medical admission. The casualty officer is concerned because Mr SA is ambivalent about a possible further suicide attempt saying that his life is a failure and that there is nothing worth living for. Before coming to see the patient, the psychiatry SHO proceeds to ask the casualty officer some routine questions.

*(For a discussion of the case study see the end of the chapter)*

While any psychiatric illness can present with self-harm or suicide intent, many patients who attempt suicide or self-harm are not previously known to mental health services. Assessments of patients who have self-harmed are very often made by non-psychiatric personnel and so it is vital that primary care clinicians are, firstly, able to detect and manage any underlying mental illness and, secondly, have a sound approach to assessing and managing risk.

## Definitions and clinical features

<u>Deliberate self-harm</u> is the <u>blanket term</u> used to mean any intentional act done in the knowledge that it was potentially harmful. Deliberate self-harm can take the form of <u>self-poisoning</u> (overdosing) or <u>self-injury</u> (cutting, slashing, burning). The motives for deliberate self-harm are vast and include emotional relief, self-punishment, attention seeking and can even be a form of self-help by way of channelling an intolerable emotional experience into a discrete physical sensation. *Suicide* is the act of intentionally and successfully ending one's own life, while

*parasuicide* (a subset of deliberate self-harm) is the term used to denote an unsuccessful suicide attempt.

Deliberate self-harm is one of the top five causes of acute medical admissions for both men and women in the UK.

## Assessment of the patient who has attempted suicide

Patients who present with self-harm have a 100-fold greater chance of completing suicide in the following year than the general population and therefore need to be assessed comprehensively. Unfortunately, psychiatry has some way to go before we are able to reliably predict the risk of someone attempting suicide. However, numerous studies have shown that certain epidemiological and clinical variables are more prevalent among those who have completed suicide (see later) and it is important to bear these risk factors in mind when assessing a patient's risk.

Remember, however, that determining suicide risk is extremely difficult, even for experienced psychiatrists and that no patient questionnaire or suicide risk scoring system has been shown to be better than thorough clinical assessment. A thorough risk assessment should include a full psychiatric history (see Ch. 26) with specific focus on:

1. Risk factors.
2. Suicide intent.
3. Mental state examination.
4. Current social support.

## Suicide risk factors

Figure 3.1 summarizes the most important epidemiological and clinical risk factors for suicide.

 Make sure you know the risk factors for suicide well; they are often asked for in exams!

### Psychiatric illness

About 90% of patients who commit suicide have a diagnosable psychiatric disorder. However, a 5-year study showed that only one-quarter of suicides in England, Wales, Scotland and Northern Ireland had been in contact with the mental health services in the year before death.

It is important to note that patients who have recently been discharged from a psychiatric hospital are a very high-risk group for suicide particularly in the first 1–2 weeks following discharge. Figure 3.2 summarizes the most important psychiatric conditions associated with suicide.

 Not only is alcohol a psychoactive depressant, but it also impairs judgement and leads to disinhibition, which probably increases the likelihood of suicidal thoughts being acted upon. The lifetime risk of suicide in problem drinkers is about 3–4%, which is 60–120 times greater than the normal population.

### Physical illness

Any disabling or unpleasant medical condition may predispose to or precipitate a suicide attempt. Many patients have co-morbid depression that potentially will respond well to treatment; however, some patients do not have a mental illness and have made a 'rational' decision to die (very rare). Most common examples are:

- Chronic painful illnesses.
- Central nervous system diseases, e.g. epilepsy, multiple sclerosis, Huntington's disease.
- Cancers, especially of the genitals or breast.
- Endocrine and metabolic conditions, e.g. Cushing's disease, porphyria.

### Recent adverse life events

Stressful life events are more common in the 6 months prior to a suicide attempt. These include: relationship break-ups, personal or family health problems, legal prosecution, financial difficulties or problems at home.

## Suicide intent

Suicide intent, which is commonly defined as *the seriousness or intensity of the wish of a patient to terminate his or her life*, is suggested by the following:

***The attempt was planned in advance*** A lethal suicide attempt usually involves days or weeks of planning the method and location of suicide. It is rarely an impulsive, spur-of-the-moment idea (the exception is the psychotic patient who impulsively responds to hallucinations or delusions). Planning is strongly suggested by the evidence of *final acts*. These include the making of a will or the leaving of a suicide note.

---

**Risk factors for suicide**

**Epidemiological factors:**
Men more likely to complete suicide (although women engage in more parasuicidal acts)
Rates highest in men aged 19 – 34 years
Divorced > widowed > single
Unemployed or retired
Social class V
Living alone, social isolation

**Clinical factors:**
Psychiatric illness (see Fig. 3.2)
Previous deliberate self-harm
Alcohol dependence
Physical illness (especially terminal illness, and debilitating or chronically painful conditions)
Family history of depression, alcohol dependence or suicide
Recent adverse life-events (especially bereavement)

**Fig. 3.1** Risk factors for suicide.

| Association between psychiatric disorders and suicide | |
|---|---|
| **Psychiatric disorder** | **Comments** |
| Depression | Most common psychiatric diagnosis (50–80% of completed suicides) Lifetime risk of suicide is 15% Risk greatest in severe illness with delusions |
| Schizophrenia | Lifetime risk of suicide is 10% High risk: young, intelligent, unemployed males with good insight and relapsing illness |
| Alcohol dependence | Lifetime risk of suicide is 3–4% High risk: elderly males, poor work record, social isolation, previous parasuicide Often have co-morbid depression |
| Personality disorders: antisocial (dissocial) and borderline personality disorders | High risk: labile mood, impulsive, aggressive, alcohol and substance misuse |
| Organic brain disease (dementia, delirium, epilepsy, head injury) | 5% of all completed suicides |
| Anxiety and eating disorders | Increased risk |

**Fig. 3.2** Association between psychiatric disorders and suicide.

*Beck's triad:* — self — world — future

### Precautions were taken to avoid discovery or rescue
For example, a patient might check into a hotel room in a distant town or ensure that no friends or family will be visiting over the ensuing hours or days.

### A dangerous method was used
Violent methods (hanging, jumping from heights, firearm use, electrocution) are more suggestive of lethal intent than overdosing. That said, use of an apparently ineffective method (e.g. taking six paracetamol tablets) might reflect lack of knowledge of the lethal dose needed, rather than a lack of intent to die. Therefore, it should be ascertained whether the method used was seen as dangerous from the patient's perspective.

### No help was sought after the act
Patients who immediately regret their action and seek help are probably less at risk than those who simply wait to die. Contrast Mr SA in the case study above with a young lady who takes a mouthful of tablets then runs downstairs to reveal to her parents what she has done.

## Mental state examination
This should be done in a calm, quiet and confidential setting, preferably when the patient has had a chance to rest and is not under the influence of drugs or alcohol. This might seem too obvious a point were it not for the unfortunate reality that patients are often referred for a psychiatric assessment while still drowsy from an overdose of sleeping tablets. Check specifically for:

- Current mood state. Is the suicide attempt regretted or is there ongoing suicidal ideation? Cognitive features of hopelessness and worthlessness are associated with higher risk of suicide.
- It is also useful to ascertain whether there are protective factors that would stop a patient from attempting suicide again. For example, a mother may have ongoing suicidal ideation, yet be adamant that she would not desert or frighten her children again.
- Undiagnosed mental illness, especially depression, schizophrenia, alcohol dependence and personality disorders. Remember that so-called 'rational' suicide is rare in western countries.

The following questions might be helpful when asking about suicidal ideation:
- Have you been feeling that life isn't worth living?
- Do you sometimes feel like you would like to end it all?
- Have you actually given some thought as to how you might do it?
- How close do you think you are to going through with your plans?
- Is there anything that might stop you from attempting suicide?

A patient may appear to be at greater risk of imminent self-harm on mental state examination if they are tired, emotionally upset or inebriated.

## Current social support

This is important to ascertain when deciding upon management. Does the patient have the resources and ability to cope if discharged? Patients with ongoing suicidal ideation can often be managed in the community if a strong social support network exists. It may be necessary to refer the at-risk patient for follow-up by the local community mental health team. Known psychiatric patients should be followed up by their care coordinator (see Ch. 30). Always inform the patient's GP of parasuicidal activity.

## Differential diagnosis

It is crucial to rule out a mental illness as a cause of a suicide attempt (see Fig. 3.2).

When assessing a patient who has self-harmed it is crucial that clinicians appear non-judgemental and empathic. Establishing a rapport with a challenging patient is a unique skill and should be a main priority.

## Discussion of case study

**Self-harm risk assessment**   Mr SA's epidemiological risk factors are that he is a young man, recently divorced, unemployed and apparently lives alone in social isolation. His clinical risk factors are that he may have alcohol use problems and has recently experienced adverse life events (divorce, financial difficulties). The evidence of final acts (suicide note) and the failure of Mr SA to seek help after the act suggest strong suicide intent. The fact that he would not have been discovered but for the landlord's timely arrival indicates a degree of forward planning, although his leaving of the door unlocked and his willingness to go to hospital after vomiting suggests some ambivalence. Mr SA had clearly consumed a significant degree of alcohol at the time of the overdose which could have clouded his judgement and given him courage which he otherwise might not have had. On mental state examination, Mr SA has ongoing suicidal ideation and cognitive features of worthlessness and hopelessness, which are known to be associated with suicide.

**Further management**   More information is necessary. The SHO should ask about all the epidemiological and clinical risk factors, specifically about: past or current mental illness (is Mr SA known to the mental health services?); previous episodes of self-harm; alcohol or substance dependence; physical illness; family history of depression, alcohol dependence or suicide and other recent adverse life events. The casualty officer has provided enough information about the lethality of the suicide attempt; however, the SHO will want to know if there was any evidence of mental illness on mental state examination, especially depression. The SHO will also be interested in Mr SA's current social support in order to try and help him formulate the most appropriate management plan.

As this is a complex risk assessment, the SHO will probably have to reassess the patient himself, especially as regards detecting mental illness on mental state examination. The SHO might ask the casualty officer to keep Mr SA overnight, so that a mental state examination can be performed in the morning when he is refreshed and no longer under the influence of alcohol. A hospital admission or follow-up by a community mental health team seems to be the most likely outcome.

**Now go on to Chapter 13 and Chapter 18 to read about affective and personality disorders and their management.**

# 4. The Psychotic Patient

Bleuler — 4 As affect loosening

Mr PP, aged 23, was assessed by his GP because his family had become concerned about his behaviour. Over the last 6 months his college attendance had been uncharacteristically poor and he had terminated his part-time work. He had also become increasingly reclusive by spending more time alone in his flat, refusing to answer the door or see his friends. After some inappropriate suspiciousness, he allowed the GP into his flat and then disclosed that government scientists had started to perform experiments on him over the last year. These involved the insertion of an electrode into his brain that detected gamma rays transmitted from government headquarters, which issued him with commands and 'planted' strange ideas in his head. When the GP asked how he knew this, he replied that he heard the 'men's voices' as 'clear as day' and that they continually commented on what he was thinking. He explained that his suspicion that 'all was not right' was confirmed when he heard the neighbour's dog barking in the middle of the night – at that point he knew 'for certain' that he was being interfered with. Prompted by the GP, Mr PP also mentioned that a man in his local pub knew of his plight and had sent him a 'covert signal' when he overheard the man conversing about the dangers of nuclear experiments. He also admitted to 'receiving coded information' from the radio whenever it was turned on. The GP found no evidence of abnormal mood, incoherence of speech or disturbed motor function. Mr PP denied use of illicit drugs and appeared physically well. After the GP discussed the case with a psychiatrist, Mr PP was admitted to a psychiatric hospital. He agreed to a voluntary admission, as he was now afraid of staying alone at home.

*(For a discussion of the case study see the end of the chapter)*

Insight ⟶ no A implicat⁰ˢ but Mx implicat⁰s.

The psychotic patient can present in many varied ways. It is often very difficult to elicit and describe specific symptoms when a patient is speaking or behaving in a grossly disorganized or even frightening fashion. Therefore, it is important to approach the psychotic patient in a logical and systematic fashion as well as to have a good understanding of the psychopathology involved.

## Definitions and clinical features

The term psychotic is classically used to describe a patient who has grossly *impaired reality testing*. This definition is not that clinically useful as 'reality testing' encompasses almost all conscious processes and so any dysfunction can present in a number of ways. Probably the narrowest clinical definition of psychosis is simply: delusions and hallucinations.

However, patients with schizophrenia and other psychotic disorders often have more symptoms than just delusions or hallucinations, e.g. psychomotor abnormalities, mood/affect disturbance, cognitive deficits and disorganization of thought and behaviour.

There are many classifications that attempt to describe all the symptoms seen in schizophrenia and psychosis. So, in order to simplify matters it is useful to approach psychotic psychopathology using four somewhat interrelated parameters:

1. Perception.
2. Thought disorder.
3. Negative symptoms.
4. Psychomotor function.

### Perceptual disturbance

*Perception* is the process of making sense of the physical information we receive from our five sensory modalities.

*Can have hallucinations in all sensory modalities* ("When you block your ears....?")

*Hallucinations* are perceptions occurring in the absence of an external physical stimulus which have the following important characteristics:

- To the patient, the nature of a hallucination is exactly the same as a *normal sensory experience* – i.e. it appears real. Therefore, patients often have little insight into their abnormal experience.
- They are experienced as *external sensations* from any one of the five sensory modalities (hearing, vision, smell, taste, touch) and should be distinguished from ideas, thoughts, images or fantasy which originate in the patient's own mind.
- They occur without an external stimulus and are not merely distortions of an existing physical stimulus (see illusions).

*Illusions* are misperceptions of real external stimuli, e.g. in a dark room, a dressing gown hanging on a bedroom wall is perceived as a person. Illusions often occur in normal people and are usually associated with inattention or strong emotion.

A *pseudohallucination* is a perceptual experience, which differs from a hallucination, in that it appears to arise in the *subjective inner space* of the mind, not through one of the external sensory organs. Patients tend to describe these sensations as being perceived with the 'inner eye' or 'mind's eye' (or ear). Examples include: distressing flashbacks in post-traumatic stress disorder or the recently bereaved widow waking up to briefly 'see' her husband sitting at the foot of the bed. Note that some psychiatrists define pseudohallucinations to mean hallucinations that patients actually recognize as false perceptions, i.e. they have insight into the fact that they are hallucinating. The former definition is probably more widely used.

According to which sense organ they appear to arise from, hallucinations are classified as auditory, visual, olfactory, gustatory or somatic. Special forms of hallucinations will also be discussed. See Figure 4.1 for an outline of the classification of hallucinations.

## Auditory hallucinations

These are hallucinations of the hearing modality and are the most common type of hallucinations in

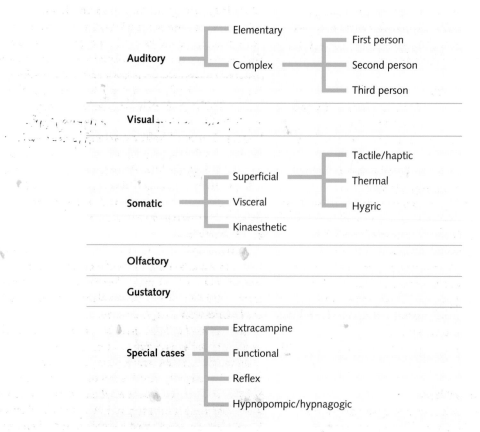

**Fig. 4.1** Outline of classification of hallucinations.

Primary sensory cortex.

induced by something else

clinical psychiatry. *Elementary hallucinations* are simple, unstructured sounds, e.g. whirring, buzzing, whistling or single words; this type of hallucination commonly occurs in acute organic states. *Complex hallucinations* occur as spoken phrases, sentences or even dialogue that are classified as:

- *Audible thoughts (first person)*: patients hear their own thoughts spoken out loud *as they think them*. When patients experience their thoughts as echoed by a voice after they have thought them, it is termed *thought echo*.
- *Second person auditory hallucinations*: patients hear a voice or voices talking directly to them. Second person hallucinations can be persecutory, highly critical, complimentary or issue commands to the patient (command hallucinations). Second person hallucinations are often associated with mood disorders with psychotic features and so will be critical or persecutory in a depressed patient or complimentary in a manic patient, i.e. mood-congruent hallucinations.
- *Third person auditory hallucinations*: patients hear a voice or voices speaking about them, referring to them in the third person. This may take the form of two or more voices arguing or discussing the patient among themselves; or one or more voices giving a *running commentary* on the patient's thoughts or actions.

erentials: organic psychoses → amphetamine psychosis

## Visual hallucinations

These are hallucinations of the visual modality and occur less frequently than auditory hallucinations in clinical psychiatry. They occur more commonly in organic brain disturbances (delirium, occipital lobe tumours, epilepsy, dementia) and in the context of psychoactive substance use (lysergic acid diethylamide (LSD), mescaline, petrol/glue-sniffing, alcoholic hallucinosis). An *autoscopic hallucination* is the experience of seeing an image of oneself in external space. The *Charles Bonnet syndrome* describes the condition where patients experience complex visual hallucinations associated with no other psychiatric symptoms or impairment in consciousness; it usually occurs in the elderly and is associated with loss of vision. *Lilliputian hallucinations* are hallucinations of miniature people or animals.

## Somatic hallucinations

These are hallucinations of bodily sensation and include *superficial*, *visceral* and *kinaesthetic* hallucinations.

*Superficial hallucinations* describe sensations on or just below the skin and may be:

- *Tactile (haptic)*: experience of the skin being touched, pricked or pinched. *Formication* is the unpleasant sensation of insects crawling on or just below the skin; it is commonly associated with long-term cocaine use (cocaine bugs) and alcohol withdrawal. Delerium Tremens
- *Thermal*: false perception of heat or cold.
- *Hygric*: false perception of a fluid, e.g. 'I can feel water sloshing in my brain'.

*Visceral hallucinations* describe false perceptions of the internal organs. Patients may be distressed by deep sensations of their organs throbbing, stretching, distending or vibrating.

*Kinaesthetic hallucinations* are false perceptions of joint or muscle sense. Patients may describe their limbs vibrating or being twisted. The fleeting but distressing sensation of free falling, just as one is about to fall asleep is an example that most people have experienced (see *hypnagogic* hallucinations below).

## Olfactory and gustatory hallucinations

These are the false perceptions of smell and taste. Note that they commonly occur together because the two senses are closely related. Remember that in patients with olfactory or gustatory hallucinations, it is important to rule out epilepsy (especially of the temporal lobe) and other organic brain diseases.

As pt. falls asleep ──────→ Hypnagogic

## Special forms of hallucination  Hypnopompic (on waking)

*Hypnagogic* hallucinations are false perceptions in any modality (usually auditory or visual) that occur as a person goes to sleep; whereas, *hypnopompic* hallucinations occur as a person awakens. These occur in normal people and are not indicative of psychopathology.

*Extracampine* hallucinations are false perceptions that occur outside the limits of a person's normal sensory field, e.g. a patient describes hearing voices from 100 miles away. Patients often give delusional explanations for this phenomenon.

A *functional hallucination* occurs when a normal sensory stimulus is required to precipitate a hallucination in that same sensory modality, e.g. voices that are only heard when the doorbell rings. A *reflex hallucination* occurs when a normal sensory stimulus in one modality precipitates a hallucination in another, e.g. voices that are only heard whenever the lights are switched on.

23

## Thought disorder

Describing the disturbance of a patient's thought form is one of the most challenging tasks facing clinicians. This problem is compounded by two factors. Firstly, it is impossible to know what patients are actually thinking – thought form has to be inferred from their speech and behaviour. Secondly, the unfortunate situation has arisen where various authors in psychiatry have described a different conceptual view of thought disorder, which has resulted in conflicting and confusing classification systems. For example, some authors classify delusions as disorders of thought form, whereas others classify them as disorders of thought content. It is probably not that important that you are able to classify and subgroup thought disorder, but rather that you have a clear understanding of the individual definitions you intend to use and are able to recognize them in the patients that you assess. In this regard, it is particularly helpful if you document and are able to cite examples of the patient's speech in their own words.

A simple classification divides thought disorders in two broad groups: *abnormal beliefs* and *disorganized thinking*.

### Abnormal beliefs

Abnormal beliefs include primary and secondary *delusions* and *overvalued ideas*. FALSE + FIXED

*Delusions*　A delusion is a false belief held with extraordinary conviction that is not accepted by other members of the patient's culture. It is important to understand the following characteristics of delusional thinking:

- To the patient, there is no difference between a delusional belief and a true belief – they are the same experience. Therefore, only an external observer can diagnose a delusion. A delusion is to ideation what a hallucination is to perception (Sims S Symptoms in the mind, 3rd edn, Saunders, Edinburgh 2002).
- The delusion is false because of faulty reasoning. A man's delusional belief that his wife is having an affair may actually be true (she may indeed be unfaithful), but it remains a delusion because the reason he gives for this belief is undoubtedly false. For example, she 'must' be having an affair because she is part of a top-secret sexual conspiracy to prove that he is a homosexual.
- It is out of keeping with the patient's social and cultural background. It crucial to establish that the belief is not one likely to be held by that person's subcultural group, e.g. a belief in the imminent second coming of Christ may be appropriate for a member of a religious group, but not for a formerly atheist, middle-aged businessman.

It is diagnostically significant to classify delusions as:

- Primary or secondary.
- Mood congruent or mood incongruent.
- Bizarre or non-bizarre.
- And according to the content of the delusion.

*Primary delusions* (autochthonous delusions) do not occur in response to any previous psycho-pathological state; their genesis is un-understandable. They may be preceded by a *delusional atmosphere (mood)* where patients have a sense that the world around them has been subtly altered, often in a sinister or threatening way. In this state a fully formed delusion has not yet developed and patients appear perplexed and apprehensive. Note that when a delusion occurs after a delusional atmosphere it is still regarded as primary – the delusional atmosphere is probably a precursor to the fully developed primary delusion. A *delusional perception* is also a primary delusion and occurs when a delusional meaning is attached to a normal perception; e.g. a patient believed he was a terrorist target because he heard an aeroplane flying in the distance. Primary delusions occur typically in schizophrenia and other primary psychotic disorders. *Secondary delusions* are the consequences of pre-existing psychopathological states, usually mood disorders – see p. 11. Many interrelated delusions that are centred on a common theme are termed *systematized delusions*.

In *mood-congruent delusions*, the contents of the delusions are appropriate to the patient's mood and are commonly seen in depression or mania with psychotic features.

*Bizarre delusions* are those which are completely impossible; e.g. the belief that aliens have planted radioactive detonators in the patient's brain. They are considered to be characteristic of schizophrenia.

Figure 4.2 lists the classification of delusions by their content. It is important that you are able to label a delusion according to its content, so take some time to familiarize yourself with this table.

## Content of delusions

| Classification | Content |
|---|---|
| Persecutory delusions * | False belief that one is being harmed, threatened, cheated, harassed or is a victim of a conspiracy |
| Grandiose delusions | False belief that one is exceptionally powerful (including having 'mystical powers'), talented or important |
| Delusions of reference | False belief that certain objects, people or events have intense personal significance and refer specifically to oneself, e.g. believing that a television newsreader is talking directly about one |
| Religious delusions | False belief pertaining to a religious theme, often grandiose in nature, e.g. believing that one is a special messenger from God |
| Delusions of love (erotomania) | False belief that another person is in love with one (commoner in women). In one form, termed *de Clérambault syndrome*, a woman (usually) believes that a man, frequently older and of higher status, is in love with her |
| Delusion of infidelity (morbid jealousy, Othello syndrome) | False belief that one's lover has been unfaithful. Note that morbid jealousy may also take the form of an overvalued idea, that is, non-psychotic jealousy |
| Delusions of misidentification | *Capgras syndrome*: belief that a familiar person has been replaced by an exact double – an impostor. *Fregoli syndrome*: belief that a complete stranger is actually a familiar person already known to one |
| Nihilistic delusions (see Cotard's syndrome, p.156) | False belief that oneself, others or the world is non-existent or about to end. In severe cases, negation is carried to the extreme with patients claiming that nothing, including themselves, exists |
| Somatic delusions | False belief concerning one's body and its functioning, e.g. that one's bowels are rotting. Also called *hypochondriacal delusions* (to be distinguished from the overvalued ideas seen in hypochondriacal disorder) |
| Delusions of infestation (Ekbom's syndrome) | False belief that one is infested with small but visible organisms. May also occur secondary to tactile hallucinations, e.g. formication (see text) |
| Delusions of control (passivity or 'made' experiences) *Note: these are all first-rank symptoms of schizophrenia* | False belief that one's thoughts, feelings, actions or impulses are controlled or 'made' by an external agency, e.g. believing that one was *made* to break a window by demons. Delusions of thought control include: *Thought insertion*: belief that thoughts or ideas are being implanted in one's head by an external agency. *Thought withdrawal*: belief that one's thoughts or ideas are being extracted from one's head by an external agency. *Thought broadcasting*: belief that one's thoughts are being diffused or broadcast to others such that they know what one is thinking |

**Fig. 4.2** Classification of delusions by content.

Note that the term 'paranoid' refers to any delusions or ideas that are unduly self-referent – typically delusions or ideas of persecution, grandeur or reference. It should not be used synonymously with the term persecutory; i.e. when a patient has a false belief that people are trying to harm him, do not say that he is paranoid, rather say that he has persecutory delusions.

25

Finally, beliefs that were previously held with delusional intensity but then become held with less conviction are termed *partial delusions*. This occurs when patients start recovering after receiving treatment.

Direct questioning about perceptual experience may alienate a non-psychotic patient and raise undue suspicion in a psychotic patient. To maintain rapport with patients begin these questions with a primer like: 'I am now going to ask you some questions which may seem a little strange, but are routine questions which I ask all patients.'

**Overvalued ideas**   An overvalued idea is a plausible belief that a patient becomes preoccupied with to an unreasonable extent. The key feature is that the *pursuit* of this idea causes considerable distress to the patient or those living around them – it is *overvalued*. Patients who hold overvalued ideas have usually had them for many years and typically have abnormalities of personality. They are distinguished from delusions by the lack of a gross abnormality in reasoning; these patients can often give fairly logical reasons for their beliefs. Overvalued ideas differ from obsessions and compulsions in that patients do not regard them as senseless or undesirable, i.e. they are ego-syntonic; whereas, patients with obsessive-compulsive disorder recognize that their thoughts or behaviours are irrational or excessive, i.e. ego-dystonic (see Ch. 7). Typical disorders that feature overvalued ideas are anorexia nervosa, hypochondriacal disorder, dysmorphophobia, paranoid personality disorder and morbid jealousy (this can also take the form of a delusion).

## Disorganized thinking

Many patients with delusions are able to communicate in a clear and coherent manner; although their beliefs may be false, their speech is *organized*. However, there is a subgroup of psychotic patients who speak in such a *disorganized* way that it becomes difficult to understand what they are saying. The coherency of patients with disorganized thinking varies from being mostly understandable in patients exhibiting *circumstantial thinking* to being completely incomprehensible in patients with a *word salad* phenomenon.

The following are important signs of disorganized thinking:

***Circumstantial and tangential thinking***   See page 10.

***Loosening of association (derailment/knight's move thinking)***   This is when the patient's train of thought shifts suddenly from one very loosely or unrelated idea to the next. In its worst form, speech becomes a mixture of incoherent words and phrases and is termed *word salad*. Loosening of association is characteristic of schizophrenia. Note that some psychiatrists, but unfortunately not all, use the term *formal thought disorder* synonymously with loosening of association.

***Neologisms and idiosyncratic word use***
Neologisms are new words created by the patient, often combining syllables of other known words. Patients can also use recognized words idiosyncratically by attributing them with a non-recognized meaning (metonyms).

***Flight of ideas***   See page 11.

***Thought blocking***   This occurs when patients experience a sudden cessation to their flow of thought, often in mid-sentence (observed as sudden breaks in speech). Patients have no recall of what they were saying or thinking and thus continue talking about a different topic.

***Perseveration***   This is when patients unnecessarily repeat a word or phrase they have previously expressed. *Palilalia* describes the repetition of the last word of their sentence; *logoclonia* describes the repetition of the last syllable of their last word. Perseveration is highly suggestive of organic brain disease.

***Echolalia***   This is when patients senselessly repeat words or phrases spoken around them by others – like a parrot.

***Irrelevant answers***   Patients give answers that are completely unrelated to the original question.

## Negative symptoms
Some psychiatrists classify schizophrenic patients according to whether they exhibit predominantly *positive* or *negative* symptoms. Positive symptoms are those that are actively *produced* and include delusions, hallucinations, loosening of association and bizarre speech or behaviour. This is opposed to

High expressed emotion = family exhibit this + poor for pt.
↳ Bad ∴ pt. requires a certain amount of stimulants.

Differential diagnosis of the psychotic patient

negative symptoms that indicate a clinical *deficit* and include marked apathy, poverty of thought and speech, blunting of affect, social isolation, poor self-care and cognitive deficits. Patients can have positive and negative symptoms simultaneously or, as often happens, develop a negative presentation after initially presenting with predominantly positive symptoms. Remember that patients with a depressed mood or those experiencing significant side-effects from psychotropic medication may also present with negative symptoms.

## Psychomotor function

Although a relatively rare phenomenon in industrialized countries, some psychotic patients will present with abnormalities of motor function. Motor system dysfunction in schizophrenia is, invariably, due to the extra-pyramidal side-effects of neuroleptic medication (see Ch. 27). However, psychotic patients can occasionally present with impressive motor signs that are not caused by psychiatric medication or a known organic brain disease. Although undoubtedly associated with the patient's abnormal mental state, the cause of this psychomotor dysfunction is far from clarified. The term *catatonia* literally means extreme muscular tone or rigidity; however, it commonly describes any excessive or decreased motor activity that is apparently purposeless and includes abnormalities of movement, tone or position. Note that catatonic symptoms are not diagnostic of schizophrenia; they may also be caused by brain diseases, metabolic abnormalities, psychoactive substances and can also occur in mood disorders. Figure 4.3 describes the common motor symptoms seen in schizophrenia.

## Differential diagnosis of the psychotic patient

Psychotic symptoms are non-specific and are associated with many primary psychiatric illnesses. They can also present secondary to a general medical condition or psychoactive substance use.

| Motor symptoms in schizophrenia | |
| --- | --- |
| Catatonic rigidity | Maintaining a fixed position and rigidly resisting all attempts to be moved |
| Catatonic posturing | Adopting an unusual or bizarre position that is then maintained for some time |
| Catatonic negativism | A seemingly motiveless resistance to all instructions or attempts to be moved; patients may do the opposite of what is asked |
| Catatonic waxy flexibility (flexibilitas cerea) | Patients can be 'moulded' like wax into a position that is then maintained |
| Catatonic excitement | Agitated, excited and seemingly purposeless motor activity, not influenced by external stimuli |
| Catatonic stupor | A presentation of *akinesis* (lack of voluntary movement), *mutism* and *extreme unresponsiveness* in an otherwise alert patient (there may be slight clouding of consciousness) |
| Echopraxia | Patients senselessly repeat or imitate the actions of those around them. Associated with *echolalia* (see above) – also occurs in patients with frontal lobe damage |
| Mannerisms | Apparently goal-directed movements (e.g. waving, saluting) that are performed repeatedly or at socially inappropriate times |
| Stereotypies | A complex movement that does not appear to be goal-directed (e.g. rocking to and fro, gyrating) |
| Tics | Sudden, involuntary, rapid, recurrent, non-rhythmic motor movements or vocalizations |

**Fig. 4.3** Motor symptoms in schizophrenia.

27

See Figure 4.4 for the differential diagnosis for the psychotic patient.

# Psychotic disorders
## Schizophrenia

There are no pathognomonic or singularly defining symptoms of schizophrenia; it is a syndrome characterized by a heterogeneous cluster of symptoms and signs. The ICD-10 has set out diagnostic guidelines based on the most commonly occurring symptom groups, which have been discussed in the preceding section (Fig. 4.5). It is important to establish that there has been a clear and marked deterioration in the patient's social and work functioning.

In the past, psychiatrists used *Schneider's first-rank symptoms* to make the diagnosis of schizophrenia. Kurt Schneider suggested that the presence of one or more first-rank symptoms in the absence of organic disease was of pragmatic value in making the diagnosis of schizophrenia. First-rank symptoms are still referred to so you should familiarize yourself with them; they are presented in Figure 4.6.

Memory aid: if you add 'bizarre delusions' and 'hallucinations coming from a part of the body' to Schneider's first-rank symptoms you will have the (a) to (d) criteria of the ICD-10 diagnostic guidelines for schizophrenia.

*Schizophrenia subtypes*   Due to the differing presentations of schizophrenia, researchers have tried to identify schizophrenia subtypes. The importance of these subtypes is that they vary in their prognosis and treatment response. The ICD-10 has coded the following subtypes, which are not necessarily exclusive:

- *Paranoid schizophrenia*: dominated by the presence of delusions and hallucinations (positive symptoms). Negative and catatonic symptoms as

---

**Differential diagnosis for the psychotic patient**

Psychotic disorders
- Schizophrenia
- Schizophrenia-like psychotic disorders
- Schizoaffective disorder
- Delusional disorder

Mood disorders
- Manic episode with psychotic features
- Depressive episode, severe, with psychotic features

Secondary to a general medical condition

Secondary to psychoactive substance use

Dementia/delirium

Personality disorder (schizotypal, borderline, schizoid, paranoid)

**Fig. 4.4** Differential diagnosis for the psychotic patient.

**Fig. 4.5** ICD-10 diagnostic guidelines for schizophrenia.

---

**ICD-10 diagnostic guidelines for schizophrenia**

*One or more of the following symptoms*:
a. Thought echo, insertion, withdrawal or broadcast
b. Delusions of control or passivity; delusional perception
c. Hallucinatory voices giving a running commentary; discussing the patient amongst themselves or 'originating' from some part of the body
d. Bizarre delusions

OR
*Two or more of the following symptoms*:
e. Other hallucinations that either occur every day for weeks or that are associated with fleeting delusions or sustained overvalued ideas
f. Thought disorganization (loosening of association, incoherence, neologisms)
g. Catatonic symptoms
h. Negative symptoms
i. Change in personal behaviour (loss of interest, aimlessness, social withdrawal)

*Symptoms should be present for most of the time during at least 1 month*
*Schizophrenia should not be diagnosed in the presence of organic brain disease or during drug intoxication or withdrawal*

*delusional experience of a normal percept⁰ (e.g. dog barks → leave town).*

---

**Schneider's first-rank symptoms of schizophrenia**

- Delusional perception
- Delusions of thought control: insertion, withdrawal, broadcast
- Delusions of control: passivity experiences of affect (feelings), impulse, volition and somatic passivity (influence controlling the body)
- Hallucinations: audible thoughts (first person or thought echo), voices arguing or discussing the patient, voices giving a running commentary

**Fig. 4.6** Schneider's first-rank symptoms of schizophrenia.
*one or more in the absence of chronic disease.*

*3rd person:*
*possible also depression.*

---

well as thought disorganization are not prominent. The prognosis is usually better and the onset of illness later than the other subtypes.

- *Hebephrenic (disorganized) schizophrenia:* characterized by thought disorganization, disturbed behaviour and inappropriate or flat affect. Delusions and hallucination are fleeting or not prominent. Onset of illness is earlier (15 to 25 years of age) and the prognosis poorer than paranoid schizophrenia.
- *Catatonic schizophrenia:* a rare form characterized by one or more catatonic symptoms (see Fig. 4.3).
- *Residual schizophrenia:* 1 year of predominantly chronic negative symptoms which must have been preceded by at least one clear cut psychotic episode in the past.

## Schizophrenia-like psychotic disorders

Throughout the history of psychiatry, researchers have speculated on the possibility that some psychotic patients with schizophrenia-like symptoms might, in fact, have a separate psychotic illness with a different mode of onset, time course and, perhaps, better prognosis. This idea was born from the observation that some psychotic episodes had an abrupt onset (without a prodromal phase), seemed to be precipitated by an acute life stress or had a duration of symptoms less than that usually observed in schizophrenia. The ICD-10 makes provision for coding of this presentation under the section, *acute and transient psychotic disorders*. The DSM-IV, on the other hand, suggests diagnoses of *schizophreniform disorder* and *brief psychotic disorder*.

## Schizoaffective disorder    *schizophrenic plus Mood!*

Schizoaffective disorder describes the presentation of both schizophrenic and mood (depressed or manic) symptoms that present in the same episode of illness, either simultaneously or within a few days of each other. The mood symptoms should meet the criteria for either a depressive or manic episode. Patients should also have at least one, preferably two,

of the typical schizophrenic symptoms – symptoms (a) to (d) as specified in the ICD-10 schizophrenia diagnostic guidelines (see Fig. 4.5). Depending on the particular mood symptoms displayed, this disorder can be coded in the ICD-10 as *schizoaffective disorder, manic type* or *schizoaffective disorder, depressed type*.

When psychiatrists talk about the *typical symptoms* of schizophrenia, they are generally referring to (a) to (d) of the ICD-10 criteria for schizophrenia (or Schneider's first-rank symptoms), e.g. delusions of control, running commentary hallucinations, etc.

## Delusional disorder

In this disorder, the development of a single or set of delusions for the period of at least 3 months is the most prominent or only symptom. It usually has its onset in middle age and expressed delusions may persist throughout the patient's life and include persecutory, grandiose and hypochondriacal delusions. Typically schizophrenic delusions, like delusions of thought control or passivity, exclude this diagnosis. Hallucinations, if present, tend to be only fleeting and are not typically schizophrenic in nature; brief depressive symptoms may also be evident. Affect, speech and behaviour are all normal and these patients usually have well-preserved personal and social skills. Rarely, patients may present with an *induced delusional disorder* (folie à deux), which occurs when non-psychotic patients with close emotional ties to another person suffering from delusions (usually a dominant figure) begin to share those delusional ideas themselves. The delusions in the non-psychotic patient tend to resolve when the two are separated.

# Mood (affective) disorders
## Manic episode with psychotic features
See Chapter 2.

## Depressive episode, severe with psychotic features
See Chapter 1.

## Psychotic episodes secondary to a general medical condition or psychoactive substance use
A medical or psychoactive substance cause of psychosis should always be sought for and ruled out. Figure 4.7 lists the medical and substance-related causes of psychotic episodes. The medical condition or substance use should predate the development of the psychosis and symptoms should resolve with treatment of the condition or abstinence from the offending substance. Absence of previous psychotic episodes or a family history of schizophrenia also supports this diagnosis.

## Delirium and dementia
Visual hallucinations and delusions are common in delirium and may also occur in dementia, particularly diffuse Lewy body dementia (see Ch. 9).

## Personality disorder
Schizotypal (personality) disorder is characterized by eccentric behaviour and peculiarities of thinking and appearance. Although there are no clear psychotic symptoms evident and its course resembles that of a personality disorder, the ICD-10 actually describes schizotypal disorder in the chapter on psychotic disorders. This is because it is more prevalent among relatives of patients with schizophrenia and,

occasionally, it progresses to overt schizophrenia. Borderline, paranoid and schizoid personality disorders also share similar features to schizophrenia without displaying clear-cut psychotic symptoms. Personality disorders are discussed in greater detail in Chapter 11.

## Algorithm for the diagnosis of psychotic disorders
See Figure 4.8.

## Assessment

### Clinical
The following questions may be helpful in eliciting psychotic phenomena on mental state examination:

*→ start w/ unusual experiences?*

#### Hallucinations
- Do you ever hear strange noises or voices when there is no one else about?
- Do you ever hear your own thoughts spoken aloud such that someone standing next to you might possibly hear them? (*audible thoughts – first person auditory hallucinations*)
- Do you ever hear your thoughts echoed just after you have thought them? (*thought echo*)
- Do these voices talk directly to you or give you commands? (*second person auditory hallucinations*)
- Do these voices ever talk about you with each other or make comments about what you are doing? (*third person auditory hallucinations/ running commentary*)

**Fig. 4.7** Medical and substance-related causes of psychotic symptoms.

| Medical and substance-related causes of psychotic symptoms | |
| --- | --- |
| **Medical conditions** | **Substances** |
| Acute intermittent porphyria | Alcohol |
| Cerebral neoplasm, infarcts, trauma, infection (including HIV, CJD, neurosyphilis, herpes encephalitis) | Amfetamines |
| | Anticholinergics |
| Endocrinological (thyroid, parathyroid, adrenal disorders) | Antiparkinsonian drugs |
| Epilepsy (especially temporal lobe epilepsy) | Cocaine |
| Huntington's disease | Corticosteroids |
| Systemic lupus erythematosus | Hallucinogens |
| Vitamin B$_{12}$, niacin (pellagra) and thiamine deficiency (Wernicke's encephalopathy) | Inhalants/solvents |
| | Organophosphates |
| | Phencyclidine (PCP) |

HIV: human immunodeficiency virus
CJD: Creutzfeldt–Jakob disease

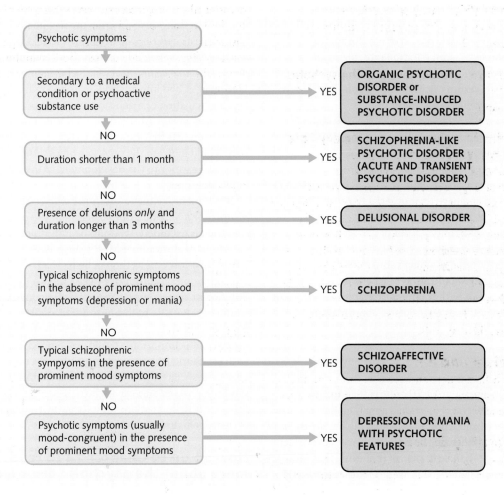

**Fig. 4.8** Algorithm for the diagnosis of a patient presenting with psychotic symptoms.

## Delusions

- Are you afraid that someone is trying to harm or poison you? (*persecutory delusions*)
- Have you noticed that people are doing or saying things that have a special meaning for you? (*delusions of reference*)
- Do you have any special abilities or powers? (*grandiose delusions*)
- Does it seem as though you are being controlled or influenced by some external force? (*delusions of control*)
- Are thoughts that don't belong to you being put into your head? (*thought insertion*)

A basic physical examination including a thorough neurological and endocrine system examination should be performed on all patients with psychotic symptoms.

## Special investigations

- It is important to obtain collateral information from the patient's GP, family and care co-ordinator (if they have one) to establish premorbid personality and functioning as well as pattern of deterioration.
- Blood investigations are performed to:
  a. Exclude possible medical or substance-related causes of psychosis
  b. Establish baseline values before administering antipsychotics and other psychotropic drugs that may alter blood composition and
  c. Assess renal and liver functioning which may affect elimination of drugs that are likely to be taken long-term and possibly in depot form.

- If the patient presents with a first episode of psychosis, a good basic screen comprises full blood count (essential when starting clozapine), erythrocyte sedimentation rate, urea and electrolytes, thyroid function, liver function tests, glucose, serum calcium, and a syphilis serology test if syphilis is suspected.
- A urine drug screen should always be done because illicit drugs both cause and exacerbate a psychosis.
- An ECG should be done in patients with cardiac problems as many antipsychotics prolong the QT interval and have the potential to cause lethal ventricular arrhythmia.
- The use of a routine EEG or CT scan to help exclude an organic psychosis (e.g. temporal lobe epilepsy, brain tumour) varies between psychiatric units; they should always be considered in atypical cases, cases with treatment resistance, or if there are cognitive or neurological abnormalities.

## Discussion of case study

Mr PP meets the ICD-10 criteria for *schizophrenia, paranoid subtype*. He has had a marked deterioration in his social and work functioning. He has *delusions of persecution* (believing he was a victim of government experiments), *thought control* (believing that ideas were being planted in his head (*thought insertion*)) and *reference* (believing that the man in pub was referring specifically to him). His claim that he knew these things after hearing the neighbour's dog bark suggests *delusional perception*. He also has *second person command hallucinations* and *third person, running commentary hallucinations*. 'Receiving coded information' from the radio might be a hallucination or a delusion of reference depending on how Mr PP described this experience subjectively. Mr PP's description that 'all was not right' could indicate the presence of a *delusional atmosphere*, prior to the development of the full-blown delusions.

It is imperative that a *substance-induced psychotic disorder* or *psychotic disorder secondary to a medical condition* is excluded. It would be important to ascertain the duration of Mr PP's psychotic symptoms. It seems as though he has had schizophrenic symptoms for over a month. If the duration of symptoms had been less than month, it would be advisable to diagnose a schizophrenia-like psychotic disorder, e.g. *acute and transient psychotic disorder*. It is important to rule out a mood disorder with psychotic features. The presence of a mood episode associated with simultaneous schizophrenic symptoms would suggest a schizoaffective episode. Prominent hallucinations militate against a diagnosis of delusional disorder.

**Now go on to Chapter 14 to read more about the psychotic disorders and their management.**

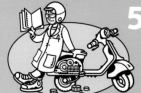

# 5. The Patient with Anxiety, Fear or Avoidance

Mrs PA, a 32-year-old divorced interior designer, was referred to a consultant psychiatrist by her family doctor because of a 6-month history of sudden, dramatic anxiety attacks accompanied by heart palpitations, profuse sweating, dizziness, a choking sensation and a fear that she was going to die. There appeared to be no logical reason for the attacks and Mrs PA described them as coming on 'out of the blue'. They reached their maximum intensity within 2 minutes and seldom lasted longer than 15 minutes, occurring two to three times a week. Because of these attacks, which occurred in any situation and at any time of day, Mrs PA had stopped going into shops or crowded public places for fear of having an attack and not being able to escape to a safe place and appearing like a 'blubbering fool'. She had started relying on her mother to accompany her on 'absolutely necessary' household excursions 'just in case' she had another attack. Her GP had booked her off work for the past 3 months, as she was too frightened to visit potential clients' houses in the event that she had another attack. Mrs PA told the psychiatrist that she had almost become housebound and felt that she was 'losing her mind'. A full physical examination, routine blood tests including: full blood count, urea and electrolytes, fasting glucose, liver functions, thyroid functions and calcium concentration as well as an electrocardiogram (ECG) revealed no abnormalities.

*(For a discussion of the case study see the end of the chapter)*

Feelings of anxiety or fear are both common and essential to the human experience. It is the very uncomfortable nature of this experience that makes anxiety such an effective alerting and therefore harm-avoiding device. However, for the same reasons, when anxiety is excessive and unchecked it can create an extremely debilitating condition. To distinguish between normal and psychopathological anxiety it is important to observe the patient's level of functioning. The Yerkes–Dodson law states that the relationship between performance and anxiety has the shape of an inverted U: mild to moderate levels of anxiety improve performance, but high levels impair it. Figure 5.1 demonstrates the Yerkes–Dodson curve.

## Definitions and clinical features

Both anxiety and fear are alerting signals that occur in response to a potential threat. Some authors suggest that *anxiety* occurs in response to threat that is unknown, internal or vague (i.e. objectless); whereas,

*fear* occurs in response to a threat from a known, external or definite object.

The experience of anxiety consists of two interrelated components: (1) *thoughts* of being apprehensive, nervous or frightened, and (2) the awareness of a *physical reaction* to anxiety (autonomic or peripheral anxiety). Figure 5.2 summarizes the physical signs of anxiety. The experience of anxiety may lead to a change in *behaviour*, particularly an *avoidance* of the real or imagined threat.

There are two patterns of pathological anxiety:
1. *Generalized (free-floating) anxiety* does not occur in discrete episodes and tends to last for hours, days or even longer and is of mild to moderate severity. It is not associated with a specific external threat or situation (i.e. free-floating) but is rather excessive worry or apprehension about many normal life events (e.g. job security, relationships and responsibilities).
2. *Paroxysmal anxiety* has an abrupt onset, occurs in discrete episodes and tends to be quite severe. In its severest form, paroxysmal anxiety presents as

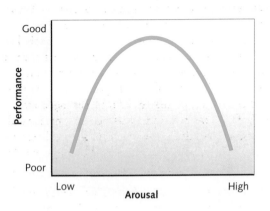

**Fig. 5.1** Yerkes–Dodson law (1908).

*panic attacks*. These are discrete episodes of short-lived (usually less than 1 hour), intense anxiety. They have an abrupt onset and rapidly build up to a peak level of anxiety. They are accompanied by strong autonomic symptoms (see Fig. 5.2), which may lead patients to believe that they are dying, having a heart attack or going mad – this increases their anxiety level and produces further physical symptoms, thereby creating a vicious cycle.

See Figure 5.3 for a comparison of panic attacks and free-floating (generalized) anxiety.

*Paroxysmal anxiety* can further be subdivided into episodes of anxiety that occur seemingly spontaneously, *without* a specific imagined or external threat (see panic disorder, later) and those episodes that occur *in response* to a specific imagined or external threat. The phobic disorders are the most common cause of paroxysmal anxiety in response to a perceived threat.

### Physical signs of anxiety

Tachycardia
Palpitations (abnormal awareness of the heart beating)
Hypertension
Shortness of breath/rapid breathing
Chest pain or discomfort
Choking sensation
Tremors, shaking
Muscle tension
Dry mouth
Sweating
Cold skin
Nausea or vomiting
Diarrhoea
Abdominal discomfort ('butterflies')
Dizziness, light-headedness, syncope
Pupil dilatation (mydriasis)

**Fig. 5.2** Physical signs of anxiety.

phobic disorders = most common cause of paroxysmal anxiety in response to a perceived threat

A *phobia* is an intense, irrational fear of an object, activity or situation (e.g. flying, heights, animals, blood, public speaking). Although they may recognize that their fear is irrational, patients characteristically avoid the phobic stimulus or endure it with extreme distress. It is the degree of fear that is irrational in that the feared objects or situations are not inevitably dangerous and do not cause such severe anxiety in most other people. In severe cases, phobic anxiety may progress to frank panic attacks.

## Differential diagnosis

When considering the differential diagnosis of anxiety you should determine:

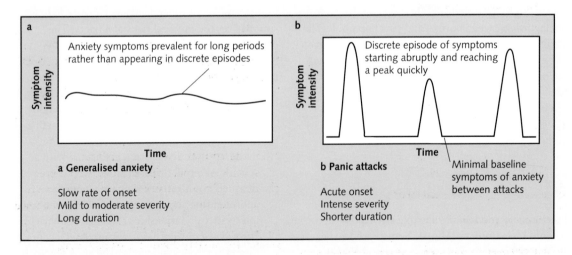

**Fig. 5.3** Graphs comparing generalized (free-floating) anxiety (A) and panic attacks (B).

- The rate of *onset*, *severity* and *duration* of the anxiety, i.e. is the anxiety generalized or paroxysmal?
- Whether the anxiety is *in response* to a specific threat or does it arise *spontaneously (unprovoked)*?
- Whether the anxiety only occurs in the context of a *pre-existing psychiatric* or *medical condition*.

Figure 5.4 presents the differential diagnosis for patients presenting with anxiety.

## Anxiety disorders

It is useful to consider the primary anxiety disorders under the headings: phobic disorders, non-situational disorders, reaction to stress and obsessive-compulsive disorder.

### Phobic disorders

Remember that:

- All phobic disorders are associated with a prominent *avoidance* of the feared situation.
- The situationally induced anxiety may be so severe as to take the form of a *panic attack*.

***Agoraphobia***   Agoraphobia literally means *fear of the marketplace*, i.e. fear of public places. In psychiatry today, it has a wider meaning that also includes a fear of entering crowded spaces (shops, trains, buses, elevators) where an immediate escape is difficult or in which help might not be available in the event of having a panic attack. At the worst extreme, patients

---

**Differential diagnosis for patients presenting with anxiety**

Anxiety disorders:
- Phobic disorders
  Agoraphobia (with or without panic disorder)
  Social phobia
  Specific phobia
- Non-situational disorders
  Generalized anxiety disorder
  Panic disorder
- Reaction to stress
  Acute stress reaction
  Post-traumatic stress disorder
  Adjustment disorder
- Obsessive-compulsive disorder

Secondary to other psychiatric disorders
(especially depression and psychosis)

Secondary to a general medical condition

Secondary to psychoactive substance use (especially alcohol use)

**Fig. 5.4** Differential diagnosis for patients presenting with anxiety.

---

may become housebound or refuse to leave the house unless accompanied by a close friend or relative.

There is a close relationship between agoraphobia and panic disorder that occurs when patients develop a fear of being in a place from where escape would be difficult in the event of having a panic attack. In fact, studies have shown that in a clinical setting, up to 95% of patients presenting with agoraphobia have a current or past diagnosis of panic disorder. Therefore, in the ICD-10 you can code agoraphobia as occurring *with or without panic disorder*.

***Social phobia***   Patients with social phobia fear social situations where they might be exposed to scrutiny by others which might lead to humiliation or embarrassment. This fear might be limited to an isolated fear (e.g. public speaking, eating in public, fear of vomiting or interacting with the opposite sex) or may involve almost all social activities outside the home.

***Specific phobia***   Specific (simple) phobias are restricted to clearly specific and discernible objects or situations (other than those covered in agoraphobia and social phobia). Examples from adult psychiatric samples in order of decreasing prevalence include:

- *Situational*: specific situations, e.g. public transportation, flying, driving, tunnels, bridges, elevators.
- *Natural environment*: heights, storms, water, darkness.
- *Blood–injection–injury*: seeing blood or an injury, fear of needles or an invasive medical procedure.
- *Animal*: animals or insects, e.g. spiders, dogs, mice.
- *Other*: fear of choking or vomiting, contracting an illness (e.g. AIDS), children's fear of costumed characters.

Patients with a phobic disorder may experience little anxiety in their daily living because they go to extreme lengths to avoid the phobic stimulus.

### Non-situational anxiety disorders

These disorders, unlike the phobic disorders, are characterized by primary anxiety symptoms that are not restricted to any specific situation or circumstance.

***Generalized anxiety disorder***   The key element of generalized anxiety disorder is long-standing, free-floating anxiety. Patients describe excessive worry about minor matters and should be apprehensive on most days for about 6 months. The ICD-10 diagnostic guidelines suggest three key elements:

1. Apprehension.
2. Motor tension (restlessness, fidgeting, tension headaches, inability to relax).
3. Autonomic overactivity (see Fig. 5.2).

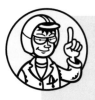 Blood–injection–injury phobias differ from others in that they are characterized by bradycardia and possibly syncope (vasovagal response), rather than tachycardia.

***Panic disorder*** Panic disorder is characterized by the presence of panic attacks that occur unpredictably and are not restricted to any particular situation (phobic disorders) or objective danger. Panic attacks are so distressing that patients commonly develop a fear of having further attacks; this is known as *anticipatory anxiety*. Anticipatory anxiety apart, patients are relatively free from anxiety symptoms between attacks.

Remember that many patients with panic disorder will also have concurrent agoraphobia, so in the ICD-10 you can code agoraphobia as occurring *with or without panic disorder*.

 Panic attacks can occur spontaneously (unprovoked) or as an extreme response to a phobic stimulus.

***Reaction to stress and obsessive-compulsive disorder*** The disorders associated with a reaction to stress and obsessive-compulsive disorder will be discussed in Chapters 6 and 7 respectively.

 Both agoraphobia and severe social phobia may result in patients becoming 'housebound' and can be difficult to distinguish. When in doubt, precedence should be given to agoraphobia.

## Other psychiatric conditions

Anxiety is a non-specific symptom and can occur secondary to other psychiatric conditions. See Figure 5.5 for examples of psychiatric problems commonly associated with anxiety.

Note that depression and anxiety are inextricably intertwined. Not only can anxiety occur secondary to a depressive disorder and vice versa, but some authors have also suggested that the two disorders are aetiologically related. About 65% of patients with anxiety also have depressive symptoms; therefore, when making a diagnosis, it is essential to decide which symptoms came first or were predominant and which were secondary. If symptoms of anxiety occur only in the context of a genuine depressive episode then depression takes precedence and should be diagnosed alone.

## Anxiety secondary to a general medical condition or psychoactive substance use

A medical or psychoactive substance cause of anxiety should always be actively sought and ruled out. Figure 5.6 lists the medical and substance related causes of anxiety. The medical condition or substance use should predate the development of the anxiety and symptoms should resolve with treatment of the condition or abstinence from the offending substance. Absence of previous anxiety or a family history of anxiety disorder also supports this diagnosis.

## Assessment

### Clinical

The following questions may be helpful in eliciting anxiety symptoms on mental state examination:

- Do you sometimes wake up feeling anxious and dreading the day ahead? (*any form of anxiety*)
- Do you worry excessively about minor matters on most days of the week? (*generalized anxiety*)
- Have you ever been so frightened that your heart was pounding and you thought you might die? (*panic attack*)
- Do you avoid leaving the house alone because you are afraid of having a panic attack or being in situation (like being in a crowded shop or on a train) from which escape will be difficult or embarrassing? (*agoraphobia*)
- Do you get anxious in social situations, like speaking in front of people or making conversation? (*social phobia*)

**Examples of psychiatric problems commonly associated with anxiety**

| Focus of anxiety | Psychiatric problem |
|---|---|
| Gaining weight | Eating disorder (see Ch. 12) |
| Having many physical complaints | Somatization disorder (see Ch. 8) |
| Having a serious illness | Hypochondriacal disorder (see Ch. 8) |
| Fear of being poisoned or killed | Delusional beliefs in paranoid schizophrenia (see Ch. 4) |
| Ruminatory thoughts of guilt or worthlessness | Depression (see Ch. 1) |
| When having an obsessional thought or resisting a compulsion | Obsessive-compulsive disorder (see Ch. 7) |

**Fig. 5.5** Examples of psychiatric problems commonly associated with anxiety.

- Do some things or situations make you very scared? Do you avoid them? (*specific phobia*)

**A basic physical examination, including a thorough neurological and endocrine system examination, should be performed on all patients with symptoms of anxiety.**

## Special investigations

The anxiety disorders can only be diagnosed when the symptoms are not due to the direct effect of a substance or medical condition. This stipulation is particularly relevant when considering diagnoses of generalized anxiety disorder and panic disorder. It is impractical to test for each of the large number of drugs and organic conditions capable of producing anxiety symptoms (see Fig. 5.6). It is, however, important to exclude any disease or substance that may be implicated through any clues in the history (e.g. past medical history and drug history) and physical examination. For example, a patient with a rapid pulse and heat intolerance should have thyroid function tests in case thyrotoxicosis is causing the anxiety symptoms. The possibility of withdrawal syndromes (e.g. alcohol, benzodiazepines, opiates) causing anxiety symptoms should also be considered.

## Discussion of case study

Repeated, unexpected episodes of short-lived intense anxiety of abrupt onset and rapidly building up to a peak level of anxiety associated with palpitations, sweating, dizziness, a choking sensation

**Medical conditions and substances that are associated with anxiety**

| Medical conditions | Substances | | |
|---|---|---|---|
| | Intoxication | Withdrawal | Side-effects of prescribed drugs |
| Cerebral trauma | Alcohol | Alcohol | Analgesics |
| Chronic obstructive airways disease | Amfetamines | Benzodiazepines | Anticholinergics |
| Congestive cardiac failure | Caffeine | Caffeine | Antidepressants (e.g. SSRIs and |
| Cushing's disease | Cannabis | Cocaine | tricyclics in first 2 weeks of use) |
| Hyperthyroidism | Cocaine | Nicotine | Antipsychotics |
| Hypoglycaemia | Hallucinogens | Other sedatives and hypnotics | Corticosteroids |
| Malignancies | Inhalants | | Sympathomimetics |
| Phaeochromocytoma | Phencyclidine | | Thyroid hormones |
| Pulmonary embolism | | | |
| Temporal lope epilepsy | | | |
| Vitamin deficiencies | | | |

**Fig. 5.6** Medical conditions and substances that are associated with anxiety.

and thoughts of being about to die, with no organic cause, suggests a diagnosis of *panic disorder*.

As is common in many patients with panic disorder, *agoraphobia* has developed as a super-added problem as evidenced by a fear of going into situations from which escape might be difficult or humiliating. Mrs PA is showing the important sign of *avoidance* of the feared situation by refusing to go out unless it is essential and then only accompanied by her mother. Note that fear of having another panic attack indicates *anticipatory anxiety*; fear of having a panic attack in a situation from which escape will be difficult or humiliating, thus resulting in avoidance of those situations indicates *agoraphobia* – Mrs PA has both.

It is important to rule out depression or other psychiatric conditions as well as medical conditions and psychoactive substance use.

**Now go on to Chapter 15 to read about the anxiety disorders and their management.**

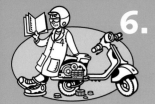

# 6. The Patient with a Reaction to a Stressful Event or Bereavement

Mrs PT, a 28-year-old divorced woman, is referred by her psychiatrist to see a cognitive-behavioural psychotherapist. She was well until 3 months ago, working night shifts as a cleaner in an inner city office block. One evening, on her way to work, two large men comered her alone at a secluded bus shelter. They pushed her violently to the ground and then proceeded to brutally rape her, threatening to 'slit her throat' if she screamed. The men ran off when they heard someone approaching, leaving Mrs PT visibly shaken but with only superficial cuts and bruises. She felt low in mood for a few days after the assault, but attempted to carry on with her job and to forget that anything had ever happened. In the month that ensued, Mrs PT avoided all attempts by her family and friends to talk about the incident and became socially withdrawn, only leaving the house when she went to work. After a month, she started having nightmares about the incident and would wake up drenched in sweat. Her work colleagues noticed that she had become 'jumpy and quick-tempered' and that sudden movements or noises easily startled her. She had also started avoiding public transportation and refused to watch any television for fear of seeing something that reminded her of the rape. Mrs PT finally sought professional help when, one night while at work, her supervisor found her lying on the floor screaming, 'Leave me alone!' repeatedly, seemingly in a trance. Later on, Mrs PT recounted to her psychiatrist how she had 'relived' the rape in her mind and how she could actually hear the voices of the men saying that they were going to kill her, just like they did on the specific night 3 months ago. The psychiatrist noticed that Mrs PT could not recall certain important aspects of the trauma.

*(For a discussion of the case study see the end of the chapter)*

It is not unusual to have some psychological symptoms after a stressful or traumatic event or bereavement. However, in some cases, these symptoms may be in excess of those usually expected and, subsequently, impair a patient's functioning. It is important to be able to distinguish between a normal reaction to a difficult life event and a specific constellation of symptoms that denote psychiatric psychopathology deserving of clinical attention.

## Definitions and clinical features

When assessing the patient who seemingly has had a pathological response to a stressful event, it is important to explore two variables: (1) the nature and severity of the *life event* and (2) the nature and severity of the *patient's reaction* to the life event.

## Nature and severity of the life event
### Stress

A psychosocial stressor is the term used for any life event, condition or circumstance that places a strain on a person's current coping skills. It is pivotal to remember that what constitutes a stress is entirely dependent on the specific person's ability to adapt or respond to a life challenge. For example, one resilient medical student may breeze through an exam period without experiencing any stress; whereas, another might feel under tremendous pressure because of a perceived or actual mismatch between their ability and the demands of the situation. Also note that the same person's coping skills vary throughout their developmental life; the death of a distant relative may be far more stressful for a middle-aged man contemplating his own mortality than for an 'invincible' adolescent.

Remember that a seemingly innocuous life event may be a significant psychosocial stressor for a vulnerable patient, e.g. change of accommodation for an elderly widow.

## Traumatic stress

A *traumatic stressor* is one that occurs outside the range of normal human experience, i.e. the stressor is of such a magnitude that it would be experienced as traumatic by almost any normal person. This type of stress occurs in situations where a person feels that their own, or a loved one's, physical integrity is under serious threat. These include natural catastrophes (earthquakes, floods), violent physical or sexual assault, fatal or near fatal car accidents, terrorist attacks, torture and military combat. Bereavement is a special case of traumatic stress that will be discussed later.

## Nature and severity of patient's reaction

Some patients are of a durable disposition and seem to weather stressful or traumatic life events with minimal symptoms whereas others seem more susceptible to the development of a diagnosable disorder. Depending on the severity of the stressor and their underlying vulnerability, patients may develop: (1) an adjustment reaction; (2) an acute stress reaction or post-traumatic stress disorder; (3) a dissociative disorder; or (4) another major mental illness like a depressive, an anxiety or a psychotic disorder.

## Adjustment reaction

This reaction encompasses a wide, non-specific range of emotional or behavioural symptoms that occur *in response* to a psychosocial stressor (significant life change or life event) to which a patient has had to adapt to or adjust. Examples include moving to a new area, changing schools or occupation, becoming a parent or being promoted. An adjustment reaction may also occur after a traumatic stressor in an individual who is resilient enough not to develop a post-traumatic stress reaction (see later). The manifestations of an adjustment reaction include mild symptoms of depression and/or anxiety and feelings of being

unable to cope. In some rarer cases, there may be disturbances of conduct, e.g. reckless driving, aggressive behaviour, truancy. Although it is assumed that the reaction would not have arisen without the original stressor, an individual's personality and vulnerability to stress play an important contributing role.

A diagnosis of *adjustment disorder* is made when a patient has an adjustment reaction that occurs within 1 month of the stressful event or life change and the duration of symptoms does not usually *exceed 6 months*. Note that a diagnosis of adjustment disorder is diagnosed by exclusion – it is made when a patient develops symptoms, after any kind of stressor, that do not meet the criteria for any other, more specific, disorder.

You should only diagnose an adjustment disorder when patients do not meet the criteria for a more specific diagnosis such as a mood, psychotic or anxiety disorder (including PTSD) or a normal bereavement reaction.

## Stress reaction

For a diagnosis of post-traumatic stress disorder (PTSD) or acute stress reaction to be made, the *stressor* must be classified as *traumatic* (see traumatic stressor above). These conditions can occur in individuals with no prior history of mental illness.

The symptoms of an *acute stress reaction* (combat fatigue, psychic shock) develop immediately after or within a few minutes of the stressor. These symptoms resolve rapidly within a few hours, or in cases where the stress continues or cannot be reversed, within 3 days. Typically, patients will experience an initial 'dazed' state followed by a narrowing of attention with an inability to process external stimuli and disorientation. This may be followed either by a period of diminished responsiveness to the extreme of a dissociative stupor or psychomotor agitation and overactivity (see Fig. 6.1 for dissociative disorders). Patients may also have amnesia for the episode – see dissociative amnesia later.

| Dissociative disorders | |
|---|---|
| Dissociative amnesia | Partial or complete memory loss for recent events of a traumatic or stressful nature not due to normal forgetfulness, organic brain disorders or intoxication (e.g. alcoholic 'blackouts') |
| Dissociative fugue | Sudden but seemingly purposeful travel beyond the individual's usual range during which self-care and normal social interaction are maintained. There are features of dissociative amnesia for personal details and in some cases a new identity may be assumed |
| Dissociative stupor | Severe psychomotor retardation characterized by extreme unresponsiveness, lack of voluntary movement and near or total mutism, not due to a physical or psychiatric disorder (that is, not due to depressive, manic or catatonic stupor) |
| Dissociative anaesthesia and sensory loss | Cutaneous or visual sensory loss that does not usually correspond to anatomic dermatomes or known neurological patterns |
| Dissociative motor disorders | Partial or complete paralysis of one or more muscle groups not due to any physical cause |
| Dissociative convulsions (pseudoseizures) | May present similarly to epileptic seizures but tongue biting, serious injury, urinary incontinence and genuine loss of consciousness are rare Absence of epileptic activity on the electroencephalogram (EEG) |
| Ganser's syndrome | Complex disorder characterized by 'approximate answers', e.g. when asked what colour the grass is, an approximate response will be 'blue' |
| Multiple personality disorder | Apparent existence of two or more personalities within the same individual. This is a rare and highly controversial diagnosis |

**Fig. 6.1** Dissociative disorders.

When assessing a patient with suspected PTSD, remember that head injuries and epilepsy are important differential diagnoses as they may present with similar symptoms and both may have been incurred at the time of the initial trauma. Alcohol and psychoactive substance intoxication or withdrawal may present similarly; this is also an important diagnostic consideration as patients with PTSD have high rates of co-morbid substance use.

The symptoms of *post-traumatic stress disorder* usually develop within 6 months of a traumatic stressor. Symptoms include all of the following:
- Repetitive *re-experiencing* of the traumatic event in the form of:

a. Flashbacks (intrusive memories, mental images or dreams of the original experience)
b. Hallucinations and illusions
c. Distress caused by internal or external cues that resemble the stressor.
  Note that, at times, patients may *dissociate* (see later) and experience the original event as though it were happening at that moment.
- *Avoidance* of stimuli associated with the stressor, amnesia for aspects of the trauma as well as emotional numbness and social withdrawal.
- Increased *arousal* (insomnia, anger outbursts, hypervigilance, poor concentration, exaggerated startle response).

### Dissociation

In clinical psychiatry, *dissociation* describes the event where a disruption occurs in the usually integrated functions of consciousness, memory, identity, perception and movement. In this rare phenomenon, memories of the past, awareness of identity, thoughts or emotions, movement and sensation, and control of behaviour become separated from the rest of an individual's personality such that they function independently or are not open to voluntary control. Hypnosis is probably the most common example of a dissociative state in a normal person. Figure 6.1 describes the most common *dissociative disorders*. The ICD-10 requires that there be some evidence of a *psychological causation* (stressful events or disturbed relationships) in association with the onset of the dissociative symptoms. Also note that this diagnosis cannot be made if there is any evidence of a physical or psychiatric disorder that might explain the symptoms. Studies have shown that a noteworthy number of patients initially diagnosed with a dissociative disorder are eventually re-diagnosed with conditions such as epilepsy, depression, schizophrenia and malingering. The psychoanalytic terms, hysteria and conversion, which are often used synonymously with dissociation, are best avoided due to their varied and vague meanings.

Depersonalization and derealization are variants of dissociation that are not necessarily pathological. *Depersonalization* is the term used to describe the experience when oneself or one's body feels somehow strange or unreal. *Derealization* is the term used to describe the experience when external reality seems strange or unreal. Depersonalization and derealization may be caused by psychiatric illness (e.g. depression, anxiety, schizophrenia), physical illness (e.g. epilepsy), psychosocial stress and substance abuse.

Before accepting the diagnosis of a dissociative disorder, a central or peripheral nervous system affliction or other psychiatric illness should be aggressively sought for and ruled out.

### Precipitation or exacerbation of an existing mental illness

The influence of a patient's environment on the development and course of their mental illness cannot be overemphasized. Considerable research has indicated that almost all forms of mental illness (e.g. depression, suicidal behaviour, psychotic illness, anxiety) can be precipitated or exacerbated by psychosocial ('life events') or traumatic stressors. However, unlike the above reactions in this group,

there need not be a direct aetiological link with the stressor involved.

## Bereavement

Note that bereavement is a unique kind of traumatic stress that is experienced by most people at some stage of their life and is therefore within the range of normal human experience. A bereavement reaction usually occurs after the loss of a loved person but can also result from other losses, like the loss of health (mental or physical), status, a national figure, or a dear pet. C. M. Parkes described the normal course of grief after bereavement as occurring in five phases – see Figure 6.2. Note that these phases of grief should not be regarded as a rigid sequence that is passed through only once. The bereaved person may pass back and forth between pining and depression repeatedly before coming to the final phase of reorganization.

The length of a normal bereavement reaction is highly variable and tends to be longer if the death was sudden and unexpected. The ICD-10 suggests that a bereavement reaction extending beyond 6 months should be coded as a form of adjustment disorder.

Although most people will meet the criteria for a depressive episode at some stage during the grieving process, normal bereavement reactions are not pathological and so no psychiatric diagnosis is made in these cases. However, patients who have been bereaved are at higher risk for developing a genuine depressive episode that will require treatment. The DSM-IV (*Diagnostic and Statistical Manual of Mental Disorders*) notes the following symptoms that are not characteristic of a normal bereavement reaction and suggest the development of a major depressive episode:

1. Guilt about things *other than* actions taken or not taken by the patient at the time of their loved one's death.
2. Thoughts of death *other than* that the patient would be better off dead or should have died with the deceased.
3. Morbid preoccupation with worthlessness.
4. Marked psychomotor retardation.
5. Prolonged and marked functional impairment.

| Alarm |
| --- |
| A highly stressed emotional state marked by physiological arousal (increased heart rate and blood pressure) |

↓

| Numbness |
| --- |
| A state of being emotionally disconnected – a form of self-protection against the acute pain of loss |

↓

| Pining |
| --- |
| A state where the bereaved are constantly reminded of, and preoccupied with, the deceased. Marked by 'pangs of grief' and intense anxiety. Hypnagogic, hypnopompic, pseudohallucinations and illusions of the deceased may occur; these are transient and always involve the dead person. |

↓

| Depression and despair |
| --- |
| A state where the bereaved have: a depressed and irritable mood, thoughts of being 'better off dead' or that they should have died with the deceased, anhedonia, loss of appetite and weight, insomnia, impaired concentration and short-term memory |

↓

| Recovery and reorganization |
| --- |
| Acceptance of loss; return of food, social, and sexual appetite; weight is regained; grief diminishes but may return for a time at anniversaries of the deceased |

**Fig. 6.2** Parkes's stages of normal bereavement.

6. Hallucinatory experiences *other than* patients thinking that they transiently see or hear the deceased.

Note that if a bereavement reaction, which is complicated by either a prolonged duration, or an abnormal quality of symptoms, does not meet the criteria for a depressive episode then a diagnosis of adjustment disorder is made.

## Differential diagnosis

The diagnosis is usually clear if you have clearly elicited the nature and severity of life event and the nature and severity of the patient's reaction. Remember that if the symptoms developed in response to a traumatic or psychosocial stressor meet the criteria for another major psychiatric diagnosis (mood disorder, psychotic disorder) then this diagnosis should be given instead of (or in clear cases of PTSD, in addition to) a diagnosis of adjustment,

acute stress or post-traumatic stress disorder. See Figure 6.3.

 The risk of developing depression increases sixfold in the 6 months that follow a stressful event.

## Discussion of case study

Mrs PT experienced a *traumatic stressor* in that she believed that her physical integrity was under immediate threat. The event was outside the range of normal human experience and thus would have been experienced as traumatic by most people. She subsequently developed *avoidance* of stimuli associated with the trauma (avoided talking or thinking about it, avoided public transportation and television), amnesia for aspects of the trauma and social withdrawal. Later on she showed signs of

| Differential diagnosis for patients presenting with a reaction to stress or trauma |
| --- |

Adjustment disorder

Acute stress reaction

Post-traumatic stress disorder

Normal bereavement reaction

Dissociative disorder

Exacerbation or precipitation of other psychiatric illness:
• Mood disorders
• Anxiety disorders
• Psychotic disorders (especially acute and transient psychotic disorders)

Malingering (see Ch. 8)

**Fig. 6.3** Differential diagnosis for patients presenting with a reaction to stress or trauma.

*increased arousal* (increased startle response, quick-tempered, 'jumpy'). Finally, Mrs PT repetitively *re-experienced* the trauma through nightmares, flashbacks and dissociation (reliving and behaving as though the trauma were occurring at that moment through mental imagery and hallucinations). All of the above suggest a diagnosis of *post-traumatic stress disorder*.

## Now go on to Chapter 15 to read about the anxiety disorders and their management.

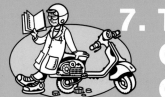

# 7. The Patient with Obsessions and Compulsions

Mr OC is 22-year-old medical student and has recently moved into his own flat. He describes a 5-month history of recurrent thoughts that he has behaved in a sexually inappropriate way towards his mother. He says that even though on one level he knows that this is near impossible, he is unable to push these thoughts away despite trying 'rigorous mental gymnastics'. The only way he is able to relieve the distress he experiences is to actually contact his mother for reassurance that his fears are not true. On most days, he physically has to go and see his mother, and will spend up to 2 hours analysing his behaviour with her until he feels reassured. Whenever he tries to stop himself from seeking reassurance, he feels a rapid escalation in anxiety, thinking that not contacting his mother is evidence that his thoughts 'might be true'. He shudders in horror when asked whether he has ever had any sexual feelings for his mother but admits that these distressing thoughts are 'obviously' his own. He is heterosexual and has recently become engaged. He is extremely embarrassed and was eventually persuaded to see his GP by his mother and fiancée when he struggled to keep up with his studies. He says that the whole thing is starting to depress him and that he has lost weight.

*(For a discussion of the case study see the end of the chapter)*

Obsessions or compulsions are terms that are often used in everyday language, e.g. 'she has an obsession with shoes' or 'he is a compulsive liar'. Psychiatrists, however, use these terms in a very specific way and it is important to elicit, recognize and understand obsessive-compulsive psychopathology.

## Definitions and clinical features

### Obsessions and compulsions

Obsessions are involuntary *thoughts*, *images* or *impulses*, which have the following important characteristics:

- They are recurrent and intrusive and are experienced by patients as unpleasant or distressing.
- They enter the mind against conscious resistance. Patients try to resist but are unable to do so.
- Patients recognize obsessions as being the product of their own mind (not from without as in *thought insertion* (see p. 25)) even though they are involuntary and often repugnant.

Obsessions are not merely excessive concerns about normal life problems and patients generally retain insight into the fact that their thoughts are irrational. In fact, patients often see their obsessions as foreign to, or against, their 'essence' (*ego-dystonic or ego-alien*), e.g. a religious man has recurrent thoughts that he has betrayed God (also, see case study).

Compulsions are repetitive *mental operations* (counting, praying or repeating a mantra silently) or *physical acts* (checking, seeking reassurance, handwashing, strict rituals) that have the following unique characteristics:

- Patients feel compelled to perform them in response to their own obsessions (see case study) or irrationally defined 'rules' (e.g. 'I must count to 10 000 four times before falling asleep').
- They are performed to reduce anxiety through the belief that they will prevent a 'dreaded event' from occurring, even though they are not realistically connected to the event (e.g. compulsive counting each night to prevent 'family catastrophe') or are ridiculously excessive (e.g. spending hours hand-washing in response to an obsessive fear of contamination).

Compulsions are experienced as unpleasant and serve no realistically useful purpose despite their tension-relieving properties. Similarly to

**Examples of the most commonly occurring obsessions and their associated compulsions in descending order**

| Obsession | Compulsion |
|---|---|
| Fear of contamination (feared object is usually impossible to avoid, e.g. faeces, urine, germs) | Excessive washing and cleaning<br>Avoidance of contaminated object |
| Pathological doubt ('Have I turned the stove off?' 'Did I lock the door?') | Exhaustive checking of the possible omission |
| Reprehensible violent, blasphemous or sexual thoughts, images or impulses (e.g. impulse to stab husband, having thoughts that one might be a paedophile)* | Act of 'redemption' (e.g. repeating 'Forgive me, I have sinned' 15 times) or seeking reassurance (see case study) |
| Need for symmetry or precision | Repeatedly arranging objects to obtain perfect symmetry |

*Patients often have these isolated obsessions without associated compulsions

**Fig. 7.1** Examples of the most commonly occurring obsessions and their associated compulsions in descending order.

obsessions, patients resist carrying out compulsions. Resisting compulsions, however, causes increased anxiety.

Obsessions and compulsions are often inextricably linked, as the desire to resist or neutralize an obsession produces a compulsive act (see Fig. 7.1 for examples of the most commonly occurring obsessions and compulsions). It can be difficult enquiring about obsessions and compulsions, especially when patients do not offer them as a presenting complaint. Figure 7.2 suggests some useful questions in eliciting these symptoms.

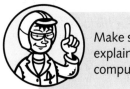 Make sure that you are able to explain what obsessions and compulsions are!

## Differential diagnosis

Obsessions and compulsions may occur as a primary illness as in *obsessive-compulsive disorder (OCD)* or may be clinical features of other psychiatric conditions. If patients have genuine obsessions or compulsions without other psychiatric symptoms then the diagnosis is invariably obsessive-compulsive disorder. For a definite diagnosis the *ICD-10* has proposed certain guidelines, as presented in Figure 7.3.

Many other psychiatric conditions may also present with repetitive or intrusive thoughts,

**Questions used to elicit obsessions and compulsions**

Do you worry about contamination with dirt even when you have already washed?
Do you have awful thoughts entering your mind despite trying hard to keep them out?
Do you repeatedly have to check things that you have already done (stoves, lights, taps, etc.)?
Do you find that you have to arrange, touch or count things many times over?

**Fig. 7.2** Questions used to elicit obsessions and compulsions.

impulses, images or behaviours. However, it is usually possible to differentiate them from OCD by applying the strict definition of obsessions and compulsions as described earlier. Also, when repetitive thoughts occur in the context of other mental disorders, the contents of these thoughts are limited exclusively to the type of disorder concerned, e.g. morbid fear of fatness in *anorexia nervosa*, ruminatory thoughts of worthlessness in *depression*, fear of dreaded objects in *phobias*. In these cases, obsessive-compulsive disorder is only diagnosed when the content of the obsessions or compulsions is unrelated to the other disorder. Figure 7.4 lists the differential diagnosis and key distinguishing features of patients presenting with obsessive-compulsive symptomatology. Figure 7.5 suggests a diagnosis algorithm that may be useful in differentiating OCD from other psychiatric conditions.

### ICD-10 diagnostic guidelines for obsessive-compulsive disorder

- Obsessions or compulsions must be present for at least 2 successive weeks and are a source of distress or interfere with the patient's functioning
- They are acknowledged as coming from the patient's own mind
- The obsessions are unpleasantly repetitive
- At least one thought or act is resisted unsuccessfully (note that in chronic cases some symptoms may no longer be resisted)
- A compulsive act is not in itself pleasurable (excluding the relief of anxiety)

### Differential diagnosis for patients presenting with obsessions or compulsions

| Diagnosis | Diagnostic features |
|---|---|
| Obsessive-compulsive disorder | At least 2 weeks of genuine obsessions and compulsions (see Fig. 7.3) |
| Depressive disorder (see Ch. 1) | Obsessive-compulsive symptoms occur simultaneously with, or after the onset of, depression and resolve with treatment<br>Obsessions are mood-congruent e.g. ruminatory thoughts of worthlessness (i.e. ego-syntonic as opposed to ego-dystonic in OCD) |
| Other anxiety disorders (see Ch. 5) | Phobias: provoking stimulus comes from external object or situation rather than patient's own mind<br>Generalized anxiety disorder: excessive concerns about real-life circumstances<br>Absence of genuine obsessions or compulsions |
| Eating disorders (see Ch. 12) | Morbid fear of fatness (overvalued idea)<br>Thoughts and actions are not recognized by patient as excessive or unreasonable and are not resisted (ego-syntonic)<br>Thoughts do not necessarily provoke, or actions reduce, distress<br>*Note: There is a higher incidence of true OCD in patients with anorexia nervosa* |
| Schizophrenia (see Ch. 4) | Thought insertion: patients believe that thoughts are not from their own mind<br>Presence of other schizophrenic symptoms<br>Lack of insight |
| Habit and impulse-control disorders: pathological gambling, kleptomania, trichotillomania (see Ch. 11) | Repetitive impulses and behaviour (gambling, stealing, pulling out hair) with no other unrelated obsessions/compulsions<br>Concordant with the patient's own wishes (therefore ego-syntonic) |
| Obsessive-compulsive (anankastic) personality disorder (see Ch. 11) | Enduring behaviour pattern of rigidity, doubt, perfectionism and pedantry<br>Ego-syntonic<br>No true obsessions or compulsions |
| Hypochondriacal disorder (see Ch. 8) | Obsessions only related to the fear of having a serious disease or bodily disfigurement |
| Gilles de la Tourette's syndrome (see Ch. 23) | Motor and vocal tics, echolalia, coprolalia<br>*Note: 35–50% of patients with Gilles de la Tourette's syndrome meet the diagnostic criteria for OCD, whereas only 5–7% of patients with OCD have Tourette's syndrome* |

**Fig. 7.4** Differential diagnosis for patients presenting with obsessions or compulsions.

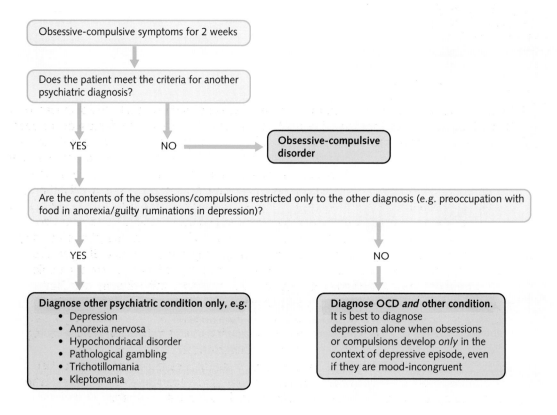

**Fig. 7.5** Algorithm for the diagnosis of obsessions and compulsions.

 You should always consider depression in patients with obsessions or compulsions because:

- Over 20% of depressed patients can have obsessive-compulsive symptoms, which occur simultaneously at or after the onset of depression. They invariably resolve with treatment of the depression.
- Over two-thirds of patients with OCD experience a depressive episode in their lifetime. Obsessions and compulsions are present before and persist after the treatment of depression.
- OCD is a disabling illness and patients often have chronic mild depressive symptoms that do not fully meet the criteria for a depressive episode. These symptoms usually resolve when the OCD is treated and the patient's quality of life improves.

## Discussion of case study

Mr OC has genuine obsessions (recurrent, intrusive thoughts that are distressing, resisted, and recognized as being from his own mind) and compulsions (repetitive reassurance seeking in response to obsessions to relieve anxiety, ridiculously excessive). He also describes symptoms of depression (depressed mood and weight loss).

His most likely diagnosis is obsessive-compulsive disorder (OCD); however, it is important to consider depression. In this case the depressed mood developed after the obsessive-compulsive symptoms. If Mr OC now met the criteria for a depressive episode then OCD and depression would be diagnosed. He most probably has mild 'reactive' depression, which will resolve when the OCD is treated (see Fig. 7.4).

**Now go on to Chapter 15 to read about obsessive-compulsive disorder and its management.**

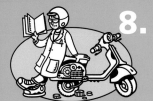

# 8. The Patient with Medically Unexplained Symptoms

Mrs SD, a 32-year-old mother of three, had consulted her family doctor at least once every 2 weeks for the past year. Mrs SD's doctor had known her for just over a year since she had moved some distance after a prolonged divorce. Her medical history, part of which was obtained from her previous GP, was considerable for someone her age and had resulted in her being unemployed. At menarche, she was diagnosed with dysfunctional uterine bleeding and dysmenorrhoea. Later, extensive investigations, which included three exploratory laparoscopies, revealed no cause for a persistent problem of upper abdominal pain with alternating diarrhoea and constipation. Three years ago Mrs SD presented with urinary frequency and dysuria. Exhaustive investigations including cystoscopy, bladder urodynamic studies and radiography were all normal. She had also been referred to various specialists including a rheumatologist for a problem of chronic neck pain that she had described as: 'the pain that has ruined mine and my kids' life!' Again, physical examination and investigations revealed no abnormalities. Mrs SD was taking up to 30 codeine tablets daily and could not sleep without two different types of sleeping tablets. Despite a difficult childhood, which featured a violent, alcohol-abusing father, and two abusive marriages that had ended in divorce, Mrs SD refused to contemplate her doctor's suggestion that there might be a psychological cause for her symptoms. However, she eventually agreed to one appointment with a psychiatrist when she developed hearing loss after her 13 year-old daughter fell pregnant.

*(For a discussion of the case study see the end of the chapter)*

Although humans have historically been recognized as consisting of the two distinct components: body (soma) and mind (or soul), most insightful doctors will testify that there is an interrelated and perhaps indivisible relationship between them. Patients with numerous physical complaints are often referred to psychiatry as a last resort because no medical cause can be found for their symptoms. Having some understanding of the mental disorders that may mimic physical illness can provide an invaluable perspective to all health practitioners.

## Definitions and clinical features

A so-called physical cause should always be sought in response to reported 'physical symptoms'. However, in certain cases, the reported symptoms:

- Do not correspond to, or are clearly not typical of, any known physical condition.
- Are associated with an absence of any physical signs or structural abnormalities.
- Are associated with an absence of any abnormalities in comprehensive laboratory, imaging and invasive special investigations.

In these cases, a so-called mental illness should be considered, especially when unexplained physical symptoms bear a close relationship with stressful life events or psychological difficulties. In this regard you need to be able to distinguish between the *somatoform disorders*, and *factitious disorder* and *malingering*.

The term 'psychosomatic' can also be used to describe physical symptoms that are presumed to be caused by psychological factors, but remember that the experience and expression of most physical symptoms are influenced by psychological factors.

## Somatoform disorders

*Soma* means body, and so the somatoform disorders are a class of mental disorders which feature symptoms that are suggestive of, or take the *form* of, a physical disorder. However, there are no detectable organic or neurophysiological abnormalities to explain these symptoms, leading to the presumption that they are caused by psychological factors. Note that these physical symptoms are not under voluntary control, i.e. they occur unintentionally, as opposed to the intentional feigning or production of symptoms in factitious disorder and malingering. *Somatization disorder* and *hypochondriacal disorder* are the most common of the somatoform disorders, but you should also be aware of *somatoform autonomic dysfunction* and *persistent somatoform pain disorder*.

 *Conversion* is a psychoanalytical term that describes the hypothetical process whereby psychic conflict or pain undergoes 'conversion' and is thus transformed into somatic or physical form to produce physical symptoms. The DSM-IV (not ICD-10) uses the term *conversion disorder* to describe the presence of one or more neurological symptoms (e.g. paralysis, blindness, sensory loss) that are not explained by any known neurological disease – this is also a type of somatoform disorder.

### Somatization disorder (Briquet's syndrome)

The essential feature of somatization disorder is *multiple, recurrent, frequently changing physical symptoms*. These include:

- *Gastrointestinal*: nausea, vomiting, diarrhoea, food intolerance, belching, regurgitation, abdominal pain, constipation.
- *Skin*: itching, burning, numbness, tingling, pain.
- *Sexual or reproductive*: loss of libido, ejaculatory or erectile dysfunction, irregular menses, menorrhagia, dysmenorrhoea.
- *Urinary*: dysuria, frequency, urinary retention, incontinence.
- *Neurological*: paralysis, sensory loss, hearing or vision loss, double vision, seizures, difficulty swallowing, impaired coordination or balance.

Note that patients should have numerous symptoms from almost all of these systemic groups, not just one or two isolated symptoms.

For the diagnosis of somatization disorder the ICD-10 suggest that all of the following be present:

- At least 2 years of symptoms with no adequate physical explanation found.
- Persistent refusal by the patient to accept reassurance from several doctors that there is no physical cause for the symptoms.
- Some degree of functional impairment due to the symptoms and resulting behaviour.

Most patients with somatization disorder will have had a long history of contact with the medical services during which numerous special investigations and operations will have been carried out – often leading to iatrogenic disease with explainable symptoms (e.g. abdominal adhesions from frequent exploratory surgery). Due to frequent courses of medication, they are very often dependent upon or abuse analgesics and sedatives.

 The 'somatic syndrome' refers to the biological symptoms of depression (see Ch. 1) and has nothing to do with somatization disorder, which is one of the somatoform disorders.

### Hypochondriacal disorder

In somatization disorder, patients express concern about numerous physical symptoms, whereas in *hypochondriacal disorder*, patients misinterpret normal bodily sensations, which lead them to believe that they have a *serious and progressive physical disease*. So patients with hypochondriacal disorder will ask for investigations to definitively diagnose or confirm their underlying disease, whereas patients with somatization disorder will ask for treatment to remove their symptoms. However, despite these repeated examinations and investigations, which reveal no abnormalities, hypochondriacal patients refuse to accept the reassurance of numerous doctors that they do not suffer from a serious physical illness.

*Body dysmorphic disorder (dysmorphophobia)* is a variant of hypochondriacal disorder that features patients being preoccupied with an imagined defect in their appearance, or, if there is a slight physical anomaly, their preoccupation is markedly excessive.

This imagined defect or deformity may concern any part of the body, e.g. a 'crooked nose' or 'ugly hands'. The preoccupation causes significant distress or impairment in functioning. Note that the psychopathology of hypochondriacal disorder (and body dysmorphic disorder) takes the form of an *overvalued idea* (see p. 26), i.e. the belief that one has a serious disease or physical defect is *overvalued*. The belief is not delusional because patients are usually open to some form of explanation and their fears are allayed, at least for a short while, after yet another special investigation has been performed.

### Somatoform autonomic dysfunction

Patients with this disorder have two types of symptoms, both concerning the autonomic nervous system. The first is characterized by objective evidence of autonomic arousal, e.g. sweating, flushing, palpitations and tremor. The second is characterized by more subjective symptoms, e.g. pains, burning, heaviness, tightness or feeling bloated. Patients then ascribe these to a particular organ or system that is largely under autonomic control, i.e. the cardiovascular system (cardiac neurosis, Da Costa's syndrome), the respiratory system (psychogenic hyperventilation and cough), the gastrointestinal system (gastric neurosis, psychogenic flatulence) and the urinary system (psychogenic dysuria and frequency). Although patients with somatization disorder may have autonomic symptoms, they also have numerous other symptoms from multiple systems and the autonomic symptoms are not attributed to only one organ or system as in somatoform autonomic dysfunction.

### Persistent somatoform pain disorder

The essential feature of this disorder is a complaint of severe and persistent pain that cannot be fully explained by any physical illness. The pain usually occurs in association with emotional difficulties or psychosocial stressors such as to suggest that they are the main causes. Although patients with somatization disorder may have symptoms of pain, they also have numerous symptoms from multiple systems and pain is not the overwhelmingly dominant symptom.

## Factitious disorder and malingering

In both factitious disorder and malingering, physical or psychological symptoms *are produced intentionally* or *feigned*. Patients may give convincing histories that fool even experienced clinicians and often manufacture signs, e.g. warfarin may be ingested to simulate bleeding disorders, insulin may be injected to produce hypoglycaemia and patients may contaminate their urine with blood or faeces. Certain patients feign psychological symptoms like hallucinations, delusions, depression or dissociation. Because there are no definitive special investigations to diagnose psychiatric disorders, these patients often go undetected and may receive large doses of psychotropic medication and electroconvulsive therapy.

Factitious disorder and malingering are differentiated by the patient's *motivation* for simulating symptoms. In factitious disorder (Münchausen's syndrome), patients are focused on the *primary internal gain* of assuming the sick role, i.e. their only aim is to be treated like a patient and to be hospitalized. In malingering, patients are focused on a *secondary external gain*; they seek the secondary consequence of being diagnosed with an illness, e.g. avoidance of military service, evading criminal prosecution, obtaining illicit drugs or obtaining financial or housing benefits.

## Differential diagnosis

The differential diagnosis for patients presenting with medically unexplained symptoms is shown in Figure 8.1.

An underlying medical condition should be ruled out when patients present with unexplained physical symptoms. Somatization disorder can resemble insidious multisystemic diseases such as systemic lupus erythematosus, multiple sclerosis, acquired immune deficiency syndrome (AIDS), acute intermittent porphyria, hyperparathyroidism, hyperthyroidism, myasthenia gravis, haemochromatosis, occult malignancy and chronic infections.

Also remember that physical complaints often occur in the context of other psychiatric conditions. Patients with *schizophrenia* may have somatic delusions or visceral somatic hallucinations. However, the explanation of these symptoms is usually quite odd and there are usually other psychotic symptoms accompanying the physical complaints. Individuals with *depressed mood* often present with numerous somatic complaints; these tend to be episodic and resolve with the treatment of the depression. Distinguishing between the *anxiety disorders* and somatization disorder can be difficult. Patients with

| Differential diagnosis for patients presenting with medically unexplained symptoms |
| --- |
| Somatoform disorders<br>• Somatization disorder<br>• Hypochondriacal disorder (including body dysmorphic disorder)<br>• Somatoform autonomic dysfunction<br>• Persistent somatoform pain disorder |
| Factitious disorder |
| Malingering |
| Other psychiatric conditions<br>• Anxiety disorders<br>• Mood disorders<br>• Psychotic disorders<br>• Dissociative disorders<br>Insidious multisystemic disease |

**Fig. 8.1** Differential diagnosis for patients presenting with medically unexplained symptoms.

*panic disorder* have multiple somatic symptoms while having panic attacks, but these resolve when the panic subsides. Patients with *generalized anxiety disorder* may also have multiple somatic preoccupations, but their anxiety is not limited to physical symptoms. *Dissociative motor disorders, dissociative convulsions (pseudoseizures)*, and *dissociative anaesthesia and sensory loss* can all present with neurological symptoms without any evidence of an organic cause. However, these symptoms are usually clearly defined and isolated as opposed to the ill-defined, multiple symptoms in somatization disorder. The difficulty in distinguishing other mental disorders from somatization disorder is illustrated by the observation that at least 50% of patients with somatization disorder have another coexisting mental illness.

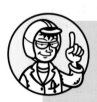

Somatization disorder usually has its onset in early adult life. The onset of multiple physical symptoms late in life is almost always due to a physical illness.

## Assessment

### Clinical

The following questions may be helpful in screening for somatoform disorders on mental state examination:

- Do you often worry about your health?
- Are you bothered by many different symptoms?
- Are you concerned that you might have a serious illness?
- Are you concerned about your facial or bodily appearance?
- Do you find it hard to believe doctors when they tell you that there is nothing wrong with you?

**A thorough physical examination with special focus on the presenting problem is imperative when dealing with somatoform complaints.**

### Special investigations

Clinicians dealing with patients with a somatoform disorder need to investigate physical complaints judiciously. It is important to take all symptoms seriously, yet excessive and needless investigations to placate an anxious patient can result in a vicious circle with a worsening of symptoms. See Figure 15.4 in Chapter 15 for guidance on how to manage these patients.

## Discussion of case study

Mrs SD has a long history of multiple, recurrent, frequently changing physical symptoms for which no physical causes have been found despite extensive investigation. She is resistant to the idea that there might be a psychological reason for her symptoms despite the association of her symptoms with psychosocial stress. Her functioning has been impaired and has probably impacted on her children's lives. Because she is focused on symptoms, not the idea that she a serious and progressive illness, Mrs SD has *somatization disorder* as opposed to *hypochondriacal disorder*. As is typical, Mrs SD has a secondary substance misuse problem (codeine and sleeping tablets). It would be important to exclude other mental illness, such as depression and anxiety, as causative factors. If there was evidence that Mrs SD intentionally produced or feigned her symptoms then *factitious disorder* or *malingering* should be considered.

**Now go on to Chapter 15 to read about the somatoform disorders and their management.**

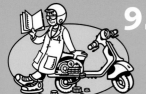

# 9. The Patient with Impairment of Consciousness, Memory or Cognition

Mr DD, aged 78, had recently been admitted to a nursing home with a diagnosis of end-stage Alzheimer's disease. His GP had referred him to a psychiatrist 6 years ago after he started experiencing difficulty remembering things. At first he would forget things like the social arrangements he had made. Later he started forgetting activities he had engaged in only the day before. His wife had noticed a gradual change in his personality in that he became increasingly withdrawn and sullen and, at times, verbally abusive. His language deteriorated to the point where he would ramble incoherently, even when there was no one else in the room. Despite having smoked for many years, Mr DD seemed unable to recognize his pipe and would stare at it quizzically for hours. He lost the ability to dress himself or complete simple multi-step tasks like making a cup of coffee. His wife discussed hospitalization with his psychiatrist when Mr DD no longer recognized her and refused to allow her to feed him. At the time of admission he was disorientated to place and time but displayed a normal consciousness level.

Two days after admission Mr DD's mental state changed dramatically. Nurses were concerned because his consciousness level was fluctuating from hour to hour. He slept through most of the day, but would wander around the ward at night looking very agitated and appeared to have visual hallucinations. The senior nurse pointed out that he had developed a productive cough.

*(For a discussion of the case study see the end of the chapter)*

The cognitive faculty of man is the most highly developed of all the species. Apart from enabling us to ponder intangible abstract concepts, our cognitive faculty is the cornerstone of basic survival. There are many temporary and progressive conditions that cause an impairment of cognitive functioning and thus result in the most debilitating deterioration in functioning. The ability to assess and evaluate cognition should therefore be a fundamental skill for all health practitioners, not just psychiatrists.

## Cognition: basic concepts and psychopathology

The term *cognition* is used in two ways by psychiatrists and psychologists. This chapter concerns cognition in its broadest sense as meaning: all the mental activities that allow us to perceive, integrate and conceptualize the world around us. These include: attention and concentration, memory, orientation, reading, writing, calculation, comprehension, learning, language, judgement,

reasoning and visuospatial ability. A narrower use of the term is found in cognitive psychology and cognitive therapy where individual thoughts or ideas are also to be referred to as 'cognitions'.

This section will discuss the basic concepts of impaired *consciousness* and *memory* and then define the three syndromes that are characterized by impaired cognitive functioning, namely: *dementia, delirium* and the *amnesic syndrome.*

## Consciousness

To be conscious is to be aware, both of objects that are perceivable and of oneself as a subjective being. Consciousness is said to be normal, heightened or lowered.

*Heightened consciousness* involves an enhanced sense of awareness or arousal: colours are brighter and more vivid, sounds seem louder and crisper, and there is a greater sense of alertness. Heightened consciousness may be induced by psychoactive stimulants (amfetamines) or hallucinogens (LSD) and may also be found in early mania (see p. 11). Heightened awareness can be on the continuum of normal experience, e.g. being in love, religious experiences, etc.

Unfortunately, the many terms describing *lowered consciousness* are muddled and confusing. Lowered consciousness needs to be distinguished from reduced wakefulness or sleep. There is a qualitative difference between the pathway from clear consciousness to sleep and the pathway from clear consciousness to coma. The difference is that the individual who is asleep can always be aroused to a state of clear consciousness with stimulation, unlike the patient with lowered or clouded consciousness. Consciousness can be seen as existing on a continuum of decreasing alertness, from clear consciousness to coma, with *clouding of consciousness* as an intermediate level in between. Figure 9.1 describes the pathway from clear consciousness to coma.

Abnormalities of consciousness often involve both a quantitative lowering of consciousness and a qualitative alteration of consciousness (the nature of awareness is altered). Most of the psychopathology described in this book concerns a qualitative alteration of awareness (e.g. hallucinations, illusions, delusions, mood changes and anxiety) and these symptoms often accompany states of quantitatively impaired consciousness, as in delirium. Two further qualitative alterations in consciousness should be clarified: *confusion* and *stupor*.

## Confusion

Patients are described as being confused when their thinking lacks its normal clarity and coherence and it can occur in a state of normal or impaired consciousness. It may be a subjective complaint by the patient or be objectively inferred from the patient's speech and behaviour. The cause of confusion is non-specific. It may be caused by a lowering of consciousness as in delirium; by a global impairment of cognitive functioning as in dementia; by the deranged thinking or perceptual abnormalities of a psychotic patient or simply when strong emotions or anxiety interfere with logical thinking.

*[handwritten annotation: akinesis / mutism / extreme unresponsiveness]*

## Stupor

This term is best used to mean a clinical presentation of *akinesis* (lack of voluntary movement), *mutism* and *extreme unresponsiveness* in an otherwise alert patient (there may be slight clouding of consciousness). Although apparently alert, the stuporous patient will initiate no spontaneous movement or speech, stare blankly and seemingly take nothing in. Psychiatric causes of stupor include schizophrenia (catatonic stupor), depression, mania and dissociative states. Organic causes of stupor include dementia, delirium, cerebral tumours or cysts, neurosyphilis, encephalitis and post-ictal states.

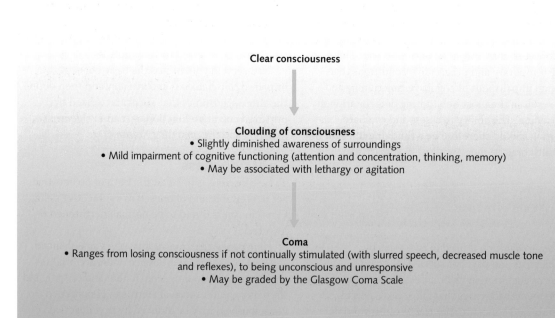

**Clear consciousness**

**Clouding of consciousness**
- Slightly diminished awareness of surroundings
- Mild impairment of cognitive functioning (attention and concentration, thinking, memory)
- May be associated with lethargy or agitation

**Coma**
- Ranges from losing consciousness if not continually stimulated (with slurred speech, decreased muscle tone and reflexes), to being unconscious and unresponsive
- May be graded by the Glasgow Coma Scale

**Fig. 9.1** The pathway from clear consciousness to coma.

The vast number of confusing terms used to describe consciousness underscores the importance of documenting a patient's state of awareness in as much detail as possible, instead of describing a complex quantitative and qualitative presentation with one word.

# Memory

The quantity of contemporary literature on memory is daunting and some of the terms used to define the types of memory have varied meanings. This section will describe the most commonly used definitions and provide a framework that has clinical applicability.

The process of retaining data is termed *storage*. Memory storage can be sensory, short-term and long-term.

### Immediate memory (also called sensory memory)
Immediate sensory information is held for less than a second, unprocessed, in the form that it was perceived by the sense organ. This allows the brain time to process the vast amount of visual (iconic memory), auditory (echoic memory) and touch (haptic memory) input it receives every second. This type of memory has limited clinical relevance.

### Short-term memory (also called primary or working memory)
Once immediate memory has been attended to, it may be transferred to a temporary memory store which has a limited capacity for 7 +/− 2 items at a time, e.g. a telephone number. This will be forgotten in 15–30 seconds if it is not rehearsed or converted into long-term memory. Short-term memory is tested clinically with the *digit span* test (see Fig. 9.2).

### Long-term memory (also called secondary memory)
All data that have been processed and understood may be added to an existing memory store. This long-term memory store is probably limitless in terms of capacity and features a duration of storage from minutes to decades.

*Recent memory*  refers to memories stored minutes, hours, days, weeks or months ago.
*Remote memory*  refers to memories stored many years or decades ago.
Note that committing a telephone number to memory for 1 hour and remembering childhood events from decades ago are both examples of long-term memory – recent and remote respectively.

Long-term memory stores may be *explicit* or *implicit*. Explicit memory (sometimes called *declarative memory*) includes all stored material of which the individual is consciously aware and can thus 'declare' to others. Implicit memory (sometimes called *procedural memory*) includes all material that is stored without the individual's conscious awareness, e.g. the ability to speak a language or ride a bicycle.

Fig. 9.2 Memory function tests.

| Memory function tests | |
| --- | --- |
| Short-term memory | **Digit span test:**<br>Ask the patient to repeat after you. Start with 2 different digits and deliver them in an even tone at a rate of one per second. If the patient repeats correctly, increase the number of digits by one each time (using different digits) until the patient's limit or digit span is reached. A normal digit span is 7 +/− 2 |
| Long-term memory | **Ability to store new memories (anterograde memory):**<br>Ask patients to commit an unfamiliar name and address to memory. Test recall 3–5 minutes later after interposition of other cognitive tests<br>**Remote memory:**<br>Ask patients about important events (personal or general knowledge) that occurred in childhood or decades ago. Correlate with collateral information<br>**Recent memory:**<br>Ask patients about events over the past few days, e.g. what they had for breakfast; what they did the day before, etc. |

Some clinicians use the term 'short-term memory' to mean recent memory (as defined in text) and the term 'immediate memory span' to mean short-term or primary memory (as defined in text). It is for this reason that many authors designate the type of memory they are referring to with the qualification: *as measured by the digit span test* (see Fig. 9.2).

*Amnesia* refers to the loss of the ability to *store* new memories or *retrieve* memories that have previously been stored. Amnesia may be caused by a physical brain affliction (e.g. head injury, dementia), or it may be secondary to some form of emotional stress (e.g. dissociative amnesia – see p. 41).

*Anterograde amnesia* occurs after an amnesia-causing event and results in the patient being unable to store new memories from the event onwards (impaired learning of new material), although the ability to retrieve memories stored before the event may remain unimpaired. Anterograde amnesia usually results from damage to the medial temporal lobes, especially the hippocampal formation.

*Retrograde amnesia* occurs after an amnesia-causing event and results in the patient being unable to retrieve memories stored before the event, although the ability to store new memories from the event onwards may remain unaffected. Retrograde amnesia usually results from damage to the frontal or temporal cortex.

Figure 9.2 describes how to clinically test the different types of memory.

Implicit memory (procedural memory) is typically preserved despite severe disruptions to explicit (declarative) memory, probably due to its independent neural location. Implicit memory is associated with the striatum and neocortex. Explicit memory is associated with the hippocampal and diencephalic structures.

## The cognitive disorders

It is useful to describe patients presenting with an impairment of cognition in terms of one of three commonly occurring syndromes: *dementia*, *delirium* and the *amnesic syndrome*.

A delirium is characterized by an acute impairment of consciousness with cognitive deficits. A dementia is characterized by multiple cognitive deficits, including memory, *without an impairment of consciousness*. An amnesic syndrome is characterized by memory impairment in the absence of other significant cognitive deficits.

Remember that identification of one of these syndromes does not mean that a final diagnosis has been made. Instead, it serves as an intermediate guide which is then used to prompt further investigation until a definitive diagnosis is reached. For example, the definitive cause of a delirium might be a subdural haematoma or hepatic encephalopathy.

### Dementia

Dementia is an acquired syndrome characterized by a global impairment of cognitive function and personality without an impairment of consciousness. It is irreversible and chronic in course with a progressive deterioration in social and occupational functioning. Symptoms should be present for 6 months before a diagnosis is made.

The following text describes the general categories of impairment in dementia:

*Memory impairment*   Impairment of memory is a common feature of dementia. Recent memory is first affected, e.g. forgetting where objects are placed, conversations and events of the previous day. With disease progression, all aspects of memory are affected, although highly personal information (name, previous occupation, etc.) is usually retained until late in the disease. Note that memory is essential for *orientation* to person, place and time and this will also be gradually affected, e.g. patients may lose their way in their own house.

*Loss of language ability (aphasia)*   Both receptive and expressive dysphasias may occur manifested by difficulty understanding commands or by vague, circumstantial speech with a reduced ability to read or write. Ultimately, patients may exhibit echolalia (repeating what is heard), palilalia (repeating their own words over and over) or become mute.

*Apraxia*  Patients may lose the ability to carry out skilled motor movements despite an intact motor and sensory function, e.g. putting a letter in an envelope.

*Agnosia*  Patients may lose the ability to recognize or identify previously familiar objects or people despite intact sensory function.

*Impairment of executive functioning*  Patients may have difficulty in planning and sequencing complex activities.

*Personality and behaviour changes*  Close family members are first to notice this. Patients may become introverted and socially withdrawn or hostile, irritable and socially disinhibited. Pre-existing personality traits may become unpleasantly accentuated.

*Psychiatric symptoms*  *Hallucinations* in all sensory modalities (visual more common) may occur in up to 30% of patients. *Delusions*, especially persecutory, may occur in up to 40% of patients. *Depression and anxiety* may occur in up to half of all demented patients. Patients with dementia are more susceptible to the development of a *delirium*.

*Neurological symptoms*  In addition to aphasia, apraxia and agnosia, 10–20% of patients will experience seizures. Primitive reflexes (e.g. grasp, snout, suck) may also be evident as well as myoclonic jerks.

The diagnosis of dementia cannot be made on the basis of memory impairment alone. It is a syndrome that includes numerous cognitive deficits including the inability to learn new complex material or adapt to novel situations, personality changes, and impaired executive functioning.

## Distinguishing the type of dementia

The term senile or late-onset dementia is used if the onset of dementia is after age 65 and presenile or early-onset dementia if at or before age 65. Figure 9.3 lists the many disease processes that can cause dementia. Alzheimer's disease (which accounts for up to 60% of all cases of dementia),

---

### Diseases that may cause dementia

Neurodegenerative
- Alzheimer's disease
- Frontotemporal dementia (includes Pick's disease)
- Dementia with Lewy bodies (DLB)
- Parkinson's disease
- Huntington's disease
- Progressive supranuclear palsy

Vascular dementia

Space-occupying lesions
- Tumours, cysts, abscesses, haematomas

Trauma
- Head injury
- Punch-drunk syndrome (dementia pugilistica)

Infection
- Creutzfeldt–Jakob disease (including 'new variant CJD')
- HIV-related dementia
- Neurosyphilis
- Viral encephalitis
- Chronic bacterial and fungal meningitides

Metabolic and endocrine
- Chronic uraemia (also dialysis dementia)
- Liver failure
- Wilson's disease
- Hyper- and hypothyroidism
- Hyper- and hypoparathyroidism
- Cushing's syndrome and Addison's disease

Nutritional
- Thiamine, Vitamin $B_{12}$, folic acid or niacin deficiency (pellagra)

Drugs and toxins
- Alcohol (see p. 69), benzodiazepines, barbiturates, solvents

Anoxia

Inflammatory disorders
- Multiple sclerosis
- Systemic lupus erythematosus and other collagen vascular diseases

Normal pressure hydrocephalus

**Fig. 9.3** Diseases that may cause dementia.

---

frontotemporal dementia including Pick's disease (which accounts for up to 20% of presenile dementia cases) and dementia with Lewy bodies (DLB) (which accounts for up to 20% of all dementia cases), all result from a *primary neurodegenerative process*.

It is important to establish the underlying type of dementia because:
- A secondary dementia-causing process (e.g. brain tumour) may be detected and possibly halted.

- The progress of certain types of dementia may be slowed with specific medication (e.g. acetylcholinesterase inhibitors in Alzheimer's disease).
- Certain drugs may be contraindicated in some dementias (e.g. antipsychotics can cause a catastrophic parkinsonian reaction in patients with dementia with Lewy bodies).
- The prognoses of the various dementias differ; this may have practical implications for patients and their families as regards final arrangements, e.g. wills.
- The patient's relatives may enquire about genetic counselling, e.g. Huntington's disease, early-onset Alzheimer's disease.

In a minority of cases the distinction will be obvious, based on other symptoms produced by the disease process, e.g. jerky movements of the face and body (chorea) and a positive family history will be indicative of Huntington's disease. In the majority of cases, the different dementias may be distinguished to some degree based on a detailed history from the patient and an informant, physical examination, relevant special investigations and follow-up over time. However, the definitive diagnosis of dementia can only be established with absolute certainty on detailed microscopic examination of the brain at autopsy – and not always then. Figure 9.4 describes the distinguishing clinical features of the various types of dementias, which account for up to 95% of all cases.

To aid the clinical distinction of dementia, some authors differentiate *cortical*, *subcortical* and *mixed* dementias based on the predominance of cortical or subcortical dysfunction – or a mixture of the two (see Fig. 9.5 for the features of cortical and subcortical dementias). Unfortunately, in advanced dementia, of whatever type, there is often a considerable overlap.

At this point you might find it helpful to read up on the aetiology and neuropathology of the various neurodegenerative dementias in Chapter 16, pp.103–108.

## Delirium

The essential feature of a delirium is an impairment of consciousness with a reduced ability to focus or maintain attention. The delirious state tends to develop over a short period of time and is transient. The following text describes the prominent symptoms of delirium:

***Impaired consciousness*** Patients may have a reduced awareness of the environment from clouding of

**Fig. 9.4** Distinguishing clinical features of the commonest types of dementia.

| Distinguishing clinical features of the commonest types of dementia | |
|---|---|
| Alzheimer's disease | Gradual onset with progressive cognitive decline<br>Diagnosis by exclusion of other causes of dementia |
| Vascular dementia (multi-infarct dementia) | Focal neurological signs and symptoms<br>Evidence of cerebrovascular disease or stroke<br>Uneven or stepwise deterioration in cognitive function |
| Dementia with Lewy bodies (DLB) | Day to day (or shorter) fluctuations in cognitive performance<br>Recurrent visual hallucinations<br>Spontaneous motor signs of parkinsonism (rigidity, bradykinesia, tremor)<br>Recurrent falls and syncope<br>Transient disturbances of consciousness<br>Extreme sensitivity to antipsychotics (induces parkinsonism) |
| Frontotemporal dementia (including Pick's disease) | Early decline in social and personal conduct (disinhibition, tactlessness)<br>Early emotional blunting<br>Attenuated speech output, echolalia, perseveration, mutism<br>Early loss of insight<br>Relative sparing of other cognitive functions |

| Features of cortical and sub-cortical dementias | | |
|---|---|---|
| Characteristic | Cortical dementia | Subcortical dementia |
| Language | Aphasia early | Normal |
| Speech | Normal until late | Dysarthric |
| Praxis | Apraxia | Normal |
| Agnosia | Present | Usually absent |
| Calculation | Early impairment | Normal until late |
| Motor system | Usually normal posture/tone | Stooped or extended posture, increased tone |
| Extra movements | None (may have myoclonus in Alzheimer's disease) | Tremor, chorea, tics |

*Cortical*: Alzheimer's disease and the frontotemporal dementias (including Pick's disease)
*Subcortical*: Parkinson's disease, dementia with Lewy bodies, Huntington's disease, progressive supranuclear palsy, Wilson's disease, normal pressure hydrocephalus, multiple sclerosis, HIV-related dementia
*Mixed*: Vascular dementias, infection-induced dementias (Creutzfeldt–Jakob disease, neurosyphilis, and chronic meningitis)

**Fig. 9.5** Features of cortical and sub-cortical dementias.

consciousness to coma. Their ability to sustain attention is reduced and they are easily distractible.

***Impaired cognitive function*** Short-term memory (primary memory) and recent memory are impaired with relative preservation of remote memory. Delirious patients are almost always disorientated to time and often to place. Orientation to self is seldom lost. Language abnormalities such as rambling, incoherent speech and an impaired ability to understand are common.

***Perceptual and thought disturbance*** Patients may have perceptual disturbances ranging from misinterpretations (e.g. a door slamming is mistaken for an explosion) to illusions (e.g. a crack in the wall is perceived as a snake) to hallucinations (especially visual and, to a lesser extent, auditory). Transient persecutory delusions and delusions of misidentification may occur.

***Psychomotor abnormalities*** Patients may be hyper- or hypoactive or fluctuate from one to the other, and may also have an enhanced startle reaction.

***Sleep–wake cycle disturbance*** Sleep is characteristically disturbed and can range from daytime drowsiness and night-time hyperactivity to a complete reversal of the normal cycle. The nightmares of delirious patients may continue as hallucinations after awakening.

***Mood disturbance*** Emotional disturbances such as depression, euphoria, anxiety, anger, fear and apathy are common.

Note that a delirium is a medical emergency and the cause should be found and treated (see Ch. 16). Figure 9.6 lists the causes of delirium.

 A physical illness should always be ruled out whenever a patient presents with prominent visual hallucinations because patients with schizophrenia and other functional psychotic disorders usually experience auditory hallucinations.

### Distinguishing between delirium and dementia

Although the syndromes of delirium and dementia both consist of memory and cognitive impairment, they differ dramatically in cause, management and prognosis. It is imperative that you understand how to differentiate between the two. Figure 9.7 summarizes the factors differentiating delirium from dementia – learn it well.

## Amnesic syndrome

While dementia is the most common cause of chronic memory dysfunction, certain brain diseases can cause a severe disruption of memory with minimal or no deterioration in global cognitive functioning (i.e.

## Causes of delirium

**Intracranial causes**

*Neurodegenerative*
- Dementia with Lewy bodies (DLB)
- Other dementias complicated by infection, anoxia etc.

*Space-occupying lesions*
- Tumours, cysts, abscesses, haematomas

*Head injury* (especially concussion)

*Infection*
- Meningitis
- Encephalitis

*Epilepsy*

*Cerebrovascular disorders*
- Transient ischaemic attack
- Cerebral thrombosis or embolism
- Intracerebral or subarachnoid haemorrhage
- Hypertensive encephalopathy
- Vasculitis (e.g. from systemic lupus erythematosus)

**Systemic causes**

*Toxic*
Alcohol (Wernicke's encephalopathy, delirium tremens – see p. 68)
Drugs (ingestion or withdrawal)
- Anticholinergics
- Anticonvulsants
- Antidepressants
- Antihypertensive drugs
- Antiparkinsonian drugs
- Antipsychotics
- Cannabis
- Cimetidine

*Systemic causes—cont'd*
- Disulfiram
- Digoxin
- Insulin
- Opiates
- Phencyclidine
- Salicylates
- Steroids
- Sedatives (benzodiazepines)

*Poisons*
- Heavy metals (lead, mercury, manganese)
- Carbon monoxide

*Metabolic and endocrine*
- Electrolyte disturbances
- Uraemia
- Hepatic encephalopathy
- Porphyria
- Hypoglycaemia
- Hyper- and hypothyroidism
- Hyper- and hypoparathyroidism
- Hyper- and hypoadrenocorticism (Cushing's syndrome, Addison's disease)
- Hypopituitarism

*Nutritional*
- Thiamine (Wernicke's encephalopathy), vitamin $B_{12}$, folic acid or niacin deficiency

Infections and sepsis

*Anoxia*
- Respiratory failure
- Heart failure

**Fig. 9.6** Causes of delirium.

| Factors differentiating delirium from dementia | | |
|---|---|---|
| **Feature** | **Delirium** | **Dementia** |
| Onset | Acute | Gradual |
| Duration | Hours to weeks | Months to years |
| Course | Fluctuating | Progressive deterioration |
| Consciousness | Impaired | Normal |
| Perceptual disturbance | Common | Occurs in late stages |
| Sleep–wake cycle | Disrupted | Usually normal |

**Fig. 9.7** Factors differentiating delirium from dementia.

 Note that dementia with Lewy bodies is the only dementia that features transient episodes of impaired consciousness as a typical feature. All other dementias do not feature an impairment of consciousness unless complicated by a delirium (i.e. as result of infection, anoxia, etc.).

aphasia, apraxia, agnosia or disturbance of executive functioning). This clinical scenario is termed the *amnesic syndrome* and usually results from damage to the hypothalamic–diencephalic system or the hippocampal region (see Fig. 9.8 for the causes of

| Causes of amnesic syndrome | |
| --- | --- |
| **Diencephalic damage** | **Hippocampal damage** |
| Vitamin B$_1$ (thiamine) deficiency, i.e. Korsakoff's syndrome *causes:*     Chronic alcohol abuse     Gastric carcinoma     Severe malnutrition     Hyperemesis gravidarum Bilateral thalamic infarction Multiple sclerosis Post subarachnoid haemorrhage Third ventricle tumours/cysts | Bilateral posterior cerebral artery occlusion Carbon monoxide poisoning Closed head injury Herpes simplex virus encephalitis |

**Fig. 9.8** Causes of amnesic syndrome.

| Differential diagnosis of cognitive impairment |
| --- |
| Dementia Delirium Amnesic syndrome Psychoactive substance intoxication or withdrawal Mental retardation (learning disability) Psychotic disorders Mood disorders Dissociative disorders Age-related cognitive decline Factitious disorder and malingering |

**Fig. 9.9** Differential diagnosis of cognitive impairment.

amnesic syndrome). The amnesic syndrome is characterized by all of the following:

- Anterograde and retrograde amnesia. The impairment of memory for past events is in reverse order of their occurrence; i.e. recent memories are the most affected.
- There is no impairment of attention or consciousness or global intellectual functioning. There is also no defect of short-term (primary or working) memory as tested by digit span.
- There is strong evidence of a brain disease known to cause the amnesic syndrome (see Fig. 9.8).

Although there is no impairment of global cognitive functioning, patients with the amnesic syndrome are usually *disorientated in time* due to their inability to learn new material (anterograde amnesia). *Confabulation* (filling of gaps in memory with fictitious details), *lack of insight* and *apathy* are also associated features.

Note that when the lesions in the hypothalamus and diencephalon are due to a thiamine deficiency,

the term *Korsakoff's syndrome* may be used. The most common cause of amnesic syndrome due to thiamine deficiency, or Korsakoff's syndrome, is chronic alcohol abuse. *Wernicke's encephalopathy* is the acute neuropsychiatric consequence of a severe thiamine deficiency and characterized by an acute onset of: (1) ophthalmoplegia (nystagmus, and abducens and conjugate gaze palsies); (2) an ataxic gait; and (3) confusion. Wernicke's encephalopathy and Korsakoff's syndrome ultimately result from the same pathological process, the former being the acute reaction and the latter, the residual defect – hence the term: *Wernicke–Korsakoff encephalopathy*. An untreated Wernicke's encephalopathy will result in a Korsakoff's amnesic syndrome in about 85% of cases. See also p. 69 and p. 110.

Due to their unimpaired intellectual functioning, tendency to confabulate and lack of insight, patients with an amnesic syndrome can appear deceptively 'normal'. This highlights the importance of obtaining collateral information as well as doing memory tests on mental state examination.

## Differential diagnosis

Figure 9.9 shows the differential diagnosis for the patient presenting with cognitive impairment.

When patients present with a significant impairment of cognitive function it is important to firstly establish their level of consciousness, and then do a comprehensive psychiatric history and mental state examination that includes a global assessment of the various domains of cognitive functioning (see MMSE later). The differentiation between and the causes of dementia, delirium and the amnesic syndrome have already been discussed. Remember that it is possible, and common, to have a delirium complicating a dementia, e.g. a patient with Alzheimer's disease develops a delirium secondary to a urinary tract infection.

*Psychoactive substance intoxication and withdrawal*, most commonly alcohol, can cause multiple cognitive deficits and a lowered level of consciousness. Remember, however, that when a psychoactive substance causes symptoms which are in excess of that which is usually associated with its intoxication or withdrawal syndrome, then substance intoxication or withdrawal *delirium* should be diagnosed. For example, the cessation of drinking in an alcohol-dependent patient can precipitate an alcohol withdrawal syndrome or, in a smaller number of cases, precipitate a life-threatening delirium. Chapter 10 discusses this in more detail.

Patients with *learning disability* characteristically have below average intellectual functioning with an impaired ability to adapt to their social environment. Unlike dementia, learning disability manifests in the developmental period (before age 18) and the level of cognitive functioning tends to be stable over time, not progressively deteriorating.

Patients with *chronic schizophrenia* may have multiple cognitive deficits, but unlike dementia, the age of onset is earlier and psychotic symptoms are present from the start. Also, the cognitive impairment in schizophrenia tends to be milder than in dementia. The disturbed behaviour, vivid hallucinations, distractibility and thought disorder of *acutely psychotic* patients may resemble a delirium. However, careful examination will reveal that the consciousness level is not lowered.

*Depressive pseudodementia* is the term used when patients present with clinical features resembling a dementia that results from an underlying depression (also called *depression-related cognitive dysfunction*). There is some debate as to whether this syndrome reflects true cognitive impairment (in which case pseudodementia is a misnomer) or whether the depression-associated psychomotor retardation, social withdrawal, difficulty thinking and poor concentration give a misleading impression of dementia in the presence of an intact cognitive faculty. In either case, the situation usually responds to antidepressant treatment. Depressive pseudodementia is differentiated from dementia by the abrupt onset of cognitive impairment with relatively normal premorbid functioning.

Memory loss, confusion and stupor can occur in the *dissociative disorders* (see p. 41), e.g. dissociative amnesia, fugue and stupor. They are distinguished from dementia and the amnesic syndrome by the lack of evidence of a physical cause and because they are usually precipitated by a psychosocial stressor.

Dementia and the amnesic syndrome must be differentiated from the normal decline in cognitive function that occurs with *ageing*. This is usually of minor severity and does not interfere with the individual's social and occupational functioning.

## Factitious disorder and malingering:
See Chapter 8.

## Assessment

### Clinical
When doing a mental state examination, a cognitive assessment should always be done. Figure 9.2 demonstrated how to test specifically for memory function. Now that you are aware of the many aspects comprising cognition, you might find the *Mini-Mental State Examination* (MMSE) a useful tool for doing a global test of cognitive functioning (see Fig. 9.10 for a description of the MMSE). This is a standardized set of questions that test the most important aspects of cognition such as orientation, registration, attention, calculation, language, executive functioning and visuospatial skills. It is often used to screen for or monitor the progress of dementia, but is very useful as a general test for assessing global cognitive ability. A score below 25/30 suggests dementia. Note that the MMSE score naturally declines with age, so that the mean score at 90 years is 23/30.

The main aim of the *physical examination* is to identify treatable underlying causes of dementia, such as hypothyroidism or a space-occupying lesion. In addition, consideration should be given to complications of dementia, such as malnutrition or falls. Cardiovascular and neurological examinations are particularly important. Evidence of hypertension or circulatory disease has obvious implications for the

| Mini Mental State Examination | | |
|---|---|---|
| **Cognitive ability tested** | **Questions** | **Maximum score** |
| 1. Orientation | What is the (year) (season) (month) (day of month) (day of week)?<br>Where are we: (country) (county) (city/town) (building) (floor level)? | 5<br>5 |
| 2. Registration | Name three common objects (e.g. 'apple', 'ball', 'table'). Now ask the patient to repeat all three. Give one point for each correct answer. Repeat them until patient learns all three. Record the number of trials needed | 3<br>Number of trials: |
| 3. Attention and calculation | *Serial 7s*: Ask the patient to subtract 7 from 100 and then again up to five times (93→86→79→72→65)<br>*OR*<br>Ask the patient to spell WORLD backwards (D→L→R→O→W) | 5 |
| 4. Recall | Ask the patient to name the three objects mentioned in 'registration' | 3 |
| 5. Naming | Ask the patient to name two objects (show a pencil) (show a watch) | 2 |
| 6. Repeating | Ask the patient to repeat: 'NO IFS, ANDS OR BUTS' | 1 |
| 7. Three stage command | Ask the patient to: 'Take this paper in your right hand, fold it in half, and put it on the floor' | 3 |
| 8. Reading | Ask the patient to read and obey the following:<br>**CLOSE YOUR EYES** | 1 |
| 9. Writing | Ask the patient to write a short sentence | 1 |
| 10. Construction | Ask the patient to copy the following drawing (overlapping pentagons): | 1 |
| | | TOTAL: /30 |

**Fig. 9.10** Mini-Mental State Examination (adapted from Folstein MF et al 1975 Mini-Mental State: a practical method for grading the cognitive state of patients for the clinician. Journal of Psychiatric Research 12:189–198).

likelihood of vascular dementia, and neurological examination may identify focal signs necessitating further investigation.

## Special investigations

Apart from HIV-testing for AIDS-associated dementia and genetic tests for Huntington's disease, there are no specific tests that are diagnostic for the neurodegenerative forms of dementia in living individuals. A number of tests are usually performed soon after the diagnosis of dementia to screen for the general medical causes of dementia or to differentiate between the different types of dementia (see Fig. 9.3).

The EEG in Alzheimer's disease reveals diffuse slowing in the early stages followed by reduced alpha and beta activity and increased theta and delta activity.

The EEG is of limited use diagnostically and is rarely used unless the clinical picture is atypical. The characteristic EEG in Creutzfeldt–Jakob disease is a slow background rhythm with paroxysmal sharp waves.

Individual units vary in their use of neuroimaging techniques to help diagnose dementia. Computed tomography (CT) and magnetic resonance imaging (MRI) are most often used to exclude other causes of cognitive impairment (e.g. tumours, haematomas). They may also be supportive, but not essential in the diagnosis of Alzheimer's disease. Magnetic resonance imaging (MRI) is particularly good at identifying small cerebral infarcts especially in the white brain matter. Figure 9.11 summarizes the CT-scan features of the main forms of dementia.

| Typical CT appearances for the main forms of dementia | |
|---|---|
| **Condition** | **CT appearance** |
| Normal ageing | Progressive cortical atrophy and increasing ventricular size |
| Alzheimer's disease | Generalized cerebral atrophy<br>Widened sulci<br>Dilated ventricles<br>Thinning of the width of the medial temporal lobe (in temporal lobe-oriented CT scans) |
| Vascular dementia | Single/multiple areas of infarction<br>Cerebral atrophy<br>Dilated ventricles |
| Frontotemporal dementia (including Pick's disease) | Greater relative atrophy of frontal and temporal lobes<br>Knife-blade atrophy (appearance of atrophied gyri) |
| Huntington's disease | Dilated ventricles<br>Atrophy of caudate nuclei (loss of shouldering) |
| Creutzfeldt–Jakob disease (CJD)<br><br>nv - new variant | Usually appears normal<br>Note that nvCJD does have a characteristic MRI picture: a bilaterally evident high signal in the pulvinar (post-thalamic) region |

**Fig. 9.11** Typical CT appearances for the main forms of dementia.

Where available, functional imaging, especially single photon emission computed tomography (SPECT), can be very helpful in differentiating the various forms of dementia.

Genetic testing is not recommended for late-onset Alzheimer's disease. Three genes may be tested for in the extremely rare families who have autosomal dominant early-onset familial Alzheimer's disease. These are amyloid precursor protein, presenilin-1 and presenilin-2. However, these three genes may only account for 30–50% of all autosomal dominant early-onset cases. See p. 103, Ch. 16 for a full discussion of the genetics of Alzheimer's disease.

Psychological investigations are used to diagnose cognitive impairment (e.g. MMSE, clock drawing test) and when investigating atypical (e.g. predominantly frontal lobe signs) or presenile presentations. Specific tests of frontal lobe functioning include the Wisconsin Card Sorting Test. Intelligence scales (e.g. Wechsler Adult Intelligence Scale) may be useful in distinguishing cases of pseudodementia. A comprehensive cognitive assessment is usually performed by a specialist clinical psychologist.

Figure 9.12 summarizes a typical dementia workup.

Similar principles apply to the investigation of *delirium*, particularly since there is invariably an identifiable organic cause. Additional investigations to consider include C-reactive protein (marker of infection), arterial blood gases, blood and urine cultures, virology, and urine drug screen. The EEG shows diffuse slowing and may be useful if encephalitis is suspected.

In addition to doing the MMSE on patients you might want to add the specific memory tests that you have already learned (Fig. 9.2) to make your cognitive assessment more comprehensive.

## Discussion of case study

Mr DD first presented with memory loss for recent events. His personality gradually changed

**Fig. 9.12** Workup of dementia.

| Workup of dementia |
| --- |

Psychiatric and medical history including review of medications and alcohol/drug use

Mental state examination

Complete physical examination with special focus on neurological examination
Physical investigations
- Urine
    Culture (exclude urinary tract infection)
    Drug and heavy metal screen
- Bloods
    Full blood count
    Urea and electrolytes, magnesium, calcium, glucose
    Liver function tests
    Thyroid function tests
    $B_{12}$ and folate
    Erythrocyte sedimentation rate (ESR)
    Syphilis serology
    HIV test if indicated
    Other screening tests if indicated (e.g. antinuclear antibodies)
- Chest X-ray
- ECG
- EEG – if indicated by history or psychiatric/physical examination, e.g. suspicion of CJD
- CT or MRI scan of the head – if indicated by history or psychiatric/physical examination
- SPECT scan – if indicated by history or psychiatric/physical examination

Psychological
- Mini-Mental State Examination (MMSE) – useful screening and monitoring tool
- Neuropsychological tests may be useful when dealing with an atypical dementia (e.g. Wisconsin Card Sorting Test for frontal lobe function) or when the diagnosis of dementia is in question (e.g. Wechsler Adult Intelligence Scale in cases of depressive pseudodementia). The Alzheimer's Disease Assessment Scale (ADAS-cog) is a comprehensive assessment scale used in research settings

Social
- Collateral information from GP, community mental health team, family
- Consider home visit to assess self-care, current driving status, risks to self

(withdrawn, prone to verbal abuse) and he also developed numerous other cognitive deficits: aphasia (rambling incoherently), agnosia (unable to recognize pipe and, later, wife), apraxia (unable to dress himself) and impaired executive functioning (unable to make a cup of coffee). This 6-year deterioration in cognitive functioning associated with a normal level of consciousness confirms the diagnosis of dementia. It is important that the type of dementia is determined; Alzheimer's disease, the commonest form of dementia, is diagnosed when other types of dementia have been excluded.

Two days after admission, Mr DD developed a delirium as evidenced by the rapid onset of a fluctuating consciousness level, disturbed sleep–wake cycle, psychomotor agitation and apparent perceptual disturbances (visual hallucinations). It is crucial that the cause of the delirium is diagnosed and treated. In this case, it could be pneumonia as Mr DD had developed a productive cough.

**Now go on to Chapter 16 to read about delirium and dementia and their management.**

Disulfiram = if drink → sick. ────→ flushing
breathing difficulties
headache
palpitat$^n$s.
nausea
vomiting

Acamprasate ──→ anti-craving

AA
CBT
Motivat$^n$al interviewing

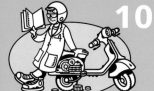

# 10. The Patient with Alcohol or Substance Use Problems

Thiamine aswell + CHLORDIAZIPOXIDE + [if at risk of fits] carbamazapine

Mr AD, aged 42, presented to his GP smelling of alcohol and complaining of depression, anxiety, marital problems and impotence. On further questioning, it transpired that he was drinking heavily, up to 10 cans of strong lager and half a bottle of whisky per day. He had been using increasing amounts over the past 2 years because alcohol no longer gave him the same feeling of well-being. Now, for the first time, he noticed that he *had* to drink in order to avoid shaking, sweating, vomiting and feeling 'on edge'. These symptoms were worse in the morning, resulting in him having two shots of whisky before breakfast. Mr AD admitted that he had neglected his family and work because keeping up his drinking habit was taking all of his time. Whereas in the past, he would vary what and when he drank, he now tended to drink exactly the same thing at the same time each day, irrespective of his mood or the occasion. Mr AD maintained that he continued to drink although he knew it was harming his liver. He was also concerned about his mental health because, on more than one occasion, he thought he saw a man-size parrot walking around the room, which he knew 'wasn't really there'. Mr AD had no previous psychiatric history or family history of psychiatric illness and was not on any medication.

*(For a discussion of the case study see the end of the chapter)*

Psychoactive substances have been used for centuries, and the use of these drugs, especially in the case of alcohol, is seen in some segments of society as socially and culturally acceptable. However, it is important to keep in mind that psychoactive substances either activate or inhibit specific parts of the brain, which can lead to a range of subjective feelings or behavioural changes. Fortunately, in most cases, these effects are innocuous; however, brain-altering substances can cause psychiatric symptoms that are indistinguishable from common psychiatric disorders such as schizophrenia and depression.

## Definitions and clinical features

The term *psychoactive substance* refers to any substance that has an effect on the central nervous system. This includes drugs of abuse or recreational drugs (including alcohol and nicotine), prescribed or over-the-counter medication and poisons or toxins.

There are a large number of different types of psychoactive substances in existence. However, whenever an external chemical or drug is added to the central nervous system, the brain only has a finite number of non-specific ways that reveal that the delicate homeostasis has been 'upset'. Therefore, in psychiatry, it is possible to describe a limited number of typical disorders or psychopathological states that may be caused by any number of different drugs.

It is useful to divide psychoactive substance related disorders into the *substance use disorders*, which describe pathological *patterns of substance use*, and the *substance-induced disorders*, which describe *pathological states directly induced by substances*. Figure 10.1 provides an overview of the substance-related disorders.

Each of the substance-induced disorders that mimic other primary psychiatric illnesses (e.g. dementia, psychotic, mood and anxiety disorders) is discussed in the differential diagnosis section in the chapters on those specific disorders. This is done so that psychoactive substances are always thought of as a potential cause of the psychiatric illness in question.

This section will introduce four new concepts specifically in relation to psychoactive substance use: substance abuse, substance dependence, substance intoxication and substance withdrawal.

## Framework of the psychoactive substance related disorders

**Substance use disorders**
- Substance abuse or harmful use
- Substance dependence (dependence syndrome)

*morbid jelousy.*

**Substance-induced disorders**
- Substance intoxication
- Substance withdrawal
- Substance intoxication delirium
- Substance withdrawal delirium (delirium tremens)
- Substance-induced dementia syndrome
- Substance-induced amnesic syndrome
- Substance-induced psychotic disorder
- Substance-induced mood disorder
- Substance-induced anxiety disorder
- Other substance-induced disorders (sexual dysfunction/sleep disorder)

**Fig. 10.1** Framework of the psychoactive substance related disorders.

## Substance abuse (misuse)

*Substance abuse* describes a maladaptive pattern of substance use that results in a failure to fulfil work, home or school obligations; physically hazardous behaviour (e.g. driving a vehicle); legal problems (e.g. arrest for disorderly conduct) and recurrent interpersonal problems (e.g. arguments/fights with spouse). *Harmful use* describes a pattern of substance use that is harmful to physical or mental health.

## Substance dependence

*Substance dependence* describes a syndrome that incorporates physiological, psychological and behavioural elements (i.e. physiological and psychological dependence). If patients exhibit either tolerance or withdrawal (see below), they may be specified as having physiological dependence. However, it is important to note that dependence does not only imply physiological dependence, and that patients can meet the criteria for the dependence syndrome without having developed tolerance or withdrawal. The dependence syndrome (ICD-10 criteria) is diagnosed if *three or more* of the following have been present together at some time during the previous year:

1. A strong desire or compulsion to take the substance.
2. Difficulties in controlling substance-taking behaviour (onset, termination, levels of use).
3. Physiological withdrawal state when substance use has reduced or ceased; or continued use of the substance to relieve or avoid withdrawal symptoms.

→ *salience/ primacy.*

4. Signs of tolerance: increased quantities of substance are required to produce the same effect originally produced by lower doses.
5. Neglect of other interests and activities due to time spent acquiring and taking substance, or recovering from its effects.
6. Persistence with substance use despite clear awareness of harmful consequences (physical or mental).

*7. early reinstatement → easily become dependent again*

 Patients are physiologically dependent on a psychoactive substance when they exhibit signs of tolerance or withdrawal.

## Substance intoxication

*Substance intoxication* describes a transient, substance-specific condition that occurs following the use of a psychoactive substance and features disturbances of consciousness, perception, mood, behaviour and physiological functions, and is closely related to dose levels.

## Substance withdrawal

*Substance withdrawal* describes a substance-specific syndrome that occurs on reduction or cessation of a psychoactive substance that has usually been used repeatedly, in high doses, for a prolonged period. It is also one of the criteria of the dependence syndrome.

 The confusion regarding use of the term 'addiction' led the World Health Organization (1964) to recommend that the term be abandoned in scientific literature in favour of the term 'dependence'.

## Alcohol-related disorders

## Alcohol use disorders

Any individual who uses alcohol can be classified into one of three categories: the social drinker, the problem drinker and the alcohol-dependent drinker:

## Social drinker

This category includes the majority of drinkers whose drinking remains within healthy limits and does not cause any harmful effects to themselves or those around them. Figure 10.2 describes how to calculate the daily intake of alcohol in units and the recommended safe intake limits.

## Problem drinker (includes substance abuse and harmful use)

This category is used when drinking causes secondary physical, psychological or social harm to the patient. The majority of problem drinkers will not necessarily be dependent on alcohol. Figure 10.3 lists the adverse physical, psychological and social consequences of drinking.

 Although many drinkers may not be suffering from alcohol dependence, they could, in fact, be problem drinkers, who might benefit from an alcohol treatment programme.

## Alcohol dependence

There are many reasons why individuals start, and continue, drinking in a problematic way. However, after a significant time of heavy, regular drinking, they may develop the *super-added* problem of alcohol dependence. This means that in addition to the original reasons which initiated their drinking, they now have an extra problem that further perpetuates it. In 1976, Edwards and Gross formulated a detailed description of *alcohol dependence syndrome* – a repeated cluster of symptoms and signs that occur in heavy drinkers (Fig. 10.4). Alcohol-dependence syndrome as described by Edwards and Gross was a strong influence on the ICD-10 described substance dependence syndrome (see above), hence their similarities. Both can be used to describe alcohol dependence, although the Edwards and Gross criteria are probably more particular to alcohol. It is important to note that alcohol dependence does not just mean physical dependence (although that is an important part of it), but describes a heterogeneous collection of symptoms, signs and behaviours which are determined by biological, psychological and sociocultural factors. Also note that the dependence syndrome is not simply said to be present or not, but is described as *degrees of dependence*. There is a difference between the

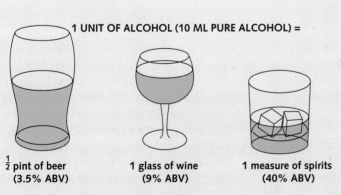

**Fig. 10.2** Safe daily alcohol limits.

**1 UNIT OF ALCOHOL (10 ML PURE ALCOHOL) =**

½ pint of beer (3.5% ABV) — 1 glass of wine (9% ABV) — 1 measure of spirits (40% ABV)

Note: this is an approximate guide only, as many beers contain 4–5% ABV and many wines 11–12% ABV
ABV, alcohol content by volume

**Safe daily alcohol limits**
Men: 3–4 units/day (<21 units/week)
Women: 2–3 units/day (<14 units/week)

Note: Alcohol can confer health benefit mainly by giving protection from coronary heart disease, but this only applies to men over 40 and postmenopausal women. The maximum health advantages are obtained by drinking 1–2 units per day.

---

### Complications of excessive alcohol use

**Psychological**
- See substance-induced disorders – Fig. 10.1

**Social**
- Absenteeism from, or poor performance at, work or school
- Legal problems (increased risk of violent crime, drink driving, alcohol-related disorderly conduct)
- Interpersonal problems (arguments with family due to alcohol)
- Financial problems (expense of drinking, unemployment)
- Vagrancy and homelessnes

*[handwritten: suicide + homocide]*

**Physical**
- *Nervous system*
  Intoxication or withdrawal delirium (delirium tremens)
  Withdrawal seizures
  Cerebellar degeneration
  Haemorrhagic stroke
  Peripheral and optic neuropathy
  Wernicke's encephalopathy/Korsakoff's syndrome
  Alcohol 'dementia'
  *[handwritten: - ataxia - nystagmus - opthalmoplegia]*
- *Gastroenterological system*
  Alcoholic liver disease (fatty liver, alcoholic hepatitis, alcoholic cirrhosis)
  Acute and chronic pancreatitis
  Peptic ulceration and gastritis
  Cancers: oropharynx, larynx, oesophagus, liver

**Physical**—*cont'd*
- *Cardiovascular system*
  Hypertension
  Arrhythmias
  Ischaemic heart disease (in heavy drinkers)
  Alcoholic cardiomyopathy
- *Immune system*
  Increased risk of infections (especially meningitis and pneumonia)
- *Metabolic and endocrine system*
  Hypoglycaemia
  Hyperlipidaemia
  Hyperuricaemia
  Hypomagnesaemia, hypophosphataemia, hyponatraemia
  Alcohol-induced pseudo-Cushing's syndrome
- *Haematological system*
  Red cell macrocytosis
  Anaemia
  Neutropenia
  Thrombocytopenia
- *Musculoskeletal system*
  Acute and chronic myopathy
  Osteoporosis
- *Reproductive system*
  Intrauterine growth retardation
  Fetal alcohol syndrome
- *Increased incidence of trauma*

**Fig. 10.3** Complications of excessive alcohol use.

dependent drinker who experiences an irksome tremor while at work and the dependent drinker who shakes so much after waking that he is unable to drink a cup of tea in the morning without spilling it.

## Alcohol-induced disorders
### Acute intoxication (including delirium)
Ingestion of significant quantities of alcohol results in transient psychological, behavioural and neurological changes, the severity of which are roughly correlated to the alcohol concentration in the brain. Low blood alcohol concentrations may produce an enhanced sense of well-being, greater confidence and relief of anxiety, which may lead to individuals becoming disinhibited, talkative and flirtatious. As blood levels increase, some drinkers may exhibit inappropriate sexual or aggressive behaviour whereas others might become sullen and withdrawn. Lability of mood is common and certain patients become maudlin and over-dramatic and may engage in parasuicidal behaviour. Incoordination, slurred speech, ataxia, amnesia (see later) and impaired

reaction times ensue followed by lowered level of consciousness, respiratory depression, coma and death.

An *alcohol intoxication delirium* (see Ch. 9) is diagnosed when there is lowered consciousness or ability to sustain attention and global cognitive impairment, which is in excess of that usually associated with alcohol intoxication.

The term *pathological intoxication* describes the sudden onset of aggressive, often violent behaviour, not typical of the individual when sober, occurring

Alcohol intoxication is a potentially life-threatening condition due to the risk of respiratory depression, aspiration of vomitus, hypoglycaemia, hypothermia and trauma (subdural haematomas, fractures, etc.).

soon after drinking small amounts of alcohol that would not produce intoxication in most people (Coid 1979). Many authors question whether such a pathological entity truly exists.

## Alcohol withdrawal (including delirium)

The development of withdrawal symptoms is one of the criteria of the dependence syndrome. The severity of alcohol withdrawal can be seen as existing on a continuum from uncomplicated withdrawal to the life-threatening withdrawal delirium (delirium tremens). Figure 10.5 summarizes the continuum of clinical features of alcohol withdrawal, from uncomplicated withdrawal to delirium. Remember, however, that uncomplicated does not mean: not serious. All withdrawal states are potentially life-threatening, as they are associated with autonomic hyperactivity and can include perceptual

Although withdrawal seizures commonly precede an alcohol withdrawal delirium, the delirium can also appear without forewarning.

disturbances and seizures – and might herald the onset of a delirium.

## Alcohol-induced dementia syndrome

Chronic, heavy alcohol use can lead to mild to moderate impairment of memory, learning, visuospatial skills and impulse control associated with cortical atrophy and ventricular enlargement. However, many authors question the legitimacy of the concept that alcohol directly causes dementia

**Fig. 10.4** Alcohol dependence syndrome (Adapted from Edwards G, Gross MM 1976 Alcohol dependence: provisional description of a clinical syndrome. British Medical Journal 1:1058–1061).

---

### Alcohol dependence syndrome (Adapted from Edwards & Gross 1976)

1. **Narrowing of repertoire**: The range of cues, internal and external, that affect drinking in a normal person influence the pattern of drinking in a dependent person less and less, i.e. drinking becomes increasingly stereotyped. The dependent person will drink the same type of alcohol at the same time each day in the same place.

2. **Increased salience of drinking**: Maintaining the stereotyped pattern of drinking is given priority over other aspects of the patient's life such as home and family life, career and previously enjoyed recreational activities.

3. **Increased tolerance to alcohol**: Increased quantities of alcohol are required to produce the same effect. Patients are able to tolerate blood alcohol levels that would incapacitate non-tolerant drinkers. Note that tolerance to alcohol can sometimes decrease considerably in patients who have been drinking heavily for many years.

4. **Withdrawal symptoms**: A fall in blood alcohol level results in withdrawal symptoms. This will occur when drinkers reduce or stop their alcohol intake. Heavier degrees of dependence may result in early morning withdrawal symptoms after a night's sleep. Withdrawal symptoms include tremors (shakes), nausea and vomiting, sweating and mood disturbances (anxiety, depression, agitation).

5. **Relief or avoidance of withdrawal symptoms by further drinking**: Dependent drinkers may need to nip off to the pub at midday, or worse, have a stiff drink in the morning or, worse still, have a drink in the middle of the night to fend off incipient withdrawal.

6. **Subjective awareness of the compulsion to drink**: Patients sometimes describe this highly subjective symptom as a 'compulsive craving' that is extremely difficult to resist.

7. **Rapid reinstatement after abstinence**: Although the dependence syndrome may take many years of heavy drinking to develop, many drinkers may rapidly redevelop dependence when they start drinking again after a significant period of abstinence. For example, within 3 days a drinker might develop severe withdrawal symptoms, and be able to tolerate vast quantities of alcohol despite 2 previous years of abstinence.

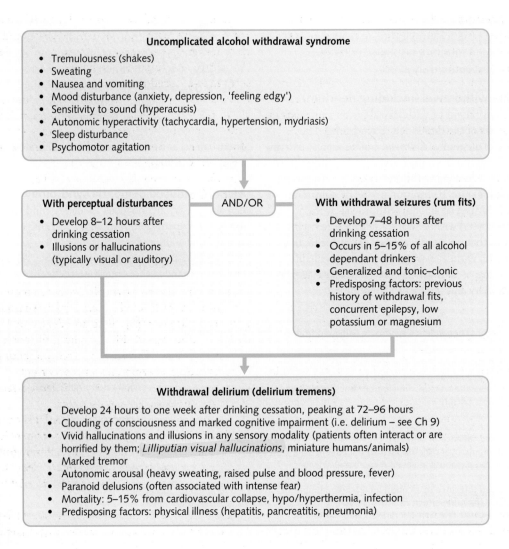

**Uncomplicated alcohol withdrawal syndrome**

- Tremulousness (shakes)
- Sweating
- Nausea and vomiting
- Mood disturbance (anxiety, depression, 'feeling edgy')
- Sensitivity to sound (hyperacusis)
- Autonomic hyperactivity (tachycardia, hypertension, mydriasis)
- Sleep disturbance
- Psychomotor agitation

**With perceptual disturbances**

- Develop 8–12 hours after drinking cessation
- Illusions or hallucinations (typically visual or auditory)

AND/OR

**With withdrawal seizures (rum fits)**

- Develop 7–48 hours after drinking cessation
- Occurs in 5–15% of all alcohol dependant drinkers
- Generalized and tonic–clonic
- Predisposing factors: previous history of withdrawal fits, concurrent epilepsy, low potassium or magnesium

**Withdrawal delirium (delirium tremens)**

- Develop 24 hours to one week after drinking cessation, peaking at 72–96 hours
- Clouding of consciousness and marked cognitive impairment (i.e. delirium – see Ch 9)
- Vivid hallucinations and illusions in any sensory modality (patients often interact or are horrified by them; *Lilliputian visual hallucinations*, miniature humans/animals)
- Marked tremor
- Autonomic arousal (heavy sweating, raised pulse and blood pressure, fever)
- Paranoid delusions (often associated with intense fear)
- Mortality: 5–15% from cardiovascular collapse, hypo/hyperthermia, infection
- Predisposing factors: physical illness (hepatitis, pancreatitis, pneumonia)

**Fig. 10.5** Clinical features of alcohol withdrawal.

because it is difficult to separate the toxic effects of alcohol from the brain damage caused by years of malnutrition, alcohol associated trauma (head injury) and the effects of multi-organ dysfunction (alcohol-induced liver and pancreatic disease). Subsequent abstinence from alcohol does lead to some improvement in cognitive functioning. See Chapter 9 for more on dementia.

## Alcohol-induced amnesia

*Alcohol-induced amnesic syndrome*, or *Korsakoff's syndrome*, occurs because of a thiamine (vitamin $B_1$) deficiency and is a common sequel to Wernicke's encephalopathy. Whereas Wernicke's encephalopathy (and progression to Korsakoff's syndrome) is treatable with prompt doses of parenteral thiamine,

only about 20% of patients with developed Korsakoff's syndrome recover. See also p. 60 and p. 110.

Episodes of anterograde amnesia or *alcoholic blackouts* can occur during acute alcohol intoxication. Memory loss may be patchy, or for a discrete block of time during which nothing can be remembered. Blackouts are common and have been experienced by two-thirds of dependent drinkers and one-third of young men in the general population.

## Alcohol-induced psychotic disorder

Both hallucinations and delusions can occur in the context of heavy alcohol consumption. A number of syndromes have been described ranging from fleeting perceptual disturbances with retained insight *(transient hallucinatory experience)* to more persistent, vivid, auditory (predominantly) or visual hallucinations with lack of insight *(alcoholic hallucinosis)* to a syndrome characterized by persecutory or grandiose delusions. These syndromes are distinguished from an intoxication or withdrawal delirium by the absence of clouding of consciousness. They do not appear to be related to schizophrenia and should clear with abstinence from alcohol.

## Alcohol-induced mood disorder

The relationship between alcohol and depression is complex. Heavy alcohol consumption may cause patients to become maudlin and dramatic which may make distinguishing true depressive illness difficult. This problem is compounded by the damage alcohol does to patients' personal lives, giving them ample reason to bemoan their existence. Many patients, however, do develop genuine depressive illness, which will require treatment in addition to abstinence from alcohol. The difficulty in these cases is deciding whether alcohol caused, or is merely associated with, the depression. Note that the lifetime risk of suicide in problem drinkers is 3–4%, which is 60–120 times greater than the normal population.

Problematic drinking is more often a consequence of mania (as a form of self-medication) rather than a persistently elevated mood state being induced by alcohol.

## Alcohol-induced anxiety disorder

Up to one-third of drinkers have significant anxiety symptoms. As in depression, establishing alcohol as a causal factor in anxiety disorders is difficult. The anxiolytic properties of alcohol often result in attempts at self-medication in patients with agoraphobia and social phobia, and alcohol withdrawal symptoms can mimic anxiety and panic symptoms. Nevertheless, alcohol use should always be considered as a direct causal factor for patients presenting with an anxiety disorder.

## Other alcohol-induced disorders

Alcohol can cause sleep disorders and sexual dysfunction, which are discussed in Chapters 21 and 22.

## Other substance-related disorders

It is beyond the scope of this book to describe the individual psychiatric consequences of each of the illicit drugs in detail, as has been done with alcohol. However, like alcohol, other substance-related disorders are classified as substance use disorders (harmful use or dependence syndrome) or substance-induced disorders (e.g. acute intoxication, psychotic disorder) – see Figure 10.1. Try to think of the many drugs of abuse in principal groups according to their characteristics and effects, namely, *opiates, stimulants, hallucinogens, depressants, cannabinoids, dissociative anaesthetics* and *inhalants* as described in Figure 10.6.

## Differential diagnosis of patients using alcohol or other drugs

Patients using psychoactive substances can present with the exact features of almost any known primary psychiatric disorder (psychotic disorders, mood disorders, dementia, delirium, amnesic disorders, anxiety disorders). Therefore, patients presenting with psychological symptoms and concurrent psychoactive drug use are a diagnostic challenge. There are three diagnostic possibilities:

1. There is a primary psychiatric disorder such as depression or schizophrenia and the patient is coincidentally using drugs or alcohol (remember that patients suffering from mental illness often use psychoactive substances to obtain relief from their symptoms).
2. The symptoms are entirely due to the direct effect of the drug and no primary psychiatric diagnosis exists.
3. Or, as is often the case, psychiatric symptoms may be due to a combination of the above, as occurs when psychoactive drugs act on patients with a *predisposing vulnerability* to the development of mental illness.

The following features suggest a drug-induced psychiatric disorder:

- The psychological symptoms are known to be associated with specific drug in question (e.g. psychotic features with amfetamine use).
- There is a temporal relationship (hours or days) between the use of the suspected drug and the development of psychological symptoms.
- There is a complete recovery from all psychological symptoms after termination of the suspected drug use.
- There is an absence of evidence to suggest an alternative explanation for psychological symptoms

**Effects of the drugs of abuse**

| Drug group | Common examples | Psychological effects | Physical effects |
|---|---|---|---|
| Opiates and morphine derivatives | Morphine, heroin or diamorphine (*smack*), codeine, methadone, dipipanone, opium | Euphoria, drowsiness, apathy, personality change | Miosis, conjuctival injection, nausea, pruritus, constipation, bradycardia, respiratory depression, coma |
| Stimulants | Amfetamine (*speed*), cocaine, crack cocaine, methylenedioxy-methamphetamine (*MDMA, Ecstasy, E*), nicotine, methylphenidate | Alertness, hyperactivity, euphoria, irritability, aggression, paranoid ideas, hallucinations (esp. cocaine – formication), psychosis | Mydriasis, tremor, hypertension, tachycardia, arrhythmias, perspiration, fever (Esp. *Ecstasy*), convulsions, perforated nasal septum (cocaine) |
| Hallucinogens | Lysergic acid diethylamine (*LSD, acid*), mescaline, psilocybin (*magic mushrooms*) | Marked perceptual disturbances including chronic flashbacks, paranoid ideas, suicidal and homicidal ideas, psychosis | Mydriasis, conjuctival injection, hypertension, tachycardia, perspiration, fever, loss of appetite, weakness, tremors |
| Central nervous system depressants | Benzodiazepines, barbiturates | Drowsiness, disinhibition, confusion, poor concentration, reduced anxiety, feeling of well-being | Miosis, hypotension, seizures, impaired coordination, respiratory depression |
| Cannabinoids | Cannabis (*dope, weed, grass*), hashish, hash oil | Euphoria, relaxation, altered time perception, psychosis | Impaired coordination and reaction time, conjuctival injection, nystagmus, dry mouth |
| Dissociative anaesthetics | Ketamine, phencyclidine (*PCP, angel dust*) | Hallucinations, paranoid ideas, thought disorganization, aggression | Mydriasis, tachycardia, hypertension |
| Inhalants | Aerosols, paint, glue, lighter fluid, petrol, benzene, gases | Disinhibition, stimulation, euphoria, clouded consciousness, hallucinations, psychosis | Headache, nausea, slurred speech, loss of motor coordination, muscle weakness, damage to brain/bone marrow/liver/kidneys/myocardium, sudden death |

**Fig. 10.6** Effects of the drugs of abuse.

(e.g. previous history of primary psychiatric illness or family history of psychiatric illness).

DRINKING DAY + WEEK?

## Assessment

### Clinical

The CAGE questionnaire is a simple tool to screen for alcohol dependence. If patients answer affirmatively to two or more questions, regard the screen as positive and go on to check if they meet the definitive criteria for the alcohol dependence syndrome.

1. Have you ever felt you ought to *cut down* on your drinking?
2. Have people ever *annoyed* you by criticizing your drinking?
3. Have you ever felt *guilty* about your drinking?
4. Have you ever needed a drink first thing in the morning to steady your nerves or get rid of a hangover (*'eye-opener'*)?

The Alcohol Use Disorders Identification Test (AUDIT), which was developed by the World Health Organization, is a 10-item screening questionnaire for problem drinking with three questions on the

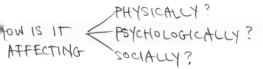
amount and frequency of drinking, four questions on harmful alcohol use and three questions on alcohol dependence. It takes 3 minutes to complete and score, and is being used increasingly in many segments of healthcare.

The *physical examination* requires an awareness of the acute and long-term effects of alcohol or substance use and should focus on:

- Evidence of acute use or intoxication (e.g. pupil constriction with opiate use; incoordination and slurred speech with alcohol use).
- Signs of withdrawal (e.g. tremulousness, sweating, nausea and vomiting, tachycardia and pupil dilatation with alcohol withdrawal).
- Immediate and short-term medical complications of substance use (e.g. head injury following alcohol intoxication, local and systemic infection caused by intravenous drug use).
- Long-term medical complications (e.g. alcohol-related liver disease, hepatitis B or C or HIV infection with intravenous drug use).

## Special investigations

Non-specific investigations are useful to exclude longer-term complications of alcohol (see Fig. 10.3) and substance misuse, and include a full blood count, urea and electrolytes, liver function tests, ECG, chest X-ray, hepatitis serology and an HIV test. If the patient is suffering from a withdrawal delirium, specific investigations may be necessary to exclude an additional complication (e.g. infection, head injury, brain abscess). A urine drug-screening test is essential whenever the use of psychoactive substances is suspected.

There is no 100% sensitive and 100% specific test for heavy drinking. Therefore, the following screening tests are only of use in a population with a high prevalence of excess alcohol consumption (to limit the false positives) and when used in combination (to improve the sensitivity and specificity):

- The *mean corpuscular volume (MCV)* measures the size of red blood cells. However, an increased MCV only has a sensitivity of 20–50% and a specificity of 55–100% for heavy drinking. Remember that due to the long life of red blood cells (120 days), the MCV may remain elevated for some time after drinking cessation.
- The raised liver enzymes, *gamma glutamyl transpeptidase (γ GT)*, *aspartate aminotransferase (AST)* and *alanine aminotransferase (ALT)* all

indicate alcohol-related liver damage. The most useful of these, γGT, only has a sensitivity of 20–90% and a specificity of 55–100% making its reliability questionable. The γGT will fall more rapidly after drinking cessation than the MCV.

- *Carbohydrate deficient transferrin (CDT)*, which is related to the protein that transports iron, is often increased in heavy drinkers. It is considered the best single screening test, but still only has a sensitivity of 60–70% and a specificity of 95%.
- *Blood alcohol concentration (BAC)*, or breath alcohol (via a breathalyser) as an indirect measure, only detects recent alcohol use. However, the finding of a high alcohol concentration (more than 100 mg/100 ml) in the absence of signs of intoxication suggests some degree of tolerance, which is likely to be indicative of chronic heavy drinking.
- Elevated *triglycerides*, *cholesterol* and *uric acid* can all be increased secondary to alcohol use, but are very non-specific and of limited clinical use.

All patients, especially young psychotic patients who are suspected of having a substance-induced psychiatric disorder, should have a urine drug-screening test. It is important to collect the urine as soon as possible because the half-lives of some drugs are short.

The sensitivity and specificity of the blood investigations as screening tests for heavy drinking may be improved when they are used in combination. For example, a measurement of MCV, γ GT and CDT in combination is far more useful than any of these in isolation.

## Discussion of case study

Mr AD is a problem drinker (alcohol causing physical, psychological and social harm). He also has the super-added problem of *alcohol dependence* as evidenced by the tolerance, withdrawal symptoms, relief of withdrawal by drinking, salience of drinking, narrowing of repertoire (Edwards and Gross criteria)

Dependence on drugs, alcohol or nicotine is associated with increased rates of psychiatric disorders (independent of other variables). The importance of this is that clinicians should screen for other psychiatric disorders when assessing individuals with dependence, especially considering that 33% of the general population (England and Wales) are dependent on nicotine, alcohol or other drugs (about 32% of the population smoke, 5% are alcohol dependent and 2% are dependent on drugs).

and also continued drinking despite awareness of harmful consequences (ICD-10 criteria). He has

physical (sexual, possibly other systems), social (marital discord, neglect of family and work) and psychological (depression, anxiety, hallucinations) complications of his alcohol use. In relation to the depression, anxiety and hallucinations, it is important to rule out a mental illness, which will require extra-clinical attention, apart from treating the alcohol dependence. The absence of family or personal history for psychiatric illness suggests that the depression, anxiety and hallucinations will resolve with abstinence. The visual hallucinations may be symptomatic of a withdrawal syndrome or be one of the perceptual disturbances sometimes caused by heavy alcohol use – in this case: *transient hallucinatory experience*, as Mr AD has retained insight.

**Now go on to Chapter 17 to read about the alcohol and substance disorders and their management.**

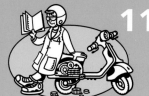

# 11. The Patient with Personality and Impulse-control Problems

The on-call psychiatrist was asked by the GP to assess Miss BP, a 27-year-old woman who had been known to the mental health services since the age of 17 with a condition that had changed little in 10 years. She lived with her mother, who had contacted the GP because Miss BP was threatening to throw herself in front of a bus. From her notes, the GP noted that Miss BP had a long history of deliberate self-harm that included self-inflicted cuts to her arms, thighs and torso and repeated overdoses. Miss BP had been sexually abused as a child by her father, who was serving a prison sentence. She had a 'love–hate' relationship with her mother, who was inclined to challenge Miss BP's promiscuous behaviour and binge drinking, which led to them having many heated arguments. Despite maintaining that all she ever wanted was love, Miss BP was unable to form any lasting relationships. She had a pattern of either idealizing or devaluing the virtues of those close to her and alternated between the extremes of helpless submissiveness and aggressive dominance. After he arrived, Miss BP told the psychiatrist that she was feeling 'more depressed than ever' because her mother had suggested that she move into her own house. With gentle questioning it transpired that she was afraid that her mother would stop caring for her if she moved out. The psychiatrist, who had known Miss BP for years, recognized that this behaviour was not unusual for her and was able to comfort her by helping her to see another perspective to her mother's suggestion. Miss BP's mood lifted and her suicidal ideation resolved.

*(For a discussion of the case study see the end of the chapter)*

People use the term 'personality' in varying contexts to mean any number of things. In fact, the term has over 100 different definitions in the psychological literature. Amid the lack of consensus on what defines personality, there is little doubt that certain people seem to experience and interact with the world in a way that is relatively different to similar individuals in their culture, and some of these people may come to the attention of health workers. The description and management of what has been arbitrarily designated 'personality disorder' is one of the most controversial subjects in psychiatry. Not only are personality disorders associated with significant distress to the sufferer, but they also place a substantial burden on healthcare, social and criminal justice agencies.

## Definitions and clinical features

The DSM-IV defines *personality traits* as enduring patterns of perceiving, thinking about and relating to the environment and oneself that are exhibited in a wide range of social and personal contexts. It is only when an individual has traits that are persistently inflexible and maladaptive, stable over time, and which cause significant personal distress or functional impairment that a *personality disorder* is said to exist.

Patients with a personality disorder do not regard their patterns of behaviour and coping style as inherently abnormal and therefore will not present with that as their primary complaint. Instead, they usually present to the healthcare services with a wide range of problems related or consequent to their abnormal personality traits, e.g. deliberate self-harm, feelings of depression or anxiety, violence or disorderly conduct, post-traumatic stress disorder, eating disorders, dissociative disorders, somatoform disorders, factitious disorders, etc. Also note that having a significant major psychiatric illness such as schizophrenia does not preclude patients from also having a personality disorder (30–60% of patients with a psychotic disorder also have a personality disorder).

The DSM-IV separates Axis II conditions (personality disorders and mental retardation) from Axis I conditions (major mental illnesses, e.g. psychotic and mood disorders) so that both are considered when diagnosing a patient with florid mental illness.

## Classification

The personality disorders can be classified into two groups according to their aetiology. The first group includes acquired personality disorders where the disordered personality clearly develops after, and is directly related to, a recognizable 'insult'. *Organic personality disorder* results when this 'insult' is some form of brain damage or disease (e.g. a brain tumour or stroke). It is characterized by social disinhibition (e.g. stealing, sexual inappropriateness) and abnormalities of emotional expression (e.g. shallow cheerfulness, aggression, apathy) and is typically seen in frontal lobe lesions. Patients can also exhibit an enduring personality change after *experiencing a catastrophic event* (e.g. concentration camp or hostage situation) or after the *development of a severe psychiatric illness*.

The second group include what is known in the ICD-10 as the *specific personality disorders* (note that this group is far more prevalent and is, therefore, simply referred to as the 'personality disorders' – as will be done for the rest of the chapter). In this group of personality disorders, it is difficult to find a direct causal relationship with any one specific thing, although genetic and environmental factors have been implicated (see Ch. 18). The specific personality disorders usually have their onset in adolescence or early adulthood and remain relatively stable over time.

Personality disorders can also be classified according to which particular maladaptive personality traits individuals display, i.e. based on clinical presentation. In this regard there are two approaches: the dimensional and categorical classification. The *dimensional approach* hypothesizes that the personality traits of patients with a personality disorder differ from the normal population only in terms of degree. Maladaptive personality traits can therefore be seen as existing on a continuum that merges into normality. The dimensional approach is used predominantly in the research of personality disorders and is measured by

personality inventories (e.g. Minnesota Multiphasic Personality Inventory – MMPI). The ICD-10 and DSM-IV primarily use the *categorical approach*, which assumes the existence of distinct types of personality disorder and therefore classifies patients into discrete categories as summarized in Figure 11.1. Despite the widespread use of the categorical approach in clinical practice, it seldom conforms to reality as there is a considerable overlap of traits and most individuals do not fit perfectly into these described categories.

In an attempt to simplify the classification of personality disorders even further, the DSM-IV has designated three personality clusters based on general similarities. *Cluster A*, which includes paranoid, schizoid and schizotypal personality disorders, describes individuals who appear odd or eccentric. *Cluster B*, which includes borderline, antisocial (dissocial), histrionic and narcissistic personality disorders, describes individuals who appear dramatic, emotional or erratic. *Cluster C*, which includes avoidant, dependent and obsessive-compulsive (anankastic) personality disorders, describes individuals who appear anxious or fearful.

 Despite the name, the majority of patients with obsessive-compulsive disorder do not meet the criteria for obsessive-compulsive personality disorder.

## Habit and impulse-control disorders

There are many psychiatric conditions which feature poor impulse control (e.g. substance-related disorders, personality disorders, psychotic disorders, mood disorders). This category of behavioural disorders includes those conditions that are not classified in other categories. They are characterized by a repeated failure to resist an impulse or temptation to perform an act that is harmful to the patient's own or others' interests. The individual may experience tension or arousal prior to the act, followed by pleasure, gratification or relief at the time of carrying out the act. Examples include pathological gambling, pathological fire setting (pyromania), pathological stealing (kleptomania) and trichotillomania (pulling out one's hair).

| Categorical classification of the personality disorders | |
| --- | --- |
| **Cluster A: 'odd or eccentric'** | |
| **Paranoid personality disorder** | Suspects others are exploiting, harming or deceiving them; doubts about spouse's fidelity; bears grudges; tenacious sense of personal rights; litigious |
| **Schizoid personality disorder** | Emotional coldness; neither enjoys nor desires close or sexual relationships; prefers solitary activities; takes pleasure in few activities; indifferent to praise or criticism |
| **Schizotypal personality disorder** | Eccentric behaviour; odd beliefs or magical thinking; unusual perceptual experiences (e.g. 'sensing' another's presence); ideas of reference; suspicious or paranoid ideas; vague or circumstantial thinking; social withdrawal |
| **Cluster B: 'dramatic, emotional, erratic'** | |
| **Borderline (emotionally unstable) personality disorder** ♀ | Unstable, intense relationships (fluctuating between extremes of idealization and devaluation); unstable self-image; impulsivity (sex, binge eating, substance abuse, spending money); repetitive suicidal or self-harm behaviour, fluctuations in mood, frantic efforts to avoid abandonment (real or imagined), transient paranoid ideation or dissociation |
| **Antisocial (dissocial) personality disorder** ♂ | Repeated unlawful or aggressive behaviour; deceitfulness; lying; reckless irresponsibility; lack of remorse or incapacity to experience guilt; often have *conduct disorder* in childhood – see p. 149 |
| **Histrionic personality disorder** | Dramatic, exaggerated expressions of emotion; attention seeking; seductive behaviour; labile shallow emotions |
| **Narcissistic personality disorder** | Grandiose sense of self-importance, need for admiration |
| **Cluster C: 'anxious or fearful'** | |
| **Dependent personality disorder** | Excessive need to be cared for; submissive, clinging behaviour; needs others to assume responsibility for major life areas; fear of separation |
| **Avoidant (anxious) personality disorder** | Hypersensitivity to critical remarks or rejection; inhibited in social situations; fears of inadequacy |
| **Obsessive-compulsive (anankastic) personality disorder** | Preoccupation with orderliness, perfectionism and control; devoted to work at expense of leisure; pedantic, rigid and stubborn; overly cautious |

*Note that the ICD-10 includes all the personality disorders described in the DSM-IV clusters above, except for schizotypal and narcissistic personality disorder. However, schizotypal disorder (similar to the DSM-IV's schizotypal personality disorder) is included in the ICD-10's chapter on psychotic disorders.*

**Fig. 11.1** Categorical classification of the personality disorders.

The term 'borderline personality disorder' is derived from the early 20th century psychoanalysts, who described a group of patients who stood 'on the borderline' between the neuroses and the psychoses.

## Assessment

### Clinical

As with all other mental illnesses, giving a patient a label of personality disorder gives those involved with their care only a limited amount of information. In fact, the clinical classification of personality

disorders is often unreliable and although psychiatrists usually agree that a patient has a personality disorder, there are often differing points of view as regards the subtype of the disorder.

A practical approach includes making a comprehensive assessment of:

- Sources of distress (thoughts, emotions, behaviour and relationships) to self and others.
- Other co-morbid mental illness.
- Specific impairments of functioning at work, home or in social circumstances.

It is usually possible to establish some idea of a patient's personality by taking a detailed history of their life focusing on the areas of education, work, forensic, relationship and sexual history. When patients are not able to describe aspects of their personality it may be useful to ask them how those close to them might describe them. It is also useful to obtain collateral information from the patient's family, teachers (including school records), employer and general practitioner, all of whom might be able to distinguish between transient and enduring patterns of behaviour.

## Self-rating instruments

In these self-report questionnaires, patients respond to numerous questions describing various personality traits – e.g. Minnesota Multiphasic Personality Inventory (MMPI), Eysenck Personality Questionnaire (EPQ), Millon Clinical Multiaxial Inventory (MCMI).

## Structured interviews

In this assessment, data are obtained from a semi-structured interview with preset questions, e.g. Structured Clinical Interview for DSM-IV Personality Disorders (SCID-II).

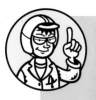 Be wary of diagnosing a personality disorder based on one interview, especially in an examination where collateral information is not available. It is better practice to tentatively identify maladaptive or inflexible personality traits that would require further assessment.

## Differential diagnosis

Almost all the mental illnesses described in this book can feature some of the behaviours that characterize the personality disorders. For example: social withdrawal, suspiciousness and eccentric ideas in schizophrenia; self-harm, low mood and poor self-image in depression; and aggression, irresponsibility and impulsivity in substance abuse or mania. The diagnostic task is also complicated by the observation that many patients with a major mental illness also have a concurrent personality disorder. Therefore, you should always consider the possibility of an underlying major mental illness (DSM-IV: Axis I) before diagnosing a personality disorder (DSM-IV: Axis II), although both can be diagnosed together. A

personality disorder should only be diagnosed when the clinical features begin in adolescence or early adulthood, are stable over time and do not only occur during an episode of a major mental illness (e.g. depressive, manic, psychotic episode).

When an individual develops a dramatic personality change after a period of normal personality functioning consider an *organic personality disorder* or a personality disorder which occurs secondary to experiencing a catastrophic event or developing a severe psychiatric illness.

 Remember that the cluster A personality disorders may present with features similar to the psychotic disorders (e.g. suspiciousness, social withdrawal and eccentric beliefs) but are differentiated by the absence of true delusions or hallucinations.

## Discussion of case study

Miss BP has a chronic condition that first presented in adolescence and has remained stable over time. She has a number of maladaptive and inflexible personality traits that have manifested as: repeated self-mutilation and suicidal behaviour; intense unstable relationships; relationships characterized by alternating idealization and devaluation; unstable self-image (alternating between submission and dominance); impulsivity (promiscuity, binge drinking), fluctuations in mood; and a desperate fear of abandonment by her mother. These characteristics are consistent with a diagnosis of borderline personality disorder. It would be important to exclude another mental illness that may co-exist with the personality disorder, such as depression or alcohol abuse/dependence. Note that there is an association between borderline personality disorder and childhood sexual abuse.

**Now go on to Chapter 18 to read about the personality disorders and their management.**

# 12. The Patient with Eating or Weight Problems

Miss ED, an 18-year-old undergraduate, eventually agreed to see a psychiatrist after much persuasion from her mother and GP. Her weight had fallen from 65 kg to 41 kg over the previous 6 months and she appeared emaciated. Her GP had measured her height at 1.65 metres and had calculated her body mass index (BMI) to be 15 kg/m². The psychiatrist saw Miss ED alone and spent some time putting her at ease and reassuring her that the interview would remain confidential. After an initial reluctance, she admitted that she was repulsed by the thought of being fat and felt that she was still overweight and needed to lose 'just a few more pounds'. She had stopped menstruating 4 months ago and had also noted that she was feeling tired and cold all the time and was finding it difficult to concentrate. The psychiatrist elicited that she only ate one small meal a day and was exercising to the point of collapse. She denied binge eating or self-induced vomiting but did admit to using 20 senna tablets daily. She reported symptoms of depression, but no suicidal ideation. Physical examination revealed a pulse rate of 50 beats per minute and fine downy hair covering her torso.

*(For a discussion of the case study see the end of the chapter)*

Many people are concerned about what and how much they eat. However, certain individuals become so morbidly concerned with their body image that their life revolves around the relentless pursuit of thinness. This life-threatening form of psychopathology needs to be distinguished from other causes of appetite and weight loss.

## Definitions and clinical features

Weight loss can be deliberately intended or occur as a secondary consequence to a medical condition, psychiatric illness or use of a substance. There are two syndromes characterized by conscious and deliberate attempts to reduce body weight: anorexia nervosa and bulimia nervosa.

### Anorexia nervosa and bulimia nervosa

A desire to be fashionably thin and shapely should be distinguished from the specific psychopathology that occurs in both anorexia and bulimia nervosa. This takes the form of an overvalued idea (see p. 26) which is characterized by a dread of fatness, resulting in patients imposing a low target weight on themselves. This desired weight might be achieved by poor caloric intake, self-induced vomiting, excessive exercise or the use of drugs (e.g. appetite suppressants, laxatives, thyroid preparations, diuretics).

In anorexia nervosa, body weight is maintained at least 15% below that expected or the body mass index (Fig. 12.1) is 17.5 kg/m² or less. There is also a generalized endocrine disturbance as evidenced by amenorrhoea in post-menarchal women; loss of sexual interest and potency in men; raised growth hormone and cortisol; and reduced $T_3$. In pre-pubertal anorectics, expected weight gain during the growth period is impaired and pubertal events (menarche, breast development) may be delayed or arrested.

In bulimia nervosa, patients usually have a normal body weight (may even be increased). The characteristic feature is a preoccupation with eating and an irresistible craving for food that results in binge eating, which is associated with a sense of lack of control and is invariably followed by feelings of shame and disgust. To counteract this caloric load, patients engage in purging (self-induced vomiting, laxative and diuretic use), fasting or excessive exercise, but can employ any number of ingenious, even dangerous, strategies (e.g. diabetic patients refusing to administer insulin).

## The body mass index (BMI)

The *body mass index* (*BMI*) relates weight to height and is used as a crude test to assess nutritional status in patients aged 16 and over.

$$BMI = \frac{weight \ (kilograms)}{height \ (metres)^2}$$

Normal: 20–25 kg/m²
Anorexia nervosa: less than or equal to 17.5 kg/m²
Medical danger: less than 13.5 kg/m²
Obesity: greater than 30 kg/m²
Gross obesity: greater than 40 kg/m²

**Fig. 12.1** The body mass index (BMI).

Figure 12.2 summarizes the ICD-10 criteria for anorexia and bulimia nervosa.

Some patients with anorexia may also engage in binge eating and purging behaviour, which is characteristic of bulimia. This does not preclude the diagnosis of anorexia; the DSM-IV terms this 'anorexia nervosa, binge eating/purging type'. The key diagnostic difference between anorexia and bulimia is that patients with anorexia are significantly underweight and have generalized endocrine abnormalities.

Women who use oral contraception may still experience menstrual bleeding, despite having a low body weight with widespread endocrine abnormalities.

## Assessment

### Clinical

It is important to define the extent of the eating disorder, yet at the same time not alienate a patient who might be ambivalent about treatment. The following are some questions that might be useful on mental state examination:

## ICD-10 criteria for anorexia and bulimia nervosa

Anorexia nervosa, *all* of the following:
1. Low body weight (BMI ≤ 17.5 kg/m²)
2. Self-induced weight loss (poor caloric intake, vomiting, exercise, etc.)
3. Overvalued idea: dread of fatness; low target weight
4. Endocrine disturbance (amenorrhoea, raised cortisol, growth hormone etc)
*Prepubertal*: failure to make expected weight gains; delayed pubertal events

Bulimia nervosa, *all* of the following:
1. Binge eating
2. Methods to counteract weight gain (vomiting, laxatives, fasting, exercise, etc.)
3. Overvalued idea: dread of fatness; low target weight

**Fig. 12.2** ICD-10 criteria for anorexia and bulimia nervosa.

### Anorexic symptoms

- Body weight and shape can be very important to some people. Do you find that you are quite concerned about your weight?
- A common way of losing weight is to eat less or to exercise a lot. Are these things that you do?
- Sometimes when women lose weight, their periods can become irregular or stop. Has this happened to you?

### Bulimic symptoms

- Are there times when you feel that your eating seems excessive or out of control?
- During these times, do you ever try to make yourself sick so that you feel better?
- Sometimes people might use pharmaceutical or street drugs to help control their weight. Have you ever had to do this?

Hypokalaemia is a potentially life-threatening complication of vomiting, as well as laxative and diuretic abuse, that usually develops insidiously. Gradual correction is safer than rapid correction so advise patients to eat high potassium foods (e.g. bananas) or to use potassium supplements. Severe hypokalaemia is an indication for hospitalization

| Medical complications of eating disorders | |
| --- | --- |
| **Related to starvation** | **Related to vomiting** |
| Emaciation | Permanent erosion of dental enamel; |
| Amenorrhoea; infertility; | dental cavities |
| reproductive system atrophy | Enlargement of salivary glands (especially |
| Constipation; abdominal pain | parotid) |
| Cold intolerance; lethargy | Calluses on the back of hands from |
| Bradycardia; hypotension; | repeated teeth trauma (Russell's sign) |
| cardiac arrythmias; heart failure | Oesophageal tears; gastric rupture |
| Lanugo: fine, downy hair on trunk; | Serious cardiac and skeletal |
| loss of head hair | cardiomyopathies from regular use of |
| Peripheral oedema | ipecacuanha syrup |
| Proximal myopathy; muscle wasting | |
| Osteoporosis; fractures | *Laboratory tests:* |
| Seizures; mild cognitive impairment; | Hypokalaemic, hypochloraemic alkalosis |
| depression | Hyponatraemia |
| | Hypomagnesaemia |
| *Laboratory tests:* | Raised serum amylase |
| Abnormal liver functions | |
| Raised urea (dehydration) | |
| Raised cortisol | |
| Raised growth hormone | |
| Reduced $T_3$ | |
| Reduced FSH and LH | |
| Hypercholesterolaemia | |
| Hypoglycaemia | |
| Hypercarotenaemia (yellowing of skin) | |
| Normocytic anaemia | |
| Leucopenia | |

**Fig. 12.3** Medical complications of eating disorders.

## Physical and special investigations

There is no diagnostic special investigation for anorexia or bulimia. However, numerous physical and metabolic changes are associated with being underweight and engaging in excessive purging as summarized in Figure 12.3. It is important to know and search for these complications because they may be associated with long-term complications or result in sudden death. Special investigations should therefore include: urea and electrolytes, full blood count, liver function tests, thyroid function tests, glucose, amylase, cholesterol and carotene level, dexamethasone-suppression test and electrocardiogram (ECG). Due to the risk of osteoporosis, a DEXA bone density scan is indicated for those patients with a 2-year history of anorexia.

## Differential diagnosis of patients with low weight

Patients with *anorexia nervosa* or *bulimia nervosa* may deny or be secretive about their symptoms, as they are often reluctant to seek treatment. Therefore, it is often difficult establishing: (1) the body image distortion associated with the overvalued idea of dread of fatness; (2) the various methods of weight loss; and (3) the presence of binge eating with associated feelings of shame and disgust. Figure 12.4 lists the other causes of significant weight loss that should be considered, especially when the onset of illness is later than adolescence or early adulthood.

*Medical causes of low weight* include malignancies, gastrointestinal disease, endocrine diseases (e.g. diabetes mellitus, hyperthyroidism), chronic infections, chronic inflammatory conditions and the acquired immunodeficiency syndrome (AIDS). Note that rare neurological syndromes associated with gross overeating include the Kleine–Levin, Klüver–Bucy and Prader–Willi syndromes.

Severe weight loss may occur in *depression*, but this is usually associated with a marked loss of appetite and interest in food. Patients with anorexia maintain their appetite until late in the disease and remain interested in food-related subjects (e.g. low calorie recipes). Note that patients with anorexia and

**Differential diagnosis for patient presenting with weight loss**

Anorexia nervosa
Bulimia nervosa
Medical causes of low weight
Depression
Obsessive-compulsive disorder
Psychotic disorders
Alcohol or substance abuse
Dementia

**Fig. 12.4** Differential diagnosis for patient presenting with weight loss.

bulimia often have co-morbid depression and that depressive symptoms may be secondary to the biological consequences of starvation and thus resolve with subsequent weight gain.

Patients with *obsessive-compulsive disorder* may lose weight when time-consuming compulsions prevent an adequate diet. Also, obsessions of contamination of food might curtail their caloric intake. As with depression, the issue is clouded by the observation that patients with anorexia also have an increased incidence of obsessive-compulsive disorder (which should only be diagnosed when they exhibit obsessions or compulsions unrelated to food or body shape). Note that obsessive-compulsive behaviour may be caused or exacerbated by significant malnutrition.

*Psychotic patients* may not eat due to delusions about food or hallucinations commanding them not to. The negative symptoms of schizophrenia (see p. 26) with self-neglect can also result in substantial weight loss.

Poor nutrition often occurs in patients with *alcohol or substance abuse* and *dementia*.

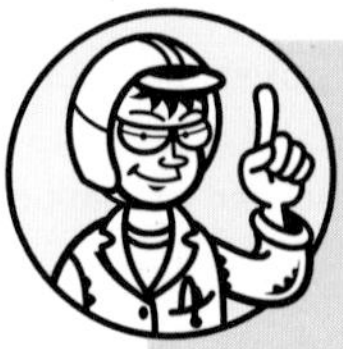

 In the differential diagnosis of weight loss, only anorexia and bulimia nervosa are associated with the overvalued idea of dread of fatness.

## Discussion of case study

Miss ED's body mass index is 15 kg/m$^2$, which is less than 17.5 kg/m$^2$ – the threshold for diagnosing anorexia nervosa. She admits to a dread of fatness and consequently pursues a target weight significantly below that which is normal or healthy. Thus, her body image distortion is an overvalued idea. Her weight loss methods include poor caloric intake, excessive exercise and laxative abuse. Dread of fatness and low body weight coupled with an endocrine disturbance (amenorrhoea) are characteristic of anorexia nervosa. The absence of binge eating precludes a diagnosis of bulimia nervosa, but Miss ED does engage in purging (use of laxatives). Medical complications include amenorrhoea, lethargy, hypothermia, mild cognitive impairment (difficulty concentrating), bradycardia and lanugo (fine downy hair on torso). The depressive symptoms may signify a co-morbid disorder or be secondary to the biological effects of malnutrition.

**Now go on to Chapter 19 to read about the eating disorders and their management.**

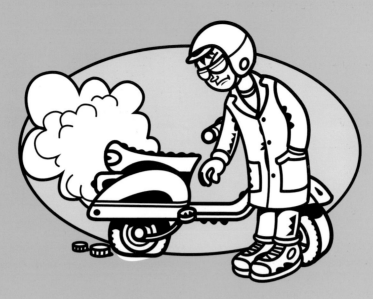

# DISEASES AND DISORDERS

# 13. The Mood (Affective) Disorders

This chapter discusses the disorders associated with the presenting complaints in Chapters 1, 2 and 3, which you might find helpful to read first:

- Depressive disorders (Ch. 1).
- Bipolar affective disorder (Ch. 2).
- Cyclothymia and dysthymia (Chs 1 and 2).
- Suicide and deliberate self-harm (Ch. 3).

## Depressive disorders

### Epidemiology
Figure 13.1 summarizes the epidemiology of the mood disorders.

### Aetiology
#### Biological and genetic factors
The monoamine theory suggests that depression is due to a shortage of noradrenaline (norepinephrine), serotonin, and possibly dopamine, and, thus, offers an explanation why antidepressants are effective in treating depression. Tricyclic antidepressants primarily prevent the reuptake of noradrenaline (norepinephrine) and serotonin, which increases their concentration in the synaptic cleft. Selective serotonin reuptake inhibitors (SSRIs) have a similar action, selectively on serotonin. Monoamine oxidase inhibitors (MAOIs) prevent noradrenaline (norepinephrine), serotonin and dopamine breakdown presynaptically, so that more is available for release. Each class of drug makes more monoamine molecules available in the synaptic cleft; these then act postsynaptically, stimulating second messenger systems. Over time this may correct intracellular abnormalities leading to a remission of symptoms.

It is likely that the monoamine theory is an oversimplification and that other neurotransmitters such as gamma aminobutyric acid (GABA) and various peptides (e.g. vasopressin) are also involved. It has been suggested that depression may be linked to abnormalities of corticosteroid regulation by the hypothalamic–pituitary–adrenal axis, or to disturbances in the lipid constituents of neuronal membranes.

Twin and family studies have shown that there is a genetic component to depression; thus, a history of depression in first-degree relatives is a significant risk factor.

#### Psychological and social factors
There is strong evidence that psychological factors may predispose to the development of depression. Families that show high expressed emotion (EE), especially in the form of critical remarks, have been shown to increase the risk of relapse in depressed patients. The risk of developing depression is increased in patients with certain personality disorders (e.g. borderline personality disorder, obsessive-compulsive personality disorder). The risk is also increased after significant adverse life events such as marital separation and job loss. Other vulnerability factors in women include:

- Having three or more children at home under the age of 14.
- Not working outside the home.
- Lacking a confiding relationship.
- Loss of a mother before the age of 11.

*?consitant w/ HPA axis theories of mice/rats.*

### Assessment, clinical features, investigations and differential diagnosis
Discussed in Chapters 1, 2 and 3.

### Management
A *biopsychosocial* approach is taken to the management of depression, which means that consideration should be given to treating biological, psychological and social aspects of the depression.

#### Treatment setting
Most patients with depression can be treated successfully in primary care, or in a psychiatric out-patient clinic. Day-hospital attendance may be helpful in patients with chronic or recurrent illness, especially if poor motivation or low self-esteem has led to a reluctance to go outside the home and make contact with others. In-patient admission may be advisable for assessment of patients with:

- Distressing hallucinations or delusions or other psychotic phenomena.
- Active suicidal ideation or planning, especially if suicide has previously been attempted or many risk factors for suicide are present (see Ch. 3).

**Epidemiology of the mood disorders**

| | Lifetime risk | Average age of onset | Sex ratio (female: male) |
|---|---|---|---|
| Recurrent depressive disorder | 10–25% (women) 5–12% (men) | late 20s | 2:1 |
| Bipolar affective disorder | 1% | 20 | Equal incidence |
| Cyclothymia | 0.5–1% | Adolescence, early adulthood | Equal incidence |
| Dysthymia | 3–6% | Childhood, adolescence, early adulthood | 2–3:1 |

**Fig. 13.1** Epidemiology of the mood disorders.

- Lack of motivation leading to self-neglect (e.g. dehydration or starvation).

Detention under mental health legislation may be necessary for patients who need admission but are unwilling to accept in-patient treatment due to reduced insight (see Ch. 29).

## Pharmacological treatment

The antidepressants are equally effective if prescribed at the correct dose and taken for an adequate length of time (with the possible exception of venlafaxine – some studies have shown greater efficacy at dose of 150 mg or greater). Clinicians therefore tend to choose an antidepressant based upon its side-effect profile after discussion with the patient. The SSRIs (sertraline, paroxetine, citalopram, fluoxetine) are usually used as first line treatments for depression, although the newer antidepressants like venlafaxine and mirtazapine can also be used. Some psychiatrists still use the older tricyclic antidepressants (amitriptyline, imipramine, lofepramine) despite their adverse side-effect profile and cardiotoxicity in overdose. Figure 13.2 summarizes some of the factors guiding the choice of an antidepressant.

Prescribed at an adequate dose for a sufficiently long period (usually 4–6 weeks), with appropriate patient education and encouragement, an antidepressant will produce a remission in 60–70% of cases (compared with 30% on placebo). When an antidepressant has brought remission of symptoms, it should be continued at full dose (i.e. at the dose that induced the remission) for at least 6 months to reduce the relapse rate. Patients with a history of recurrent depressive disorder may need to take antidepressants for a longer period, perhaps even

**Choosing an antidepressant**

The antidepressants all have a similar efficacy for the treatment of depression. Therefore, the choice of which drug to prescribe depends on:

- Their side-effects: SSRIs have a more favourable side-effect profile over TCAs. Also, side-effects should be matched to a patient's lifestyle, e.g. the weight gain caused by mirtazapine may be preferable to the sexual dysfunction caused by the SSRIs; some patients benefit from the sedation caused by some antidepressants, e.g. amitriptyline, trazodone, mirtazapine (see Ch. 27).
- Previous good response to a specific drug: this is usually re-prescribed.
- Safety in overdose: SSRIs are safer in overdose than TCAs.
- For severe depression requiring hospitalization, antidepressants that affect both noradrenaline (norepinephrine) and serotonin may be preferable, i.e. TCAs and high-dose venlafaxine (SSRIs may be slightly less effective in hospitalized patients).
- Atypical depression (i.e. hypersomnia, overeating, and anxiety) may respond preferably to MAOIs.
- Associated psychiatric symptoms, e.g. patients with obsessions or compulsions may respond preferably to the SSRIs or clomipramine.
- Concomitant physical illnesses, e.g. TCAs are contraindicated in patients with a recent myocardial infarction, or arrhythmias.

SSRI, selective serotonin reuptake inhibitor; TCA, tricyclic antidepressant; MAOI, monoamine oxidase inhibitor

**Fig. 13.2** Choosing an antidepressant.

lifelong in severe cases. The prophylactic effect of antidepressants of reducing relapse has been demonstrated for up to 5 years (with imipramine).

Treatment often fails due to inadequate dose of drug, duration of treatment or poor compliance; therefore, these factors should always be ruled out. However, when a patient has not responded to an antidepressant at the correct dose for the length of treatment the following strategies may be employed (often in this order):

- Increasing the dose of the current antidepressant (e.g. increasing fluoxetine from 20 mg to 40 mg).
- Change to another antidepressant within the same class (e.g. from fluoxetine to sertraline).
- Change to another antidepressant from a different class (e.g. from sertraline (SSRI) to venlafaxine (SSNRI)).
- Consider augmenting the current antidepressant with lithium or another antidepressant (usually done by a psychiatrist). Pindolol (a beta-blocker), tri-iodothyronine ($T_3$) and L-tryptophan have also been used as augmenting agents in treatment-resistant depression.
- Consider other treatment modalities such as psychotherapy and ECT.

A depressive episode with psychotic features usually requires the adjunctive use of antipsychotic medication.

- Patients may respond idiosyncratically to different antidepressants of the same class (e.g. SSRIs), so it is worthwhile trying a different antidepressant from within the same class.
- Depressed patients who are treated with tricyclic antidepressants are often prescribed inadequate doses. A dose of greater than 125 mg per day is required to treat depression.

## Psychological treatment

Both drug treatments and psychotherapy are effective in the treatment of an acute depressive episode and in the prevention of relapse. Psychotherapeutic approaches (see Ch. 28) may be used as an alternative to medications or in combination with them. Options include:

- Cognitive-behavioural therapy (CBT): cognitive therapy identifies distorted or illogical thoughts (cognitions) and assumptions and then attempts to replace them with more 'reality-based' thinking and behaviours. Behaviour therapy involves behavioural experiments (testing irrational thoughts against reality), target setting and activity scheduling. Requires between six and 20 sessions. See p. 195.
- Interpersonal therapy (IPT): identifies interpersonal problems resulting from grief, role disputes, role transitions or interpersonal deficits and attempts to modify these. See p. 196.
- Psychodynamic therapy: see p. 194.
- Family and marital interventions may be useful for family or marital discord.
- Mindfulness-based cognitive therapy: helps patients to disengage or become mindful of their depressive ruminations instead of trying to 'solve' them – decreases the risk of recurrence if used in recovered patients.

Studies have shown that cognitive-behavioural therapy (CBT) can be as effective as antidepressants in treating moderate depressive episodes. Also, patients who receive CBT following standard antidepressant treatment have significantly lower rates of relapse 4 years later than patients receiving standard clinical treatment alone (35% versus 70%).

## Electroconvulsive therapy (ECT)

Indications for ECT in depression include:

- Poor response to adequate trials of antidepressants.
- Intolerance of antidepressants due to side-effects.
- Depression with severe suicidal ideation.
- Depression with psychotic features, severe psychomotor retardation or stupor.
- Depression with severe self-neglect (poor fluid and food intake).
- Previous good response to ECT.

## Course and prognosis

Depression is self-limiting, and without treatment a first depressive episode will generally remit within 6 months to 1 year. However, the course of depression is often chronic and relapsing and at least 60% of patients may have a further depressive episode, with the risk of future episodes increasing with each relapse.

Depression is one of the most important risk factors for suicide; rates of suicide are over 20 times greater in patients with depression compared with those in the general population.

## Bipolar affective disorder

### Epidemiology
Figure 13.1 summarizes the epidemiology of the mood disorders.

### Aetiology
#### Biological and genetic factors
The monoamine hypothesis is as applicable to elevated mood as it is to low mood, with manic episodes thought to be associated with increased central noradrenaline (norepinephrine) or serotonin.

Evidence from twin studies has shown a strong genetic component to the aetiology of bipolar affective disorder (more pronounced than in depression) and many patients have a positive family history. Concordance rates in monozygotic twins range from 65 to 75%; whereas, rates for dizygotic twins are 14%.

Significant life events and severe stresses may provoke the onset of a first manic or hypomanic episode (e.g. there is an increased risk of manic episodes in the early postpartum period). However, there are no personality traits strongly associated with the development of bipolar affective disorder.

### Assessment, clinical features, investigations and differential diagnosis
Discussed in Chapters 1, 2 and 3.

### Management
Management considerations include:
- Treatment of an acute manic or hypomanic episode.
- Treatment of an acute depressive episode.
- Maintenance treatment (prevention of relapse).

### Treatment setting
The initial treatment setting depends on the presentation and severity of illness. A manic episode may necessitate a period of hospitalization in cases of:
- Reckless behaviour endangering the patient or others around them.
- Significant psychotic symptoms.
- Impaired judgement, e.g. sexual indiscretions, overspending.

- Excessive psychomotor agitation with risk of self-injury, dehydration and exhaustion.
- Thoughts of harming self or others.

Detention under mental health legislation is often necessary in patients with reduced insight. Bipolar patients may also require hospital admission for depressive episodes for reasons outlined on p. 85.

### Pharmacological treatment
The mainstay of acute and maintenance treatment of bipolar illness are the **mood stabilizers**, which include lithium and the anticonvulsants (sodium valproate/valproic acid and carbamazepine). Although lithium and semisodium valproate (Depakote®) are licensed in the UK for acute mania, they may not provide the immediate behavioural control needed in acutely manic patients. So the initial treatment of acute mania usually requires antipsychotic medication in the form of an atypical antipsychotic such as olanzapine, or a typical antipsychotic such as haloperidol. Benzodiazepines, e.g. lorazepam or diazepam, are often given concurrently as they work synergistically to control agitation. These drugs are then tapered off as the initial phase of mania has subsided and the mood stabilizers begin to take effect.

**Lithium** and **carbamazepine** are licensed in the UK for the prophylaxis of bipolar affective disorder, although **sodium valproate** is often used off-licence by psychiatrists for the same purpose. In general, maintenance treatment for the prophylaxis of bipolar affective disorder is indicated in patients who have had more than one episode.

Before commencing lithium, patients should be provided with information on its potential side-effects and toxicity and the need for periodic blood tests (usually 3-monthly) to assess the plasma level (see Ch. 27).

Liver and haematological functioning should be assessed before and soon after starting patients on valproate or carbamazepine. Research is emerging that atypical antipsychotics such as olanzapine and clozapine may also be effective in preventing relapse.

Carbamazepine is particularly effective in patients with rapid cycling bipolar affective disorder, i.e. four or more mood episodes (depressive, manic or mixed) per year.

In depressive episodes associated with bipolar affective disorder, antidepressants should be used with the utmost caution owing to their tendency to push mood beyond normal and provoke hypomanic or manic episodes. In cases where their use is necessary it is prudent to make concurrent use of a mood stabilizer. Lithium, olanzapine and the newer anticonvulsant lamotrigine also appear to have antidepressant properties in bipolar illness.

Approximately half of all bipolar patients who discontinue lithium will have a recurrence of mania within 5 months. In addition, in some patients, discontinuation of lithium leads to recurrent mood swings that cannot be controlled by the reintroduction of lithium. This emphasizes the need for patient education about rigid compliance as well as the correct selection of patients for lithium treatment.

## Psychological treatment
Psychotherapy is performed much less commonly in bipolar affective disorder than in unipolar depression; however, it may play a supportive role and help to improve compliance.

## Electroconvulsive therapy (ECT)
Although ECT may precipitate a manic episode in bipolar patients, it can be an effective antimanic agent, superior even to lithium, especially in severe mania and mixed states – 80% of patients can be expected to show a marked improvement.

## Course and prognosis
The prognosis is generally poor as more than 90% of patients who have a single manic episode go on to have future episodes. The frequency of episodes varies considerably, but averages out to four mood episodes in 10 years. Between 5% and 15% of patients have four or more mood episodes (depressive, manic or mixed) within a year, which is termed *rapid cycling* and is associated with a poor prognosis. Completed suicide occurs in 10–15% of patients.

## Dysthymia and cyclothymia

### Aetiology
The extent to which the aetiologies of dysthymia and cyclothymia resemble those of depression and bipolar affective disorder is unclear. There are biological similarities between dysthymia and depression; for example, REM latency is decreased in both conditions. Genetic studies link cyclothymia and bipolar affective disorder, as up to a third of patients with the former have a positive family history of the latter.

### Epidemiology and course
Figure 13.1 summarizes the epidemiology of the mood disorders. Both dysthymia and cyclothymia have an insidious onset and a chronic course, often beginning in childhood or adolescence. A significant number of patients with cyclothymia will go on to suffer more severe affective disorders, most notably bipolar affective disorder. Dysthymia may coexist with depressive episodes ('double depression'), anxiety disorders and borderline personality disorder.

### Assessment, clinical features, investigations and differential diagnosis
Discussed in Chapters 1, 2 and 3.

### Treatment
The two conditions may be treated pharmacologically with the same drugs used in depressive and bipolar affective disorder, but antidepressants should be used with caution in cyclothymia owing to their occasional tendency to turn mild depressive symptoms into hypomania. Psychological therapy may be useful for both conditions.

- What are the epidemiological differences between recurrent depressive disorder and bipolar affective disorder?
- How does the monoamine theory of depression relate to antidepressants?
- Name four vulnerability factors for depression.
- When would you consider hospitalization for a depressive or manic episode respectively?
- What is the role of psychological therapies in the treatment of depression?
- What strategies would you employ when a patient does not respond to 4 weeks of treatment with an SSRI?
- What medications may be used to augment antidepressants in treatment-resistant cases?
- What is the initial treatment of the acutely manic patient?
- What are the advantages and disadvantages of the use of ECT in bipolar affective disorder?
- How would you counsel patients regarding their prognosis after one manic episode?
- What is the relationship between cyclothymia and bipolar affective disorder?

## Suggested further reading

Anderson I M, Edwards J G 2001 Guidelines for choice of selective serotonin reuptake inhibitor in depressive illness. Advances in Psychiatric Treatment 7: 170–180

Clark A 2001 Proposed treatment for adolescent psychosis. 2: Bipolar illness. Advances in Psychiatric Treatment 7: 143–149

Keck P 2002 Clinical management of bipolar disorder. URL: http://www.medscape.com/ viewprogram/135

MacHale S 2002 Managing depression in physical illness. Advances in Psychiatric Treatment 8: 297–306

Porter R, Linsley K, Ferrier N 2001 Treatment of severe depression – non-pharmacological aspects. Advances in Psychiatric Treatment 7: 117–124

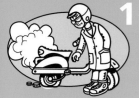

# 14. The Psychotic Disorders: Schizophrenia

Among the psychotic disorders, the main ones that should be distinguished are schizophrenia, delusional disorder, schizoaffective disorder, and acute and transient psychoses. This chapter will concentrate on schizophrenia, the most prevalent and widely researched disorder in this group.

## Schizophrenia

### History
Ideas about the disorder we now term schizophrenia crystallized towards the end of the last century. The concept of this disorder has evolved during this century. Important landmarks in the definition of this disorder are:

- 1893: Emil Kraepelin separated affective psychoses (e.g. mania) from non-affective psychoses; he gave the term 'dementia praecox' to clinical conditions resembling the main forms of schizophrenia.
- 1911: Eugen Bleuler coined the term 'schizophrenia' ('splitting of the mind'); his description placed more emphasis on thought disorder and negative symptoms than on positive symptoms.
- 1959: Kurt Schneider defined first-rank symptoms, which now comprise criteria (a)–(d) of the ICD-10 classification (Figs 4.5 and 4.6).
- 1970 to the present: the main international classification systems, ICD-10 and DSM-IV, have further clarified the diagnostic criteria. The main distinction between ICD-10 and DSM-IV is that the latter specifies a 6-month duration of symptoms and places a large emphasis on social or occupational dysfunction.

### Epidemiology
- The *incidence* ranges from 5 to 50/100 000 individuals per year.
- The *prevalence* varies geographically but is approximately 1%.
- The *lifetime risk* is approximately 1% (see also Fig. 14.1).

- The *age of onset* is between late teens and mid 30s. Women have a later age of onset. Men: 18–25 years; women: 25–35 years.
- Men have a slightly higher incidence than women, although comparisons are difficult due to the differing ages of onset between genders.
- There is an increased prevalence in lower socioeconomic classes (classes IV and V). The *social drift* (impairment of functioning caused by schizophrenia results in a 'drift' down the social scale) and *social causation* (poor socioeconomic conditions contribute to the development of schizophrenia) theories attempt to explain this.
- Similarly, there is an increased prevalence in urban (inner city) compared to rural areas. Social drift and social causation theories apply here too.
- The incidence rate is higher for immigrants, especially African-Caribbeans in the UK.

### Aetiology
The aetiology of schizophrenia involves a complex interaction of biological and environmental factors.

dysbindin
COMT

### Genetic
There is a strong tendency for schizophrenia to run in families. Figure 14.1 shows the lifetime risk of developing schizophrenia, if relatives have schizophrenia. Twin studies show a higher concordance rate for monozygotic twins (50%) than for dizygotic twins (10%). Evaluation of adoption studies provides further supporting evidence for a genetic factor: babies adopted away from schizophrenic parents to non-schizophrenic parents retain their increased risk, whereas the risk is not increased when babies are adopted to schizophrenic parents from non-schizophrenic biological parents. The mechanism for this inheritance is unknown although several candidate genes are emerging.

### Developmental factors
Strong evidence is now emerging that schizophrenia is associated with complications during pregnancy

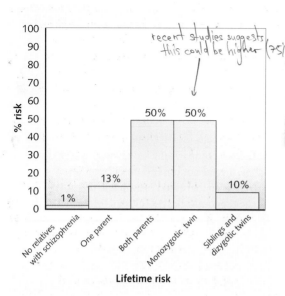

*recent studies suggests this could be higher (75%)*

**Lifetime risk**

**Fig. 14.1** Lifetime risk of developing schizophrenia if relatives have schizophrenia.

If schizophrenia was entirely a genetic disease, the concordance rate for monozygotic twins would be 100%. A concordance rate of 50% suggests that although there is a significant genetic factor involved, there must be an environmental factor contributing to its development as well.

and birth. In addition, the observation that more schizophrenics are born in late winter or spring has led to the theory that schizophrenia is linked to second-trimester influenza infection.

### Brain abnormalities

Increasingly sophisticated neuroimaging techniques are starting to consistently identify structural and functional abnormalities associated with schizophrenia; the findings may be secondary to the disorder itself or its treatment. They include:

- Ventricular enlargement (appears to be associated with negative symptoms).
- Reduced brain size (frontal and temporal lobes, hippocampus, amygdala, parahippocampal gyrus).

Furthermore, schizophrenics have been found to perform worse at specific tests of frontal lobe function and demonstrate 'soft' neurological signs, e.g. abnormalities of stereognosis or proprioception.

### Neurotransmitter abnormalities

Based largely on the effects of the conventional antipsychotics, which block dopamine $D_2$ receptors, the dopamine hypothesis suggests that schizophrenia is secondary to overactivity of the mesolimbic dopamine pathway in the brain. Furthermore, drugs that potentiate this pathway (e.g. amfetamines, antiparkinsonian drugs) are known to cause psychotic symptoms. The recent identification of several dopamine receptor subtypes and successful use of clozapine, which has little affinity for the $D_2$ receptor, but is a strong antagonist of $D_1$, $D_4$ and $5\text{-}HT_2$ receptors, suggests a more complex mechanism than previously thought.

### Life events

Stressful life events occur more frequently in the month before a first psychotic episode or relapse, and may, therefore, precipitate the illness. However, it may be that the early stages of the illness itself cause the stressful events.

### Expressed emotion

When family or carers become *over-involved*, *over-critical*, or *hostile* towards a schizophrenic patient, he or she is more likely to relapse. This interaction has been termed 'high expressed emotion' and exerts an influence if contact is greater than 35 hours a week.

## Assessment, clinical features, investigations and differential diagnosis

Discussed in Chapter 4.

## Management

There is no known cure for schizophrenia. Management is aimed at improving symptoms and preventing relapse. Long-term medication is the mainstay of treatment, although psychosocial treatment is also very important.

### Treatment setting

The initial treatment setting depends on the presentation and severity of illness. Hospitalization is often necessary in cases of first episode psychosis and when there is a significant risk that psychotic symptoms may lead to harm to self or others or self-neglect. Detention under mental health legislation is often necessary in patients with reduced insight.

*(handwritten top notes)*

2 receptors typicals → 95% have extrapyramidal side-effects (tardive diskinesia, Parkinsonism, dystonia, akathesia)
+ weight gain (less w/quitiapine).
HT2+ ← atypicals → 90% no extrapyramidal but metabolic syndrome
D2

*(handwritten)* → also because it requires gradual start over many months, and when pt stops for 48hrs; need to begin at baseline once more.

When patients are stable, they are managed in the community with the help of a care coordinator and regular follow-up in a psychiatric out-patient clinic.

## Pharmacological treatment

Typical antipsychotics (e.g. haloperidol) have traditionally been the first-line treatment for schizophrenia. However, in June 2002, the National Institute for Clinical Excellence (NICE) recommended the use of atypical antipsychotics (e.g. olanzapine, risperidone) as first-line treatments for newly diagnosed patients and for patients on typical antipsychotics who experience either inadequate symptom control or unsatisfactory side-effects.

Typical antipsychotics (first-generation or conventional) have been used since the 1950s. They are effective at treating positive symptoms (delusions, hallucinations, disorganized thinking) but may fail to treat, or even worsen, negative symptoms (apathy, poverty of thought and speech). They are also associated with extra-pyramidal side-effects (EPSE – parkinson-like symptoms, acute dystonia, akathisia), tardive dyskinesia (24% of patients), neuroleptic malignant syndrome and hyperprolactinaemia. Parkinsonism and acute dystonias (e.g. oculogyric crisis) should be promptly treated with anti-cholinergics, e.g. procyclidine.

Atypical antipsychotics (second-generation or novel) have been used in the UK since 1990. They are at least as effective as the typical antipsychotics in treating positive symptoms and may improve negative symptoms, mood symptoms, and perhaps cognition as well. They are less likely to cause EPSE and tardive dyskinesia and thus lead to improved compliance. Clozapine, quetiapine and, to a lesser extent, olanzapine are prolactin sparing. Despite these major benefits, several side-effects have emerged that may limit the utility of some of these medications, e.g.:

*(handwritten) ↑ weight*

- Agranulocytosis: clozapine
- Diabetes, weight gain, lipid abnormalities: clozapine, olanzapine and quetiapine
- Increased prolactin levels (galactorrhoea, sexual dysfunction, osteoporosis): risperidone and amisulpride

*(handwritten) quetiapine = prolongs QT*

With the exception of clozapine, which is indicated for treatment-resistant schizophrenia, no atypical has been consistently shown to be more effective than any other.

*Treatment resistant schizophrenia (TRS)* is defined as a lack of satisfactory clinical improvement despite the sequential use of at least two antipsychotics for 6–8 weeks, one of which should be an atypical. In these instances, patients should be started on clozapine at the earliest opportunity. Clozapine is not used as a first-line medication due its potential to cause life-threatening agranulocytosis in just less than 1% of patients. Thus, regular haematological monitoring is obligatory and patients are required to be registered with a monitoring service. Clozapine will benefit over 60% of treatment-resistant patients.

Compliance with medication is poor in schizophrenia, with up to 80% of patients failing to comply. This frequently leads to relapse. Compliance can be increased by the use of depot intra-muscular medication (atypical preparations now available, e.g. risperidone), which is administered 2–4 weekly; increased social support and patient education.

The length of treatment requires careful consideration as single episodes cannot be predicted and most patients with schizophrenia relapse. After a first episode, treatment may be gradually stopped after 6–8 months; for most patients, antipsychotics are a long-term, perhaps lifelong, treatment.

*(handwritten) pretty good for -ve symptoms !! but v.strict dosing + agranulocyt*

## Other medical treatments

Benzodiazepines can be of enormous benefit in short-term relief of behaviour disturbance, insomnia, aggression and agitation, but they do not have any specific antipsychotic effect.

Antidepressants and lithium are sometimes used to augment antipsychotics in treatment-resistant cases, especially when there are significant affective symptoms, as is the case in schizoaffective disorders, or post schizophrenia depression.

ECT is now rarely used in schizophrenia. The usual indication is the rare case with severe catatonic symptoms.

*(handwritten) Aside: carbamazapine (Hyperthyroidism) can also cause agranulocytosis*

The duration of untreated illness prior to starting effective antipsychotic medication has been shown to be the most important predictor of relapse. In addition, the prognosis improves when patients are treated early with appropriate medication. This underscores the importance of early detection and treatment of schizophrenia.

*(handwritten bottom)* RESPIRADONE = good atypical 1st line.

## Psychological treatments

Until recently, psychotic disorders were thought to be unresponsive to psychological interventions, but increasing evidence points towards their value in augmenting drug treatments:

- Cognitive-behavioural therapy has been shown to be effective in reducing symptoms in schizophrenia. It is also useful for helping patients with poor insight come to terms with their illness, thereby increasing compliance with medication.
- Family psychological interventions focus on alliance building, reduction of expressions of hostility and criticism (expressed emotion), setting of appropriate expectations and limits, and effecting change in relatives' behaviour and belief systems. Family intervention has been shown to reduce relapse and admission rates.
- Schizophrenia can be a devastating condition and is associated with significant social morbidity. Therefore, the importance of support, advice, reassurance, and education to both patients and carers cannot be overemphasized.
- Social-skills training can improve social competence and help with adaptive functioning in the community.
- Psychodynamic psychotherapy is generally not used in schizophrenia.

## Social treatments

Issues beyond drug and psychological treatment should be addressed to enable successful rehabilitation into the community; these include financial benefits, occupation, accommodation, daytime activities, social supports, and support for carers. A variety of agencies can provide these services, notably, health services, social services, local authorities, local support groups, and national support groups (SANE, MIND).

All patients with schizophrenia should be assessed for the care-programme approach (CPA) to achieve optimum coordination in the delivery of services. Community psychiatric nurses (CPNs), consultant psychiatrists, occupational therapists, psychologists or social workers are appointed as care coordinators. Their primary role is to coordinate the multifaceted aspects of patients' care and to monitor mental state and compliance with medication.

After discharge from hospital and during exacerbation of symptoms, some patients benefit from attending a day hospital, which provides structure and social support during the day.

Assertive community treatment has been shown to reduce hospital admissions and time spent in hospital.

## Acute behaviour disturbance

Severe psychomotor agitation or aggressive behaviour frequently occur in acutely ill psychotic patients. Note that in patients who are not well known, it is vital that the correct diagnosis is established. Many other conditions, for example mania, delirium, alcohol and substance withdrawal and dementia, can present with acute aggression and agitation, all of which require special consideration. The algorithm in Figure 14.2 describes the principles of acute management.

Lorazepam is the only benzodiazepine that has reliable rate of absorption from muscle tissue and therefore should always be used, if at all possible, when benzodiazepines are given intra-muscularly. Other advantages include its relatively short half-life (10–20 hours) and its lack of active metabolites during elimination (no accumulation).

## Course and prognosis

The course of schizophrenia is highly variable and difficult to predict for individual patients. In general, the disorder is chronic, showing a relapsing and remitting pattern. About **20%** have a **single lifetime episode** with no further relapses. However, more than **50%** of patients have a **poor outcome** characterized by **repeated psychotic episodes** with hospitalizations, depression and suicide attempts.

About **10%** of schizophrenic patients will **successfully complete suicide**. Those most at risk are young men who have attained a high level of education and who have some insight into their illness. The periods soon after the onset of illness and in the months following discharge from hospital are particularly vulnerable.

The lifespan for schizophrenic patients is on average 10 years shorter than for the general population. Causal factors include suicide, increased smoking, socioeconomic deprivation, neglect of diet, and accidents.

| All interventions should occur simultaneously and early |

**Environmental interventions**

- Create a calm environment
  -Turn off TV/radio
  -Remove other patients to another room
- Remove objects that can be used as weapons e.g. chairs, ashtrays etc.
- Get help from trained staff

**Behavioural interventions**

- Talk slowly and softly
- Never turn your back to the patient
- Place yourself between the exit and the patient
- Be aware – eye contact may help establish a rapport, or may seem threatening
- Innocuous questions about sleeping and eating may prove a useful distraction
- Convey a genuine sense of concern
- Allow patient to verbalize feelings but cut short if anger is escalating
- Restraint may be necessary with removal to a safer secluded area

**Medica interventions**
Consider another cause of the agitation, e.g. alcohol withdrawal

**Accepting oral medication**

Benzodiazepine e.g. lorazepam 0.5–2 mg, diazepam 10–30 mg

**+/−**

Atypical antipsychotic, especially dispersible preparations, e.g. olanzapine 10–20 mg, risperidone 4–8 mg

**OR** - Consider a typical antipsychotic, e.g. haloperidol 5–10 mg
**Caution**:
- Acute dystonia
- QT prolongation
- Akathisia – may increase agitation/ aggression
- Reduces seizure threshold

**Refusing oral medication**

Intramuscular lorazepam 0.5–2 mg

**+/−**

Intramuscular haloperidol 5–10 mg
**Caution**: side-effects

**Note**: Intramuscular fast-acting atypical antipsychotics are probably preferable – but not yet available in the UK

**Note**: Rapid tranquillization may in exceptional circumstances require intravenous benzodiazepines and antipsychotics

**Fig. 14.2** Acute management of the agitated or aggressive patient.

The overall prognosis for schizophrenia appears to be better in developing as opposed to developed countries; the reasons are unclear but may reflect better extended-family social support or greater social acceptance once recovered. The factors associated with a good prognosis are:

- Female sex.
- Married.
- Older age of onset.
- Abrupt onset of illness (as opposed to insidious onset).
- Onset precipitated by life stress.
- Short duration of illness prior to treatment.
- Good response to medication.
- Paranoid subtype, as opposed to hebephrenic subtype (see p. 28–29).

- Absence of negative symptoms.
- Illness characterized by prominent mood symptoms or family history of mood disorders.
- Good premorbid functioning.

 Patients with an early age of onset of schizophrenia tend to have a worse outcome. They are more often male, have more prominent negative symptoms, more evidence of cognitive impairment and more evidence of structural brain abnormalities.

- Why is there an increased prevalence of schizophrenia in lower socioeconomic classes?
- What are the epidemiological and prognostic differences between men and women with schizophrenia?
- What is your response to parents who ask you whether their other child will also develop schizophrenia?
- What is the relevance of expressed emotion in families with a member who has schizophrenia?
- Why are atypical antipsychotics the first-line treatment for schizophrenia?
- Define treatment-resistant schizophrenia and its management.
- What is the value of lorazepam in the treatment of schizophrenia?
- What types of symptoms in schizophrenia are associated with a good prognosis?

## Suggested further reading

Birchwood M, Spencer E, McGovern D 2000 Schizophrenia: early warning signs. Advances in Psychiatric Treatment 6: 93–101

Clark A F 2001 Proposed treatment for adolescent psychosis. 1: Schizophrenia and schizophrenia-like psychoses. Advances in Psychiatric Treatment 7: 16–23

Seeman M V, Seeman P S 2002 Choosing an antipsychotic and why. URL: http://www.medscape.com/viewprogram/2014

Spencer E, Birchwood M, McGovern D 2001 Management of first-episode psychosis. Advances in Psychiatric Treatment 7: 133–142

Zimbroff D L 2003 Clinical management of agitation. URL: http://www.medscape.com/viewprogram/2311

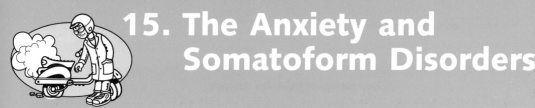

# 15. The Anxiety and Somatoform Disorders

This chapter discusses the most important disorders associated with the presenting complaints in Chapters 5, 6, 7 and 8, which you might find helpful to read first.

## Anxiety disorders

### Epidemiology

The anxiety disorders are the most prevalent of all the psychiatric disorders with a combined 1-year prevalence rate of 12–17%. Epidemiological data collected from different countries have shown varying prevalence rates for the individual anxiety disorders (see Fig. 15.1 for the epidemiology of the anxiety disorders). It is important to remember that anxiety disorders are usually underdiagnosed in primary care settings, or only recognized years after onset.

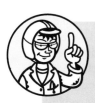

In clinical settings, over **95%** of patients who present with **agoraphobia** also have a current diagnosis or a past history of **panic disorder**.

Anxiety disorders tend to be more common in women than men apart from social phobia and obsessive-compulsive disorder where the prevalence is about equal.

### Aetiology
#### Genetic and biological factors

Genetic factors are thought to play some role in the development of most anxiety disorders.

Panic disorder and obsessive-compulsive disorder appear to be the most heritable anxiety disorders, with more than a third of those affected having a first-degree relative who has had the same diagnosis. The genetic contribution to generalized anxiety disorder is less clear-cut, but there is an association between this diagnosis and having relatives who abuse alcohol.

Biological factors have been the subject of considerable interest in anxiety disorders. Defects in neurotransmitter systems such as abnormal receptors may contribute to the development of specific disorders (e.g. generalized anxiety disorder: serotonin or GABA systems; panic disorder: serotonin, noradrenaline (norepinephrine), or GABA systems). Obsessive-compulsive disorder is associated with hypersensitivity of some serotonin receptors.

#### Social and psychological factors

Anxiety disorders have been linked to **stressful life events**. In post-traumatic stress disorder a significant traumatic event is essential to the diagnosis. Psychosocial stressors may also precede the onset of symptoms in other anxiety disorders.

Some psychiatrists take the view that anxiety disorders are predominantly psychological in origin. Cognitive-behavioural theories suggest that symptoms are a consequence of inappropriate thought-processes and overestimation of dangers, as in the case of panic attacks:

- A cognitive model of the panic attack suggests that an attack may be initiated when a **susceptible individual misinterprets** a **normal body stimulus**. For example, a patient may become aware of their heart beating. Instead of dismissing this as normal, they may assume that it is under excessive pressure and that something could be physically wrong. This fear activates the sympathetic nervous system, producing a real increase in the rate and strength of the heart beat. A vicious cycle ensues in which the perception of increasing cardiac effort convinces the sufferer that they are on the point of collapse or a myocardial infarction. The resulting **crescendo of symptoms may proceed to a full-blown panic attack** involving several of the panic symptoms listed in Figure 5.2 (p. 34).

A psychoanalytical perspective may view anxiety as arising from unresolved conflicts from childhood psychosexual development.

| Epidemiology of the anxiety disorders | | | |
|---|---|---|---|
| Anxiety disorder | One-year prevalence* | Usual age of onset | Sex ratio (female:male) |
| Generalized anxiety disorder | 2.8% | Variable: childhood to late adulthood | 2–3:1 |
| Panic disorder (with or without agoraphobia) | 3.9% | Late adolescence to mid-30s | 2–3:1 |
| Social phobia | 3.7% | Mid-teens | About equal |
| Specific phobia | 4.4% | Childhood to adolescence | 2:1 |
| Post-traumatic stress disorder | 3.6% | Any age – after trauma | 2:1 |
| Obsessive-compulsive disorder | 2.1% | Adolescence to early adulthood | Equal |

**Fig. 15.1** Epidemiology of the anxiety disorders. (One year prevalence rates from Narrow et al 2002. Revised pervalence estimates of mental disorders in the United States. Archives of General Psychiatry 59:115–123)

## Assessment, clinical features, investigations and differential diagnosis

Discussed in Chapters 5, 6 and 7.

## Management

Pharmacological and psychological treatments are both effective in the treatment of anxiety disorders and should therefore be used in partnership wherever possible. Figure 15.2 summarizes the most important concepts in treating anxiety disorders. It is important that you familiarize yourself with this table, as anxiety disorders are common in primary care settings and can often be managed there.

### Pharmacological treatment

- Selective serotonin reuptake inhibitors (**SSRIs**) are considered first-line treatments for most anxiety disorders due to their proven efficacy and tolerable side-effect profile. **Venlafaxine** (SSNRI) has a similar side-effect profile and also has proven efficacy in generalized anxiety disorder.
- Despite their proven efficacy in anxiety disorders, tricyclic antidepressants (TCAs) are generally considered second-line treatments to the SSRIs owing to their increased frequency of adverse effects, e.g. dry mouth, sedation, postural hypotension, tachycardia, etc. Clomipramine has proven efficacy in obsessive-compulsive disorder (OCD).
- Restlessness, jitteriness and an initial increase in anxiety symptoms may occur in the first few days of treatment with either the SSRIs or the TCAs, which may hamper compliance in already anxious patients. This can be managed by titrating the dose up slowly or by using benzodiazepines in combination with antidepressants during the first few weeks of treatment. Also note that the anxiolytic effect of the benzodiazepines is immediate in comparison to the latency period of 2–4 weeks (up to 6 weeks in OCD) with the antidepressants.
- Benzodiazepines are only used in acute anxiety (e.g. panic attacks) and in treatment-resistant cases owing to the risk of dependency and withdrawal reactions. They should not be used in patients with a history of benzodiazepine abuse.
- The monoamine oxidase inhibitors (MAOIs), despite being effective in some conditions, are not considered first-line owing to the possibility of severe side-effects and interactions with other drugs or food components (cheese reaction).

### Psychological treatment

- Cognitive-behavioural therapy (CBT) has proven efficacy in most anxiety disorders and often has a synergistic effect with medication.
- CBT is the first-line treatment for specific phobias, mainly in the form of behaviour therapy, which may involve systematic desensitization, flooding or modelling (see Ch. 28).
- In panic disorder, cognitive-behavioural therapy may involve helping the sufferer to understand that panic attacks may start from a misinterpretation of a normal stimulus, leading to a 'vicious cycle' of spiralling fear and sympathetic activation. When the patient understands this model, the therapist may encourage the patient to break the cycle by promoting rejection of the assumption that the original stimulus (e.g.

**Treatment of anxiety disorders**

| Anxiety disorder | Pharmacotherapy | Psychotherapy |
|---|---|---|
| Generalized anxiety disorder | First line:<br>  SSNRI (venlafaxine)<br>  SSRI (paroxetine)<br>Second line (as effective but less well tolerated):<br>  TCA (imipramine)<br>Treatment-resistant cases:<br>  Consider benzodiazepines (diazepam), hydroxyzine and buspirone | CBT<br>Psychodynamic therapy<br>Relaxation techniques |
| Panic disorder and agoraphobia | First line:<br>  SSRIs (citalopram, paroxetine, fluoxetine, sertraline, fluvoxamine)<br>Second line (as effective but less well tolerated):<br>  TCA (clomipramine, imipramine)<br>Treatment-resistant cases:<br>  Consider: benzodiazepines (diazepam, clonazepam, alprazolam), venlafaxine, reboxetine, mirtazapine and MAOIs (phenelzine)<br>Acute panic attacks:<br>  Benzodiazepines (alprazolam, lorazepam) | CBT (including exposure therapy for agoraphobia) |
| Social phobia | First line:<br>  SSRIs (paroxetine, sertraline, fluvoxamine)<br>Second line (as effective but less well tolerated):<br>  MAOI (phenelzine) – caution side-effects<br>Treatment-resistant cases:<br>  Consider benzodiazepines (clonazepam), venlafaxine, nefazodone, gabapentin | CBT (including exposure therapy) |
| Specific phobia | Pharmacotherapy is not standard treatment | CBT (desensitization, flooding or modelling) |
| Obsessive-compulsive disorder | First line:<br>  SSRIs (sertraline, fluoxetine, fluvoxamine, paroxetine, citalopram)<br>Second line (as effective but less well tolerated):<br>  Clomipramine<br>Treatment-resistant cases:<br>  Consider antipsychotics, pindolol, clonazepam | CBT (including exposure therapy, and response prevention)<br>Family therapy |
| Post-traumatic stress disorder | First line:<br>  SSRIs (sertraline, fluoxetine, paroxetine)<br>Second line (as effective but less well tolerated):<br>  TCA (amitriptyline, imipramine)<br>Treatment-resistant cases:<br>  Consider MAOI (phenelzine), lamotrigine | Systematic desensitization<br>CBT<br>Psychodynamic therapy<br>Eye movement desensitization and reprocessing therapy (EMDR) |

*Note: psychological debriefing after the trauma is not effective and may be harmful*
*Note: the first and second line drugs in parentheses are those that have proven efficacy from double-blind randomized control trials.*
*SSRI: selective serotonin reuptake inhibitor; TCA: tricyclic antidepressant; SSNRI: selective serotonin noradrenaline (norepinephrine) reuptake inhibitor; MAOI: monoamine oxidase inhibitor; CBT: cognitive-behavioural therapy.*

**Fig. 15.2** Treatment of anxiety disorders.

palpitations) is indicative of impending physical dysfunction (e.g. heart attack).

- Effective treatments in post-traumatic stress disorder include systematic desensitization, eye movement desensitization and psychodynamic therapy.

- Other therapies commonly used in anxiety disorders include supportive, psychodynamic, and family therapies (see Ch. 28).
- Counselling may be helpful for patients who are experiencing stressful life events, illnesses or bereavements.

Inhibition of serotonin uptake seems to be the essential component of effective drug therapy for obsessive-compulsive disorder as evidenced by the efficacy of the SSRIs and clomipramine. Clomipramine, which predominantly inhibits serotonin reuptake, is more effective than the other tricyclic antidepressants with predominant noradrenaline (norepinephrine) reuptake inhibition (e.g. desipramine, nortriptyline).

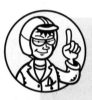

Beta-blockers are sometimes used for anxiety because they reduce autonomic anxiety symptoms (palpitations, tremor, etc.). Although they have been shown to reduce performance anxiety (not the same as social phobia) in musicians, they should be used with caution in other anxiety disorders due to their propensity to lower blood pressure and induce postural hypotension (patients with anxiety disorders frequently suffer from postural hypotension anyway).

## Course and prognosis

The prognoses of the anxiety disorders vary greatly between individuals.

- Generalized anxiety is likely to be chronic, but fluctuating, often worsening during times of stress.
- Depending on treatment, up to one-half of panic disorder patients may be symptom-free after 3 years, but one-third of the remainder have chronic symptoms that are sufficiently distressing to significantly reduce quality of life. Panic attacks are central to the development of agoraphobia, which usually develops within 1 year after the onset of recurrent panic attacks.
- The course of social phobia is usually chronic, although adults may have long periods of

remission. Life stressors, e.g. a job promotion, may exacerbate symptoms.

- The long-term prognosis of specific phobias is less well known, but it is thought that simple phobias that persist from childhood are less likely to remit than those that begin in response to distress in adulthood.
- Approximately half of the patients with post-traumatic stress disorder will recover fully within 3 months. However, a third of patients are left with moderate to severe symptoms in the long term. The severity, duration and proximity of a patient's exposure to the original trauma are the most important prognostic indicators.
- The majority of patients with obsessive-compulsive disorder have a chronic fluctuating course, with worsening of symptoms during times of stress. About 15 % of patients show a progressive deterioration in functioning.

## Somatoform disorders

The somatoform disorders: somatization disorder, hypochondriacal disorder (including body dysmorphic disorder), somatoform autonomic dysfunction, persistent somatoform pain disorder, and factitious disorder and malingering were discussed in Ch. 8. This section will focus on somatization disorder and hypochondriacal disorder.

### Epidemiology

Figure 15.3 presents the epidemiological data for somatization disorder and hypochondriacal disorder.

### Aetiology

The aetiology of somatoform disorders is poorly understood, although episodes often follow the appearance of a stressor.

Somatization disorder may, in part, be due to genetic factors, as up to one-fifth of sufferers' first-degree female relatives also have the condition. Theories of a biological aetiology include the suggestion that physical symptoms result from a failure to regulate cytokines (e.g. interleukins). Psychological models suggest that the symptoms are unconsciously produced as a substitute form of communication.

Patients with hypochondriacal disorder may have a lower threshold for suspecting illness or may subconsciously covet the gains to be had from adopting the sick role.

**Epidemiology of somatization disorder and hypochondriacal disorder**

| Anxiety disorder | Lifetime prevalence | Usual age of onset | Sex ratio |
|---|---|---|---|
| Somatization disorder | 0.2–2% | Before age 25, often in adolescence | Far more common in women (about 10:1) |
| Hypochondriacal disorder | 1–5% | Early adulthood | Occurs in both men and women |

**Fig. 15.3** Epidemiology of somatization disorder and hypochondriacal disorder.

## Assessment, clinical features, investigations and differential diagnosis

Discussed in Chapter 8.

## Course and prognosis

Both somatization disorder and hypochondriacal disorder tend to have a chronic episodic course, with waxing and waning symptoms often exacerbated by stress. Good prognostic features in hypochondriacal disorder include acute onset, brief duration, mild hypochondriacal symptoms, the presence of genuine physical co-morbidity and the absence of a co-morbid psychiatric disorder.

## Treatment

Pharmacotherapy will only alleviate symptoms when the patient has an underlying drug-responsive condition such as an anxiety disorder or depression. Both individual and group psychotherapy may be useful in reducing symptoms by helping patients to cope with their symptoms and develop alternative strategies for expressing their emotions. Figure 15.4 summarizes the role of the general practitioner in managing patients with somatoform disorders.

**Role of the general practitioner in managing patients with somatoform disorders**

- Arrange to see patients at regular fixed intervals, rather than reacting to the patient's frequent requests to be seen
- Increase support during times of stress for the patient
- Take symptoms seriously, but also encourage patients to talk about emotional problems, rather than just focusing on physical complaints
- Limit the use of unnecessary medication, especially those that may be abused (e.g. benzodiazepines, opiates)
- Treat coexisting mental disorders, e.g. anxiety, depression
- Limit special investigations (especially invasive, costly investigations) to those absolutely necessary
- Have a high threshold of referral to specialists
- If possible, arrange that patients are only seen by one or two doctors in the practice to help with containment and to limit iatrogenic harm
- Help patients to think in terms of coping with their problem, rather than curing it
- Involve other family members and carers in the management plan
- Consider referral to a psychiatrist or psychotherapist

**Fig. 15.4** Role of the general practitioner in managing patients with somatoform disorders.

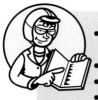

- What are the key epidemiological differences between generalized anxiety disorder and obsessive-compulsive disorder (OCD)?
- How does the cognitive model account for panic attacks?
- When are benzodiazepines indicated in the treatment of anxiety?
- Which anxiety disorders are treated with SSRIs as a first-line pharmacological option?
- Why is clomipramine effective in treating OCD?
- What are the treatment options for patients with a specific phobia?
- What is the role of medication in treating hypochondriacal disorder?

## Suggested further reading

Bandelow B, Zohar J, et al 2002 World Federation of Societies of Biological Psychiatry (WFSBP). Guidelines for the pharmacological treatment of anxiety, obsessive-compulsive and posttraumatic stress disorders. World Journal of Biological Psychiatry 3: 171–199

Lingford-Hughes A, Potokar J, Nutt D 2002 Treating anxiety complicated by substance misuse. Advances in Psychiatric Treatment 8: 107–116

Rosenbaum J F, Fredman S 2002 Treatment of anxiety disorders with comorbid depression. URL: http://www.medscape.com/viewprogram/1925

Sanderson W C, Rego S A 2000 Empirically supported psychological treatment of panic disorder and agoraphobia. URL: http://www.medscape.com/viewprogram/350

# 16. Dementia and Delirium

This chapter discusses the disorders associated with the presenting complaints in Chapter 9, which you might find helpful to read first.

## Dementia

### Epidemiology

The overall prevalence of dementia is approximately 0.3% of the total UK population, rising sharply with increasing age. Figure 16.1 illustrates the increasing prevalence of dementia with age. The prevalence in persons aged 65 or over is approximately 5% and in those over 80 about 20%. The term senile or late-onset dementia is used if the onset of dementia is after age 65 and presenile or early-onset dementia if at or before age 65.

The relative proportions are:

- Alzheimer's disease, approximately 30–60% of cases.
- Vascular dementia, approximately 10–30%.
- Combined Alzheimer's and vascular dementia, approximately 10–30%.
- Dementia with Lewy bodies, approximately 15%.
- Frontotemporal dementia, which includes Pick's disease, is the most common form of primary degenerative dementia, after Alzheimer's disease, that affects the middle-aged, accounting for up to 20% of presenile dementia cases.

### Aetiopathology (each type of dementia will be discussed separately)

#### Alzheimer's disease (AD)

Alzheimer's disease (AD) is classified as:

- Early-onset AD, or presenile AD, if the onset of dementia is before age 65.
- Late-onset AD, or senile AD, if the onset of dementia is after age 65.

Some authors further divide AD into:

- Familial type: when numerous family members are affected.
- Sporadic types: when no other family members are affected.

Late-onset sporadic AD is the commonest form of AD and accounts for up to 90% of cases. Note that 'familial' does not mean 'genetic': there may be a genetic factor involved, or multiple family members may have been exposed to something in the environment that contributed to the development of dementia. Similarly 'sporadic' does not mean 'not genetic': there is strong evidence that suggests that genetic factors play a significant role in 'sporadic AD'. Nevertheless, the onset of familial AD generally occurs earlier than the onset of sporadic AD.

At present, the cause of most cases of AD is unknown. It appears to be a combination of multifactorial genetic risk factors and, as yet, uncertain environmental factors. **Increased production and deposition of β-amyloid** appears to be the central pathological process in the so-called *amyloid cascade hypothesis*.

*Amyloid cascade hypothesis*

#### Genetic factors

*Late-onset AD.* It is not clear how much genetic factors contribute to the risk of developing late-onset AD (sporadic or familial). What is clear is that genetic factors are the largest single risk factor, and family studies have shown a threefold-increased risk of developing AD in the first-degree relatives of sufferers. The most important gene associated with late-onset AD is the gene that codes a protein involved in cholesterol metabolism called apolipoprotein E (ApoE), which occurs in three different alleles. Individuals who inherit one copy of the ApoE 4 allele are at an increased risk of developing AD, and those with two copies are at even greater risk. Also, individuals with increasing ApoE4 alleles tend to develop AD at a younger age. However, other environmental and genetic factors must be involved because having two ApoE 4 alleles does not guarantee the development of AD, and many patients with AD have no copies of the allele at all.

*Early-onset AD.* Some forms of early-onset familial AD are inherited in an autosomal dominant fashion. From studies of the rare families affected, three genes have thus far been isolated:

- Amyloid precursor protein – chromosome 21.
- Presenilin-1 – chromosome 14.
- Presenilin-2 – chromosome 1.

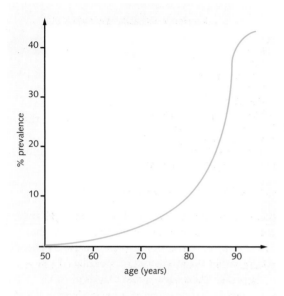

**Fig. 16.1** Graph showing increasing prevalence of dementia with age.

Note that these genes that have been isolated thus far may only account for 30–50% of all autosomal dominant cases. These autosomal dominant dementias present between the ages of 30 and 60 years, sometimes as early as age 28 when there is a mutation at presenilin 1.

Note that adults with trisomy 21 (Down's syndrome) invariably develop neuropathological changes similar to AD by middle age and many will develop dementia. This has been attributed to triplication and over-expression of the gene for amyloid precursor protein (APP).

You should be aware of four genes in Alzheimer's disease – one in late-onset AD, and three in early-onset autosomal dominant AD:
- In late-onset AD, the gene coding for the ApoE 4 allele increases an individual's susceptibility to develop AD.
- In early-onset AD, the possession of one of the three genes: amyloid precursor protein, presenilin-1 and presenilin-2, virtually guarantees that an individual will develop AD.

Do not forget that late-onset sporadic AD accounts for the overwhelming majority of all AD cases.

*Neurotransmitter abnormalities*  The *cholinergic hypothesis* states that many of the cognitive, functional and behavioural symptoms in AD are due to a reduction in brain acetylcholine activity, secondary to the degeneration of cholinergic neurons in the nucleus basalis of Meynert and other nuclei projecting to the hippocampus and mesial temporal region. Evidence for this theory comes from studies of physostigmine, a powerful inhibitor of acetylcholinesterase (acetylcholinesterase inactivates acetylcholine in the cholinergic synapse), which was shown to improve memory in healthy individuals. This led to the development of cholinesterase inhibitors in the symptomatic treatment of mild to moderate AD.

*Environmental factors*  There is no consistent evidence to confirm the role of toxins, viruses, and autoimmune factors in the aetiology of AD. Aluminium is related to AD in dialysis patients, but it has not been shown to increase the risk for the general population. Poor educational attainment appears to increase risk, but this relationship may equally be explained by other factors such as social class, nutrition, and delayed detection in the well educated. Postmenopausal hormone replacement therapy (HRT) appears to be a protective factor.

*Neuropathology*  The gross pathology is characterized by generalized atrophy of the brain, with widened sulci and enlarged ventricles – most marked in the frontal and temporal lobes.
  The microscopic findings include:
- Intracellular *neurofibrillary tangles* resulting from abnormal phosphorylation of tau protein.
- Granulovacuolar degeneration (intracellular cytoplasmic vacuoles).
- Extracellular senile plaques consisting of a central core of β-amyloid, aluminium and silica.
- *Amyloid deposition* in the walls of blood vessels.

## Vascular dementia
The cause of vascular dementia is presumed to be multiple cortical infarctions or many small infarctions in the white matter (Binswanger's disease) resulting from widespread cerebrovascular

disease. On occasions, vascular dementia can arise from a single infarct. As with both Alzheimer's disease and cerebrovascular disease, vascular dementia is closely associated with increasing age. In rare cases, the disease is linked to a dominant gene on chromosome 19 (cerebral autosomal dominant arteriopathy). The risk factors for developing vascular dementia are the same as for cerebrovascular disease in general and are summarized in Figure 16.2.

## Dementia with Lewy bodies (DLB)

Little is known about the cause of dementia with Lewy bodies. Allelic variation on the apolipoprotein E gene of chromosome 19 may be linked. Lewy bodies are neuronal inclusions composed of abnormally phosphorylated neurofilament proteins aggregated with ubiquitin and $\alpha$-synuclein. The Lewy bodies found in the paralimbic and neocortical structures of patients with DLB are identical to those found in the basal ganglia of patients with Parkinson's disease. Lewy bodies are also found in the brains of patients with Alzheimer's disease and Down's syndrome. Remember from Chapter 9 that parkinson-like motor features may be a core feature of DLB.

## Frontotemporal dementia

The cause of the frontotemporal dementias is unknown. They are associated with bilateral atrophy of the frontal and anterior temporal lobes (atrophied paper-thin gyri known as 'knife-blade atrophy') and degeneration of the striatum. There are three main histological types (60% – microvacuolar; 25% – Pick's type; 15% – microvacuolar/Pick's type combined with histological signs of motor neuron disease). Pick's bodies are intraneuronal masses of cytoskeletal elements.

Only a minority of patients with frontotemporal dementia exhibit the Pick-type histological changes, hence the term 'frontotemporal dementia' is preferred to 'Pick's disease'.

## Huntington's disease

Huntington's disease has autosomal dominant inheritance with complete penetrance. It is caused

---

### Risk factors for vascular dementia

- Male
- Smoking
- Previous stroke
- Hypertension
- Diabetes
- History of myocardial infarct
- Carotid artery stenosis
- Valvular disease
- Hypercholesterolaemia
- Hypercoagulation disorders

**Fig. 16.2** Risk factors for vascular dementia.

by a gene on the short arm of chromosome 4 that contains an excessive number of trinucleotide (CAG) repeat sequences, usually more than 40, which results in production of the abnormal protein 'Huntingtin'. The length of the abnormal trinucleotide repeat sequence is inversely correlated to the age of onset of the disease.

## Parkinson's disease

Like Huntington's disease, Parkinson's disease is also a disease of the basal ganglia and is often associated with a subcortical form of dementia (see Fig. 9.5, p. 59). About 30% of patients with Parkinson's disease will develop dementia. The three classic symptoms of Parkinson's disease are resting tremor, rigidity and bradykinesia (poverty of movement).

## Creutzfeldt–Jakob disease (CJD) and other prion-related diseases

A prion is a proteinaceous particle that does not contain DNA or RNA. This agent, which seems to be infectious although structurally simpler than any virus, is able to cause a severe and invariably fatal disease of the brain. All the prion-related disorders result in a spongiform degeneration of the brain in the absence of an inflammatory immune response, associated with the deposition of the prion protein (PrP) in the form of amyloid sheets.

Most cases of CJD appear to be sporadic affecting people in their 50s, although it can be transmitted iatrogenically (e.g. infected corneal transplants and surgical instruments). It presents with a rapidly progressing dementia with cerebellar ataxia and myoclonic jerks over a time course of 6–8 months. The EEG characteristically shows stereotyped sharp wave complexes.

New variant CJD (nvCJD) is thought to be secondary to the ingestion of BSE-infected (bovine spongiform encephalopathy) beef products. It typically presents in young adults with mild psychiatric symptoms such as depression and anxiety before the development of ataxia, dementia and finally death over a period of 18 months. There are no characteristic EEG changes, although nvCJD may have a characteristic MRI picture: a bilaterally evident high signal in the pulvinar (post-thalamic) region.

Other prion diseases include kuru (prion transmitted by cannibalism of neural tissue, described in the highland tribes of New Guinea) and Gerstmann–Straussler syndrome (autosomal dominant condition caused by mutation of PrP gene on chromosome 20).

### HIV-related dementia

Infection with the human immunodeficiency virus (HIV) is thought to cause direct damage to the brain in addition to the complications of HIV infection, such as opportunistic infections (cerebral cytomegalovirus infection, cryptococcocis, toxoplasmosis, tuberculosis, syphilis) and cerebral lymphoma. HIV encephalopathy presents clinically as a subcortical dementia and neuropathological examination shows diffuse multifocal destruction of the white matter and subcortical structures.

## Assessment, clinical features, investigations and differential diagnosis

Discussed in Chapter 9.

## Management

There is no cure for any of the neurodegenerative forms of dementia. Although the prognosis is invariably poor, considerable improvements in the quality of patients' lives are possible through a variety of psychosocial and pharmaceutical approaches. The principles of management are:

- Treating the underlying cause if possible (e.g. hypothyroidism, modifying vascular risk factors).
- Treating associated disorders or complications (e.g. aggression, chest infections, incontinence).
- Addressing functional problems that result (e.g. kitchen skills, financial management, social isolation).
- Providing advice and support for carers.
- Symptomatic treatment with cholinesterase inhibitors when indicated.

### Specific management strategies

- Family practitioners have a central role in the diagnosis and management of dementia.

Dementia sufferers should, however, be referred as soon as possible to their local psychogeriatric service where appropriate management and support can be provided

- Assessment and treatment can usually be done in a primary care or out-patient setting. It may be necessary to admit patients with end-stage dementia or severe behavioural problems to a nursing home or specialist dementia unit.
- Disturbed behaviour such as aggression or agitation may be treated with antipsychotics (especially atypical antipsychotics) or benzodiazepines. Psychotic and depressive symptoms may be treated with antipsychotics and antidepressants. Low doses are essential since the elderly may show greater susceptibility to parkinsonian side-effects. All of these drugs may worsen cognitive function, particularly those with strong anticholinergic effects. Be wary of treating a patient with dementia with Lewy bodies with antipsychotics due to the risk of a catastrophic parkinsonian reaction.
- The cholinesterase inhibitors, donepezil, rivastigmine and galantamine, have been licensed for use in the treatment of mild to moderate Alzheimer's disease in the UK and are recommended by the National Institute for Clinical Excellence (NICE) for those patients with dementia whose Mini-Mental State Examination score (MMSE) is above 12. Up to half the patients given these drugs will show a slower rate of cognitive decline and possible improvement in neuropsychiatric symptoms (e.g. apathy, hallucinations, agitation), but they should be discontinued in those thought not to be responding. Cholinesterase inhibitors have also shown promise in the treatment of dementia with Lewy bodies (DLB) and may soon be licensed as first-line treatment.
- Memantine (Ebixa®), an N-methyl-d-aspartate (NMDA) receptor antagonist, is a new class of anti-Alzheimer's drug that has been shown to be effective in individuals with moderate to severe Alzheimer's disease. It protects against excess glutamate and subsequent high intracellular calcium by blocking NMDA receptors, thereby preventing the influx of calcium.
- Assessment of functioning in the form of activities of daily living (ADL) scales is useful in focusing on, and developing, patients' remaining skills and

resources. Reality orientation and reminiscence therapies have been used to reduce confusion and stimulate remote memories. Practical social interventions such as memory aids (e.g. calendars, notebooks) may be helpful in the early stages of dementia.

- Benzodiazepines should be used with caution in patients with dementia, as they seem particularly vulnerable to their adverse effects such as sedation, with the risk of falls, and marked confusion.
- Remember that 50% of patients with dementia with Lewy bodies (DLB) will have a <u>catastrophic reaction to antipsychotics (even atypicals) precipitating irreversible parkinsonism, impaired consciousness</u>, severe autonomic symptoms and a two- to threefold increase in mortality. Benzodiazepines and cholinesterase inhibitors are safer in this group of patients. This exemplifies the need to exercise caution when prescribing antipsychotics and the importance of differentiating the various types of dementia.

## Course and prognosis

The course of dementia is invariably progressive and fatal. Successful treatment of medical causes such as hypothyroidism or hydrocephalus usually arrests rather than resolves the cognitive decline. The duration of survival from the time of diagnosis for the various forms of dementia is:

- Alzheimer's disease: 7–9 years.
- Vascular dementia: variable, usually less than Alzheimer's disease.
- Dementia with Lewy bodies: 1–2 years.
- Frontotemporal dementia: 8–11 years.
- Huntington's disease: 12–16 years.
- Creutzfeldt–Jakob disease: 6–8 months (new variant CJD: 18 months).

# Delirium

## Epidemiology

Most research into the epidemiology of delirium concentrates on the elderly, who, along with infants and young children, are more vulnerable to this disorder. The prevalence in hospitalized, medically ill patients ranges from 10% to 30%. Between 10% and 15% of patients over the age of 65 are delirious on admission and 10–40% develop a delirium during hospitalization. Patients with dementia are at an increased risk of developing a delirium; in fact, up to two-thirds of cases of delirium occur in patients with dementia.

## Aetiology

An underlying medical or drug-related cause of delirium, as discussed in Chapter 9 (see Fig. 9.6) is usually identified. The exact pathophysiological mechanisms for delirium remain unclear, but postulated mechanisms include:

- Alterations in cholinergic and noradrenergic neurotransmitter systems.
- Interruption of the blood–brain barrier.

## Assessment, clinical features, investigations and differential diagnosis

Discussed in Chapter 9.

## Management

Delirium can be highly distressing for patients and anxiety provoking for medical ward staff who are not used to dealing with agitated patients. General principles of management are as follows:

- Hospitalization is essential.
- Vigorously investigate and treat any underlying medical condition.
- To limit confusion and foster trust, try to ensure that the patient is nursed by the same staff consistently.
- Merely the physical presence of a reassuring person is often enough to calm a distressed patient.
- Maximize visual acuity (e.g. glasses, appropriately lit environment) and hearing ability (e.g. hearing aid, quiet environment) to avoid misinterpretation of stimuli.
- Encourage a friend or family member to remain with the patient to help comfort and orientate them.

- Clocks, calendars and familiar objects may be helpful with orientation.
- Typical antipsychotics, especially low dose haloperidol, are generally effective in treating delirious symptoms, in part due to their sedative qualities, but perhaps also due to their effects on the dopamine–acetylcholine balance.
- Avoid sedative medication if possible, particularly drugs with a powerful anticholinergic effect (e.g. phenothiazines). The use of benzodiazepines requires caution, as they tend to be less effective at managing delirious symptoms than antipsychotics except in alcohol- or substance-related delirium in which they are highly effective. They may be very effective in managing the common problem of insomnia.

The specific management of delirium tremens is outlined in Chapter 17.

 Remember that delirium is not a final diagnosis: this syndrome indicates the presence of a very serious medical condition that should be managed on a medical, not psychiatric, ward.

## Course and prognosis

The average duration of a delirium is 7 days. In-patients who develop delirium have an increased mortality, with elderly patients having up to a 75% chance of dying during that admission. This is unsurprising given the often serious nature of the underlying medical conditions.

- What is the prevalence of the three most common forms of dementia?
- Name four genes associated with Alzheimer's disease.
- Explain how cholinesterase inhibitors work with reference to the cholinergic hypothesis of Alzheimer's disease.
- What are the microscopic findings on the post-mortem brain of a patient with Alzheimer's disease?
- What are four modifiable risk factors for the development of vascular dementia?
- What is the genetic abnormality in Huntington's disease?
- Describe the clinical picture and give three examples of subcortical dementias.
- How does Creutzfeldt–Jakob disease (CJD) differ from new variant CJD (nvCJD) in terms of age of onset, time course and findings on special investigations?
- What are the advantages and potential dangers of using antipsychotics in dementia?
- In what sort of patients with dementia are cholinesterase inhibitors effective?
- How would you suggest the nurse in charge of a surgical ward manage a patient with delirium?
- What pharmacological therapy is useful in delirium?

## Suggested further reading

McCullagh C D, Craig D, et al 2001 Risk factors for dementia. Advances in Psychiatric Treatment 7: 24–31

Meagher D 2001 Delirium: the role of psychiatry. Advances in Psychiatric Treatment 7: 433–443

British Journal of Psychiatry 2002 Old age psychiatry papers. British Journal of Psychiatry 180: 116–167

Tangalos E G 2003 Transforming long-term care for Alzheimer's disease. URL: http://www.medscape.com/viewprogram/2410

Treloar A, Beck S, Paton C 2001 Administering medicines to patients with dementia and other organic cognitive syndromes. Advances in Psychiatric Treatment 7: 444–450

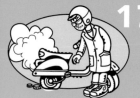

# 17. Alcohol and Substance-related Disorders

This chapter discusses the disorders associated with the presenting complaints in Chapter 10, which you might find helpful to read first. Alcohol-related disorders will be presented first followed by other psychoactive substances.

## Alcohol disorders

### Epidemiology

Prevalence rates vary considerably depending on the geographical location, the age group surveyed and how drinking problems are defined.

- The prevalence of alcohol dependence (ICD-10 definition) in England and Wales is about 5% (8% of men and 2% of women).
- In 2001, it is estimated that in Great Britain there were around 18 100 drink drive casualties of all severities – 6% of all road casualties, the highest level since 1990 (Department for Transport: Road Accidents Great Britain 2001, Casualty Report).
- In 2001, 27% of men in Great Britain, and 15% of women aged 16 or over had drunk more than 21 and 14 units a week respectively (General Household Survey 2001).
- In 2001, 39% of men in Great Britain drank more than four units of alcohol on at least one day in the previous week, with 21% drinking more than eight units on at least one day. In the same year 22% of women in Great Britain drank more than three units on at least one day in the previous week, with 10% drinking at least six units (General Household Survey 2001).

Remember that the safe daily alcohol limits are not more than 3–4 units/day for men and 2–3 units/day for women (see Fig. 10.2, p. 67). It is best to advise patients in terms of daily benchmarks of consumption rather than weekly units. Note that 39% of men and 21% of women in Great Britain are exceeding these limits.

### Aetiology

The causes of alcohol dependence are multifactorial and are determined by biological, psychological and sociocultural factors.

### Genetic and biochemical factors

Strong evidence shows a genetic component to alcohol abuse. Family studies show an increased risk of dependence among relatives of dependent individuals. Twin studies indicate that monozygotic twins have a higher concordance rate than dizygotic twins, and adoption studies also indicate a heritable component. The nature of this influence is unclear. It may operate at the level of heritable personality characteristics or it might relate to the body's inherited biochemical susceptibility to alcohol and its consequences. For example, 50% of east-Asian populations have a deficiency in one of the aldehyde dehydrogenase enzymes, leading to flushing and palpitations after small quantities of alcohol; this may explain reduced rates of consumption and dependence in these cultures.

From a biochemical perspective, chronic alcohol consumption produces decreasing activity of gamma aminobutyric acid (GABA) systems and increasing activity of glutamate systems. Both of these changes increase the likelihood of neuroexcitability and withdrawal seizures on cessation of drinking.

### Psychological factors

Behavioural models explain dependence in terms of operant conditioning where:

- *Positive reinforcement* occurs when the pleasant effects of alcohol consumption reinforce drinking behaviour, despite adverse social and medical consequences.
- *Negative reinforcement* occurs when continued drinking behaviour is reinforced by the desire to avoid the negative effects of the alcohol withdrawal syndrome.

An alternative behavioural explanation is the observational learning theory (modelling), which suggests that patterns of drinking are modelled on the drinking behaviour of relatives or peers. Family studies support the idea that drinking habits follow those of older relatives.

The presence of psychiatric (anxiety, mania, depression and schizophrenia) or physical illness appears to increase the risk of problem drinking. There is also evidence linking alcohol dependence with antisocial and borderline personality traits.

## Social and environmental factors

The cultural attitude towards alcohol affects the prevalence of alcohol-related problems (e.g. lower rates in Jewish societies as opposed to Mediterranean countries). Alcohol is also greatly affected by price; less alcohol is consumed and there are fewer alcohol-related illnesses in countries where it is expensive. There is also an association between certain occupations and deaths from alcohol-induced liver cirrhosis. The highest-risk professions are members of leisure and catering trades (publicans especially), doctors, journalists and those involved with shipping and travel. Furthermore, higher rates of dependence are noted in unskilled workers and the unemployed compared to the higher social classes; this may be partly explained by the 'social drift' caused by alcohol dependence (see p. 91).

The frequency of significant life events increases the risk of harmful drinking. Although the anxiolytic properties of alcohol are often used as a means of coping with stress ('tension reduction' hypothesis), the social and physical complications of heavy drinking often lead to even further stress.

## Assessment, clinical features, investigations and differential diagnosis

Discussed in Chapter 10.

## Management

The management of alcohol-related problems ranges from the early recognition of a drinking problem with subsequent advice concerning reduction of drinking, which can be undertaken by a general practitioner, to in-patient detoxification with subsequent long-stay rehabilitation, which usually takes place under the auspices of a specialist alcohol advisory service and, if needed, a medical team.

### The treatment of alcohol withdrawal

All clinicians working with problem drinkers need to be able to recognize alcohol dependence because the threat of experiencing withdrawal symptoms may be a barrier to the reduction of alcohol consumption and the withdrawal syndrome itself is associated with significant morbidity and mortality. Not all patients who are dependent will experience significant withdrawal symptoms. Therefore, a thorough assessment of the severity of potential withdrawal syndrome is required (see Ch. 10). The treatment of the withdrawal syndrome is commonly termed *detoxification*. The following points are important in this regard:

- It should be possible to safely and effectively detoxify the majority of patients in the community as an out-patient over the course of 1 week.
- Contraindications to community detoxification include severe dependence, a history of withdrawal seizures or delirium tremens, an unsupportive home environment and a previous failed community detoxification. In these cases, in-patient detoxification is advised.
- In order to ameliorate severe symptoms and reduce the risk of developing seizures or a delirium, a drug with cross-tolerance to alcohol is prescribed, usually in the form of the benzodiazepine, chlordiazepoxide (diazepam and lorazepam are also effective). Initially, high doses are given (up to 40–60 mg four times daily), but this is tapered down over 5–7 days. Note that although clomethiazole (Heminevrin®) has been used in the past, it should be avoided due to its potential fatal interaction with alcohol in patients who continue drinking.
- In order to avert a Wernicke's encephalopathy, it is wise to give thiamine (vitamin $B_1$) supplements orally (100 mg daily).

Figure 17.1 summarizes the treatment of delirium tremens (and Wernicke's encephalopathy).

The treatment of alcohol dependence involves more than 'detoxification'. Detoxification treats the withdrawal syndrome (only one component of dependence) which involves ameliorating withdrawal symptoms and pre-empting or treating more serious complications such as withdrawal seizures or delirium. The management of dependence involves addressing all the psychological, biological and sociocultural factors that have led to its development.

| Management of delirium tremens |
| --- |

**Emergency hospitalization essential**
Vigorous search for a medical complication, e.g.:
- Infection (especially pneumonia)
- Head injury
- Liver failure
- Gastrointestinal haemorrhage
- Wernicke's encephalopathy*

**Medication:**
- Large doses of a drug with cross-tolerance to alcohol, e.g. benzodiazepines (oral chlordiazepoxide up to 400 mg daily) – i.v. therapy seldom needed. Also treats seizures
- Only use antipsychotics (e.g. haloperidol) for severe psychotic symptoms (risk of lowering seizure threshold)
- Large doses of parenteral (intramuscular or slow intravenous) thiamine – two Pabrinex® ampoules twice daily for 5 days. Oral thiamine is not adequate*

**Monitoring of temperature, fluid, electrolytes and glucose:**
- Risk of hyperthermia, dehydration, hypoglycaemia, hypokalaemia, hypomagnesaemia

**General principles for managing a delirium (see p. 107)**

* Wernicke's encephalopathy can occur in the context of delirium tremens, or in isolation. Treatment is with large doses of parenteral thiamine (as listed under medication, above).

**Fig. 17.1** Management of delirium tremens.

 Delirium tremens is a medical emergency that is not uncommon on medical and surgical wards. It has a mortality of about 5% emphasizing the need for prompt recognition and appropriate treatment. Make sure that you know the symptoms (Ch. 10) and management well.

## Maintenance after detoxification
### Pharmacological therapy
- Disulfiram (Antabuse®): blocks alcohol oxidation, leading to an accumulation of acetaldehyde. This causes unpleasant symptoms of anxiety, flushing, palpitations, headache and a choking sensation within 20 minutes of alcohol consumption. The drug is usually taken orally, although surgical implants are available. It is contraindicated in patients with compromised cardiorespiratory function.
- Acamprosate (Campral®): enhances GABA transmission and appears to reduce the likelihood of relapse after detoxification by reducing craving. Some patients find it helpful.

*Psychosocial interventions*   Not all interventions are suited to all patients and the care package needs to be tailored accordingly. The various forms of psychosocial intervention that have been shown to be effective in managing alcohol problems include:
- Motivational interviewing (Miller & Rollnick) and the application of Prochaska & DiClemente's *stages of change* model, which moves patients through a cycle of change from 'precontemplation' to 'contemplation' to 'determination' to 'action' to 'maintenance'.
- Cognitive behaviour therapy (cue exposure, relapse prevention work, behavioural contracting).
- Group therapy.
- Alcoholics anonymous: 12 step programme (Al-Anon and Al-Ateen support the families and teenage children of alcoholics respectively).
- Social support: social workers, probation officers and citizen's advice agencies may be able to help with homelessness, criminal charges and debt.
- Primary prevention: increasing the cost of alcohol through taxation appears to be the most effective strategy in reducing overall consumption. Limiting availability, curtailing advertising and health education seem less effective measures.

## Course and prognosis
Alcohol dependence has a variable course and is characterized by many relapses. However, the prognosis is not as poor as is often thought, as highly functioning individuals show a higher than 65% 1-year abstinence rate following treatment. Good prognostic indicators include being in a stable relationship, employment, having stable living conditions with good social supports and having good insight and motivation. The studies that have followed up dependent drinkers for many years have demonstrated varying outcomes and indicated that there is no average outcome. Alcohol-dependent individuals have a 3.6-fold excess mortality compared with age-matched controls. The lifetime risk of suicide is 3–4%, which is 60 to120 times greater than that of the general population.

## Other psychoactive substances

### Epidemiology

- The prevalence of drug dependence in the general population varies according to age; 6.7% of those aged 16–24 years are dependent compared with 0.5% of those aged 55–64 years (all ages – 2.1%).
- The number of problem drug misusers who presented to drug treatment agencies and general practitioners for treatment in England in 2001/02 increased by around 8% over the previous year and of those:
  a. about one-third (35%) were under 25 and about two-thirds (65%) were aged 25 and over
  b. around a quarter (26%) of users were female and around three-quarters (74%) were male, i.e. a male-to-female ratio of 3:1
  c. heroin was the most frequently reported main problem drug, accounting for nearly three-quarters of users (73%). The next most frequently reported main drugs of misuse were cannabis (8%), crack (5%) and cocaine, amfetamines and methadone (each 3%) (Department of Health, Provisional statistics from the national drug treatment monitoring system in England, 2001/02).
- Although heroin is the most frequently reported problem drug, cannabis is the most commonly consumed illegal drug (used by 5% of the population).
- Among 11–15-year-olds in England in 2001, cannabis was the most frequently reported illicit drug used in the last year (used by 13%) (Department of Health, Drug use, smoking and drinking among young people in England in 2001).

The penalties applicable to offences involving drugs are graded broadly according to the *harmfulness attributable to a drug when it is misused* and for this purpose the Misuse of Drugs Act (1971) classifies drugs into three groups according to their perceived dangerousness:

- *Class A* includes: heroin (diamorphine), morphine, pethidine, methadone, dipipanone, cocaine, lysergic acid diethylamine (LSD), phencyclidine, methylenedioxymethamfetamine (MDMA, Ecstasy) and all injectable class B substances.
- *Class B* includes: oral amfetamines, cannabis, codeine and barbiturates.
- *Class C* includes: most benzodiazepines, buprenorphine, meprobamate, pemoline and dextropropoxyphene.

### Aetiology

The aetiological factors for illicit-drug dependence are not well understood, although they would appear to be related to a mixture of biopsychosocial factors. The operant conditioning model described in the alcohol section also applies to other psychoactive substances. Similarly, price, availability, and cultural attitudes appear to be key factors influencing the use of illicit substances. In addition, social deprivation, a family environment of substance abuse, conduct disorder in childhood, antisocial personality disorder, and severe mental illness all increase the likelihood of substance-misuse problems.

The introduction of harsher legal penalties for suppliers and users of illicit drugs, and increased education about the effects of drug use, have not resulted in a decrease in illicit-drug use over the last 30 years.

### Assessment, clinical features, drug classification and differential diagnosis

Discussed in Chapter 10.

### Management

As with the management of alcohol dependence, management involves more than treating physical dependence with detoxification, but also concerns the maintenance of abstinence and the addressing of the psychological, biological and sociocultural factors that led to substance dependence in the first place.

A detailed management of substance abuse is beyond the scope of this book; however, specific key points on the treatment of some individual substances will be mentioned.

#### Opiates

- Patients should be given education about harm minimization, including the risks of using contaminated injecting equipment (HIV, hepatitis

B and C, infective endocarditis, etc.) and unsafe sexual behaviour.

- Clean needles and injecting equipment, hepatitis B vaccination and condoms should be offered.
- Withdrawal is distressing although not life-threatening and may be attempted rapidly in mild to moderate dependence. The symptoms may be ameliorated by lofexidine, a centrally acting α-adrenoceptor agonist that reduces sympathetic outflow.
- Maintenance treatment of opiate use can be offered to patients with severe dependence by converting to the longer-acting oral opiate methadone. It helps stabilize the user's life and prevents the complications of injecting. Before prescribing potentially fatal doses of methadone, opiate dependence should be proven by a urine drug screen. Serious respiratory depression may result if the patient is not already tolerant to opiates.
- Methadone may be prescribed indefinitely, but the aim should be gradual reduction with long-term abstinence.
- Sublingual buprenorphine (Subutex®), a partial opiate agonist, is also used as substitution therapy for patients with moderate dependence. The dose is then gradually reduced to avoid a precipitous withdrawal syndrome. Note that because it is only a partial agonist, it may precipitate withdrawal in patients who are dependent on high doses of opiates (more than 30 mg methadone daily).
- Once detoxified, naltrexone (an opiate antagonist) is sometimes used to block the euphoriant effects of any continued opiate use. It induces withdrawal if the patient is still dependent.
- Psychological interventions are integral to good therapeutic outcomes and include motivational interviewing, cognitive-behavioural therapy (including relapse prevention) and social support.

## Benzodiazepines

As with alcohol, caution must be exercised when attempting a withdrawal from benzodiazepines as it is potentially fatal and may include hallucinations, convulsions and delirium. Patients are initially converted from short-acting (e.g. lorazepam, temazepam) to long-acting compounds (usually diazepam). Doses are then reduced very slowly by a small amount every few weeks, depending on what the patient can tolerate.

## Cocaine and amfetamine

Both cocaine and amfetamine can be stopped abruptly. Antidepressants may help the depressed mood that follows withdrawal from heavy use. Psychotic disorders induced by these drugs benefit from symptomatic treatment with short courses of benzodiazepines or antipsychotics.

- What are safe levels of alcohol consumption and how many people in the UK exceed those limits?
- How does the operant conditioning model of behavioural theory explain alcohol and substance abuse?
- What does detoxification aim to treat and how does that differ from the treatment of dependence?
- What are the differences in the principles of management of community detoxification and delirium tremens?
- What are the three most commonly encountered drug problems in patients presenting for treatment?
- What non-drug management strategies are employed in the treatment of intravenous heroin dependence?
- What is the role of methadone in treatment of opiate dependence?
- How is benzodiazepine withdrawal similar to alcohol withdrawal?

## Suggested further reading

Baigent M F 2003 Physical complications of substance abuse: what the psychiatrist needs to know. Current Opinion in Psychiatry 16(3): 291–296. Available from URL: http://www.medscape.com/viewarticle/452724

Edwards G, Marshall E J, Cook C C 1997 The treatment of drinking problems: a guide for the helping professions, 3rd edn. Cambridge University Press, Cambridge

McIntosh C, Ritson B 2001 Treating depression complicated by substance misuse. Advances in Psychiatric Treatment 7: 357–364

Miller WR, Rollnick S 1991 Motivational interviewing preparing people to change addictive behaviour. Guilford Press, New York

Prochaska JO, DiClemente CC, Norcross JC 1992 In search of how people change; applications to addictive behaviours. American Psychologist 47:1102–1114

Raistrick D 2000 Management of alcohol detoxification. Advances in Psychiatric Treatment 6: 348–355

British Journal of Psychiatry 2001 Substance misuse papers. British Journal of Psychiatry 178: 101–128

Swadi H 2000 Substance misuse in adolescents. Advances in Psychiatric Treatment 6: 201–210

→ N.B XXY = Klinefelter's syndrome

(XYY = an aneuploidy (specifically a trisomy) of the sex chromosime in which a human male receives an extra Y chromosome, prod. a 47, XYY karyotype

PHENOTYPE = "normal"
KARYOTYPE = 97% of pts. do not know their karyotype.

# 18. The Personality Disorders

This chapter discusses the disorders associated with the presenting complaints in Chapter 11, which you might find helpful to read first.

## Personality disorders

### Epidemiology
Epidemiological research in personality disorders is made difficult by poor case definitions and the lack of consensus regarding the correct diagnostic instruments. The prevalence of any personality disorder in community surveys ranges from 4% to 13%, although it varies according to the population group sampled. It is higher in patients consulting general practitioners (10–30%), even higher in psychiatric out-patient clinics (30–40%) and higher still in psychiatric in-patient (40–50%), parasuicidal samples (40–80%) and prisons (50–80%). Figure 18.1 describes the prevalence of the individual disorders and their relevant epidemiology.

### Aetiology
Although the aetiology of personality disorders is unknown and many theories abound, both environmental and genetic factors seem to be important. The genetic evidence includes:

- Twin studies: monozygotic twins show a higher concordance for personality disorders than dizygotic twins.
- The cluster A personality disorders (especially schizotypal) are more common in the relatives of patients with schizophrenia.
- Depressive disorders are more common in the relatives of patients with borderline personality disorder.
- Individuals with XYY chromosomes show increased antisocial behaviour independent of other variables.

Some authors have suggested that schizoid personality disorder might be a neurodevelopmental disorder, possibly within the autistic spectrum. There is also evidence that children with minimal brain damage are at risk for personality disorders, especially antisocial personality disorder which may also be associated with electroencephalogram (EEG) abnormalities.

The finding of low levels of the serotonin metabolite 5-HIAA (5-hydroxyindoleacetic acid) in aggressive or suicidal patients as well as the observation that SSRIs can sometimes result in personality changes (e.g. increased threshold for rejection) indicates that neurotransmitters might have a significant influence on personality.

Early adverse social circumstances are associated with the development of dependent and borderline personality disorders (e.g. parental deprivation, impaired attachment). There is also an association between borderline personality disorder and childhood sexual abuse.

Psychoanalytical theory has attempted to explain personality disorders as arising from the failure to successfully progress through the stages of psychosexual development with the subsequent development of characteristic defence mechanisms (e.g. *projection* in paranoid personality disorder; *splitting* in borderline personality disorder).

### Assessment, clinical features, classification and differential diagnosis
Discussed in Chapter 11.

### Management
There is considerable debate concerning how personality disorders should be managed and by whom (please see suggested further reading). What is clear is that, at present, the management of personality disorders falls predominantly within the domain of the healthcare establishment and to a lesser extent the criminal justice agencies.

A multidisciplinary approach is often essential as psychological, social and biological treatment modalities all have an important role. A comprehensive assessment should be made of sources of distress (thoughts, emotions, behaviour and relationships) to self and others, other co-morbid mental illness and specific impairments of functioning at work or home. If at all possible, a formulation of realistic goals of treatment should be discussed and agreed with patients.

| Epidemiology of personality disorders | | |
|---|---|---|
| Personality disorder | Prevalence in general population | Comments |
| Paranoid | 0.5–2.5% | More common in males and lower socioeconomic class individuals<br>More common in relatives of patients with schizophrenia |
| Schizoid | 0.5–1.5% | More common in males and offender populations<br>May be more common in relatives of patients with schizophrenia |
| Schizotypal | 3% | More common in relatives of patients with schizophrenia<br>May be slightly more common in males |
| Borderline (emotionally unstable) | 2% | More prevalent in younger age groups and females<br>Most severe in mid-20s with improvement in late 30s<br>Associated with poor work history and single marital status<br>Co-morbid with depression, substance abuse, bulimia and anxiety. There is a 9% suicide rate<br>High users of mental health services |
| Antisocial (dissocial) | 3% males<br><1% females | Far more common in men<br>Highest prevalence in 25–44 year-olds<br>Associated with school drop-out, conduct disorder and urban settings<br>Very high prevalence in prisons and forensic settings<br>Highly co-morbid with substance abuse |
| Histrionic | 2–3% | Recent research shows equal gender ratio (previously thought to be more common in women)<br>Associated with parasuicide |
| Narcissistic | <1% | More common in males and forensic settings |
| Dependent | 1–2% | Co-morbid with borderline personality disorder |
| Avoidant (anxious) | 1–5% | Equal gender ratio<br>Co-morbid with social phobia |
| Obsessive-compulsive anankastic) | 1–2% | More common in white, male, highly educated, married and employed individuals |

**Fig. 18.1** Epidemiology of personality disorders.

Hospital admission may sometimes be helpful in times of crisis. However, it may be constructive to come to an agreement with patients regarding the aims and duration of admission.

Psychosocial interventions include:

- Assistance with social problems such as housing, finances, employment and disturbed relationships.
- Supportive psychotherapy provides patients with an authority figure during times of crisis and focuses on acceptance and helping patients with their dependence needs.
- Cognitive behavioural therapy may target specific symptoms or behaviours, e.g. depression, anxiety, anger and deliberate self-harm.

- Cognitive analytic therapy (CAT) has shown some promise in patients with borderline personality disorder.
- Dialectical behaviour therapy (DBT) is a promising intervention for borderline personality disorder and has been shown to reduce parasuicidal behaviour and time spent in hospital; and improve patient engagement and social and global functioning.
- Assertive community outreach (ACT) programmes, which are often used for chronic schizophrenic and bipolar patients, also show promise in the treatment of personality disorders.
- Group or individual psychodynamic psychotherapy – see p. 194.

- Certain highly motivated patients derive benefit from treatment in a therapeutic community.

Although the treatment of personality disorders is challenging, it is helpful to take a longitudinal approach, bearing in mind that symptoms can improve with time and that significant clinical improvement is possible.

*Pharmacological treatments* are used to treat specific symptoms as opposed to treating the underlying personality:

- Mood stabilizers such as lithium and carbamazepine may be useful in treating aggression, impulsivity and mood instability.
- Antipsychotics may be of some use in treating the psychotic symptoms that sometimes are experienced by schizotypal and borderline personality disorder patients. Low dose flupentixol has also been shown to reduce parasuicidal behaviour. Antipsychotics are also sometimes used to help with impulsivity, agitation and aggression.
- Antidepressants may be useful in treating depressive symptoms. SSRIs may help with obsessive-compulsive symptoms as well as impulsivity and self-harm behaviour.
- Benzodiazepines should be used with caution as abuse may lead to dependence. They may,

however, be used to alleviate acute anxiety or to sedate an acutely agitated or aggressive patient.

Although pharmacological therapy may alleviate specific symptoms (e.g. depression, anxiety) in personality disordered patients, it is unlikely to have any long-term effect on maladaptive personality traits.

## Course and prognosis

It is important to remember that patients with personality disorder have a greater incidence of other mental illnesses such as depression, anxiety and schizophrenia. Furthermore, these tend to be more severe and have a worse prognosis than if the personality disorder was not present. Patients with personality disorder (especially cluster B) also have higher rates of suicide and accidental death than the general population. The course of personality disorders is not as dire as is often portrayed. Half of all borderline personality patients will show clinical recovery at 10–25-year follow-up. Patients with antisocial personality may also improve with time especially if they have formed a relationship with a therapist. Schizotypal and obsessive-compulsive personality disorders tend to be stable over time, although schizotypal patients may go on to develop schizophrenia

- What are the differences and similarities in epidemiology between borderline and antisocial personality disorders?
- Name three psychosocial interventions that are showing promise in the treatment of personality disorder.
- What are the roles of antipsychotics and benzodiazepines in the treatment of personality disorder?
- How are personality disorders and other mental illnesses related in terms of prognosis?

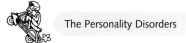 

## Suggested further reading

Adshead G 2001 Murmurs of discontent: treatment and treatability of personality disorder. Advances in Psychiatric Treatment 7: 407–415

Davison S E 2002 Principles of managing patients with personality disorder. Advances in Psychiatric Treatment 8: 1–9

Palmer R L 2002 Dialectical behaviour therapy for borderline personality disorder. Advances in Psychiatric Treatment 8: 10–16

British Journal of Psychiatry 2003 Ramifications of personality disorder in clinical practice. British Journal of Psychiatry 182(Suppl. 44): s1–s35

Winston A P 2000 Recent developments in borderline personality disorder. Advances in Psychiatric Treatment 6: 211–217

# 19. Eating Disorders

This chapter discusses the disorders associated with the presenting complaints in Chapter 12, which you might find helpful to read first.

## Anorexia and bulimia nervosa

### Epidemiology
Both anorexia and bulimia nervosa are far more common in women and have a male-to-female ratio of 1:10. The incidence rates for the detection of cases by GPs in Britain in 1993 were 4.2 per 100 000 population for anorexia nervosa, and 12.2 per 100 000 for bulimia nervosa. Although more cases of both disorders have been identified over recent years, the evidence for a rising incidence is not conclusive. Figure 19.1 summarizes the epidemiology of both anorexia and bulimia nervosa.

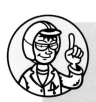 Anorexia nervosa is 5–10 times less common, and tends to have an earlier age of onset, than bulimia nervosa. It was previously thought to have an increased prevalence in higher socioeconomic classes; however, a number of studies have produced conflicting results.

### Aetiology
The cause of neither anorexia nor bulimia has been clarified, but both biological and psychosocial factors have been implicated.

#### Anorexia nervosa
*Genetic/biological factors* Twin studies have shown a higher concordance rate for monozygotic (55%) than dizygotic twins (24%). First-degree relatives have a higher incidence of eating disorders (5%), as well as mood disorders, which suggests an association between the two disorders. Abnormalities of serotonin metabolism have been implicated as serotonin suppresses food consumption, and one study found an increased concentration of a serotonin metabolite (5-HIAA) in anorectics.

*Environmental/ psychological factors* Western culture's obsession with thinness and the mass media's portrayal of the 'ideal woman' seems to influence young girls' perception of their own body image. Families of anorectics may be characterized by overprotection, enmeshment (overinvolvement with lack of differentiation between parent and child), conflict avoidance and rigidity (resistance to change). Another theory maintains that sexual maturity represents a conflict for anorectics, which results in them attempting to avoid menstruation and changes in body shape that are associated with puberty.

#### Bulimia
*Genetic/biological factors* The role of genetic factors is unclear. Serotonin, noradrenaline (norepinephrine) and plasma endorphins have all been implicated, although many neurotransmitter abnormalities occur secondary to weight loss and purging.

*Environmental/psychological factors* A past history of dieting, which frequently triggers binge eating and increases the risk of developing bulimia by eightfold, is always present. Up to half of bulimics have a history of anorexia. Family relationships seem to be more conflictual than in anorexia. Perfectionism, low self-esteem and high neuroticism scores are common. Alcohol and substance abuse, personality disorders and depression are associated conditions.

### Assessment, clinical features, investigations, complications and differential diagnosis
Discussed in Chapter 12.

### Management considerations in anorexia
Ambivalence towards treatment coupled with the psychological consequences of starvation (poor concentration, depression, lethargy) make patients with anorexia a difficult group to treat. Therefore treatment should be collaborative and a therapeutic

**Epidemiology of anorexia and bulimia nervosa**

| Disorder | Prevalence | Age of onset | Socioeconomic class |
|---|---|---|---|
| Anorexia nervosa | 0.5% of schoolgirls/university students; 4–6% of ballet dancers/models<br>Increased prevalence in Western cultures | Mid- to late adolescence | Initially thought to be more prevalent in higher socioeconomic classes; however, several studies do not support this (still debated) |
| Bulimia nervosa | 1–3% of young women | Late adolescence to early adulthood | Equal socioeconomic class distribution |

**Fig. 19.1** Epidemiology of anorexia and bulimia nervosa.

alliance should be established early on. Motivational interviewing (Miller & Rollnick 1991) and the application of Prochaska & DiClemente's (1992) *stages of change* model are helpful in engaging patients and overcoming treatment resistance. The degree of severity of anorexia determines the level of care:

- Patients who simply diet excessively can be treated with education about nutrition and weight monitoring by a GP or nurse. Voluntary organizations and self-help groups may also be helpful.
- The treatment of choice in patients with anorexia nervosa is some form of brief out-patient psychotherapy with the encouragement of family involvement. Furthermore, weight should be monitored and medical complications (see p. 81) actively sought for. In these cases, a multidisciplinary approach is needed, involving the GP, a general adult or child psychiatrist, a psychotherapist and possibly a community psychiatric nurse. Figure 19.2 summarizes the various forms of psychosocial therapy interventions.
- There should be low threshold for referral to a specialized eating disorder unit, especially in patients who are resistant to out-patient treatment, and those who have severe anorexia or poor prognostic factors (see Fig. 19.3).
- Hospitalization is necessary for certain medical (e.g. body mass index less than 13.5 kg/m$^2$, rapid weight loss, severe electrolyte abnormalities, syncope) and psychiatric (risk of suicide, social crisis) indications. In rare cases, when patients lose insight into the dangerousness of their condition and the ability to make rational decisions about medical treatment, it may be necessary to enforce compulsory admission and life-saving treatment under mental health legislation. In severe cases, nasogastric or intravenous feeding may be necessary.

The use of psychotropic medication is limited, and should be instituted cautiously, in patients who are underweight. SSRIs may be useful for treating co-morbid depression and obsessive-compulsive disorder. Fluoxetine may be helpful in maintaining weight gain and preventing relapse.

Although patients with anorexia frequently have depression and obsessive-compulsive disorder as co-morbid illnesses, starvation-induced malnutrition itself may lead to depression, obsessional symptoms, sleep disturbances and a lack of concentration. The use of medication should be restricted to severe symptoms and those that do not improve with weight gain.

In England and Wales, the Mental Health Act only makes provision for the compulsory treatment of mental illness (not physical illness). However, food is considered by the Mental Health Act to be treatment for mental illness because it leads to a direct improvement in the psychological symptoms (impaired decision-making) caused by starvation-induced weight loss. Therefore, in certain cases, patients may be force-fed under the Mental Health Act.

**Fig. 19.2** Psychosocial therapy options for anorexia nervosa.

| Psychosocial therapy options for anorexia nervosa | |
|---|---|
| **Therapy type** | **Comments** |
| Psychoeducation about nutrition and weight | Advice on balanced eating and dangers of excessive exercising<br>Educate about the complications of starvation, bingeing and purging<br>Educate about the nature of anorexia (body image disturbance, starvation–hunger–bingeing relationship)<br>Results of special investigations may be used to motivate |
| Nutritional management and weight restoration | Negotiation of target weight<br>Eating plan: amount of calories per day; 3 meals/day with snacks in between to avoid hunger<br>Teach shopping and cooking skills if necessary |
| Cognitive-behavioural therapy (CBT) | 20–24 sessions with 'top up' as necessary<br>May explore issues of control, low self-esteem and perfectionism |
| Interpersonal therapy (IPT) | Focuses on improving social functioning and interpersonal skills |
| Family therapy | May be very effective for adolescents still living with parents, and for onset of illness before 18 years<br>May expose attachment patterns and interpersonal difficulties |
| Psychodynamic psychotherapy | Reserved for specialists in eating disorders |

## Management considerations in bulimia

Patients with bulimia tend to be more motivated to improve and are usually of a healthy weight. The treatment is predominantly psychological, ranging from psychoeducation, self-help manuals and self-help groups in mild cases, to cognitive-behavioural therapy or interpersonal psychotherapy in more serious cases. Specialist eating disorder input or in-patient care may be necessary in severe cases. Tricyclic antidepressants and SSRIs (fluoxetine licensed at 60 mg) have been shown to reduce bingeing and purging behaviour, but psychotherapy remains the treatment of choice. Co-morbid substance abuse and depression is common and should be managed as indicated.

## Prognosis

*Anorexia*  The course of anorexia is variable. Up to 50% of patients recover and return to normal weight, eating and menstruation. Note that studies have shown that up to 25% of patients go on to develop normal weight bulimia. About a third of patients fail to recover. The mortality from anorexia

is over 10%; half of these deaths are due to the complications of starving and about a third due to suicide. The factors that are associated with a poorer prognosis are described in Figure 19.3, and indicate that the more severe the illness the poorer the outcome.

*Bulimia*  The course of bulimia is also variable, although generally better than anorexia with 50–70% of patients recovering after 2–5 years. There is no increased mortality. Poor prognostic factors include severe bingeing and purging behaviour, low weight and co-morbid depression.

| Poor prognostic factors in anorexia nervosa |
|---|
| Long duration of illness<br>A late age of onset<br>Very low weight<br>Associated bulimic symptoms<br>Personality difficulties<br>A poor family relationship<br>Poor social adjustment |

**Fig. 19.3** Poor prognostic factors in anorexia nervosa.

- In which population groups is anorexia nervosa more prevalent?
- How does anorexia nervosa differ from bulimia nervosa in terms of prevalence and age of onset?
- What observations have been made about the families of patients with anorexia and bulimia nervosa?
- What is the role of SSRIs in the treatment of patients with anorexia and bulimia nervosa?
- What is the treatment of choice in patients with anorexia?
- What are the indications for hospitalization in patients with anorexia?
- What are the poor prognostic factors in anorexia and bulimia nervosa?

## Suggested further reading

Connan F, Treasure J 2000 Working with adults with anorexia nervosa in an out-patient setting. Advances in Psychiatric Treatment 6: 135–144

Daee A, Robinson P, Lawson M, Turpin J A, Gregory B, Tobias J D 2002 Psychologic and physiologic effects of dieting in adolescents. Southern Medical Journal 95(9): 1032–1041. Available from URL: http://www.medscape.com/viewarticle/442892

Miller WR, Rollnick S 1991 Motivational interviewing: preparing people to change addictive behaviour. Guilford Press, New York

Prochaska JO, DiClemente CC, Norcross JC 1992 In search of how people change; applications to addictive behaviours. American Psychologist 47:1102–1114

Sharp C W, Freeman C P L 1993 The medical complications of anorexia nervosa. British Journal of Psychiatry 162: 452–462

Tamburrino M B, McGinnis R A 2002 Anorexia nervosa: a review. Panminerva Medica 44: 301–311

# 20. Disorders Related to Menstruation, Pregnancy and the Puerperium

This chapter will discuss disorders specific to the female reproductive cycle and include:

- Premenstrual syndrome.
- Psychiatric considerations in pregnancy.
- Puerperal disorders including postnatal blues, depression and psychosis.
- Mental illness in the menopause.

## Premenstrual syndrome

### Clinical features

The premenstrual syndrome (PMS) has been defined as the recurrence of symptoms during the premenstruum, with their absence in the postmenstruum (Dalton 1984). The symptoms of PMS tend to occur in the 10 days prior to menstruation and remit in the 2 weeks following menstruation. Over 150 symptoms have been implicated, but mood symptoms in the form of depression (71%), irritability (56%) and tiredness (35%) predominate. Physical symptoms such as headache (33%), abdominal bloating (31%) and breast tenderness (21%) are also fairly common.

### Epidemiology/aetiology

Up to 40% of women report experiencing some symptoms of PMS and one study detected cyclical symptoms in up to 80% of women. However, only about 5% of women have severe symptoms that interfere with their work or lifestyle. The prevalence is higher in women over the age of 30 years, multiparous women (prevalence increases with parity), women who do not use oral contraception and women who experience significant degrees of psychosocial stress. Genetic, hormonal/biological and psychosocial factors have been implicated in the aetiology (good relationships have a protective effect).

### Management

The management of PMS is mainly non-specific and includes reassurance, psychosocial counselling or support, stress management, healthy eating (limiting fluctuations in blood sugar), exercise and abstaining from caffeine or alcohol in the week before menstruation. The evidence for pharmacological therapy is limited but oral contraception, progesterone supplementation, serotonergic antidepressants (clomipramine, fluoxetine), mefenamic acid, diuretics, bromocriptine and vitamins (pyridoxine) are sometimes helpful. Studies show that PMS also responds well to placebo.

## Psychiatric considerations in pregnancy

- Pregnancy is generally a time of mental well-being; the development of new psychiatric illnesses is unusual and women with a history of mental illness do not have an increased risk of episodes during pregnancy, unlike in the puerperium.
- There is evidence of an increased incidence of adverse life events in the weeks and months prior to a spontaneous abortion (miscarriage). At a month following miscarriage, up to 50% of women have a diagnosable depressive disorder (four times normal) with features typical of a bereavement (see p. 42).
- There appears to be no significant increase in the rates of mental illness following a termination of pregnancy (TOP), especially since society's attitude toward abortion has become more accepting.
- In patients who are on psychiatric medication or who require psychiatric medication during pregnancy, a judgement needs to be made, in conjunction with the patient, regarding the risk of relapse or withholding pharmacological treatment against the risk of the medication-induced teratogenic or adverse effects.
- In pregnancy, lithium and benzodiazepines are probably teratogenic. Tricyclic antidepressants have been used extensively and appear to be safe, although they have been associated with adverse effects in neonates (tachycardia, muscle spasms, convulsions). The SSRIs have not been used as extensively, but there have not been any adverse reports from the most often used: fluoxetine and paroxetine. Antipsychotics have no established

125

teratogenic effects, but may cause extra-pyramidal side-effects in neonates.

 *Pseudocyesis* is the rare condition in which a non-pregnant woman has the signs and symptoms of pregnancy, e.g. abdominal distension, breast enlargement, cessation of menses, slight enlargement of the uterus etc. *Couvade syndrome* describes the condition in which men develop typical pregnancy-related symptoms during their partner's pregnancy, like morning sickness and vague abdominal pains in mild cases, to experiencing the pain of labour and childbirth in severe cases. Both of these conditions are psychosomatic and should be distinguished from *delusion of pregnancy*, which is the delusion of being pregnant, without the physical symptoms. Pseudocyesis and delusion of pregnancy may occur together.

## Menopause

Mild psychological symptoms may understandably accompany the changes that occur with the menopause, but there is little evidence that the menopause itself leads to an increased incidence of mental illness. It should be remembered that this is a time associated with other psychosocial stressors like children leaving home and a growing awareness of ageing. There is no clear psychiatric indication for hormone replacement therapy (HRT) and its use for psychological symptoms is still controversial. Nevertheless, some women, especially those with cyclical depression, have obtained symptomatic improvement from HRT. HRT should never substitute treatment with recognized antidepressants for genuine depression.

## Puerperal disorders

The puerperium, unlike pregnancy, is a relatively high-risk period for the relapse of a pre-existing mental illness as well as for the development of a new mental illness. There are three conditions that you should consider when evaluating the woman with psychological symptoms in the puerperium:

- Postnatal blues.
- Postnatal depression.
- Puerperal psychosis.

## Postnatal blues

This very common condition, which occurs in about 50% of postpartum women, is also called 'maternity blues', 'baby blues' and 'third day blues'. It occurs within the first 10 days post-delivery and is characterized by episodes of weepiness associated with mild depression or emotional lability, anxiety and irritability that peak between the third and fifth day. The absence of a link between postnatal blues and life events, demographic factors or obstetric events suggests an underlying biological cause (e.g. a precipitous fall in progesterone post-delivery). Postnatal blues is a self-limiting condition that resolves spontaneously and usually only requires reassurance. However, an apparent bad case of postnatal blues may herald the onset of postnatal depression.

## Postnatal depression

### Clinical features

Postnatal depression (PND) usually develops within 3 months after delivery and typically lasts between 2 and 6 months. The symptoms are similar to a non-puerperal depressive episode, that is, low mood, loss of interest or pleasure, fatiguability and suicidal ideation (although suicide is rare). Note, however, that sleeping difficulties, weight loss and decreased libido can be normal for the first few months following delivery. Additional features of PND may include:

- Anxious preoccupation with the baby's health, despite a relatively healthy baby, often associated with feelings of guilt and inadequacy.
- Reduced affection for the baby with possible impaired bonding.
- Obsessional phenomena, which often involve recurrent, intrusive thoughts of harming the baby (note that it is crucial to ascertain whether these are regarded as repugnant (ego-dystonic), as obsessions usually are, or whether they pose a potential risk).

- Infanticidal thoughts (thoughts of killing baby), which are different from obsessions in that they are not experienced as repugnant (i.e. they are ego-syntonic), may be seriously entertained, and, worryingly, may involve planning.

## Epidemiology

The prevalence of depression in postnatal women is about 10%. Studies have shown that this is similar to that found in the general population of women. There is no association with socioeconomic class or parity.

## Aetiology

Psychosocial factors are strongly linked to the development of PND, with recent stressful life events, lack of close confiding relationships, a young maternal age and marital strife all implicated. A previous history of depression, particularly PND and postnatal blues, is an important risk factor. Among those women with history of depressive disorder, obstetric complications during delivery are associated with an increased rate of PND. Evidence indicates that biological factors are not as important as they are in postnatal blues and puerperal psychosis.

## Management

The treatment of choice in most cases of PND is counselling, e.g. supportive counselling, mother-and-baby groups, relationship counselling. For more severe cases, antidepressant medication is necessary. Antidepressants may be transmitted in small quantities to the baby via breast milk; however, unless bottle-feeding is preferred (e.g. to allow the duty of feeding to be shared), breast-feeding need not necessarily stop. As in pregnancy a judgement needs to be made, in conjunction with the patient, regarding the risks versus benefits of medication. Figure 20.1 summarizes the information available about the use of psychotropic medication in breast-feeding mothers. Mothers with severe PND with suicidal/infanticidal ideation may require hospital admission, and, in these cases, admission with the baby to a mother-and-baby unit is preferable. Electroconvulsive therapy (ECT) may be a highly effective treatment when indicated and usually results in a rapid improvement, which is important when mother and baby are separated. Remember that the assessment of the infant's well-being is an additional part of the comprehensive psychosocial and risk assessment.

| Psychiatric medication in breast-feeding mothers | |
| --- | --- |
| Drug group | Comments |
| Tricyclic antidepressants | Amounts transmitted in breast milk are too small to be harmful<br>Low-dose amitriptyline appears safe<br>Clomipramine may be used for obsessional phenomena<br>Avoid doxepin – accumulation of metabolite |
| SSRIs | Little information available. Manufacturer advises caution<br>Fluoxetine is excreted in very small amounts, but has a long half-life and thus may accumulate<br>Paroxetine and sertraline: less than 1% of the daily dose excreted in breast milk; short half-life |
| Lithium | Risk of neonatal lithium toxicity as breast milk contains 40% of maternal lithium concentration.<br>Avoid if possible |
| Antipsychotics | Only small amounts excreted but possible effects on developing nervous system<br>Avoid high doses due to risk of lethargy in infant<br>Only use when benefit outweighs risk; consider bottle-feeding |
| Benzodiazepines and other hypnotics | Avoid. May cause lethargy in infant |

**Fig. 20.1** Psychiatric medication in breast-feeding mothers.

## Prognosis

Most women respond to standard treatment; however, some patients have a protracted course. They should be followed up closely and may need long-term treatment. Woman who develop PND without a pre-existing history of depression are at risk for future episodes of PND but not for non-puerperal depression.

Note that PND is associated with disturbances in the mother–infant relationship, and studies have shown that this can lead to problems with the child's cognitive and emotional development.

- Pregnancy has been shown to be a time of decreased psychiatric morbidity, whereas the incidence of psychiatric illness in puerperium is exceptionally high. In primiparous women, there may be up to a 35-fold increased risk of developing a psychotic illness and needing hospital admission within the first month of childbirth. This emphasizes the importance of close vigilance in the postpartum period, especially in women with a prior, or family, history of mental illness.
- Despite the increased rate of depression, postnatal suicide is rare. The suicide rate in the year following childbirth is one-sixth the rate for a matched control group. Note, however, that suicide is far more common than infanticide and, therefore, becomes a particular concern when infanticidal thoughts are present.

## Puerperal psychosis

## Clinical features

The postpartum period is an extremely high-risk period for the development of a psychotic episode. These episodes characteristically have a rapid onset,

usually between day 4 to 3 weeks post-delivery and almost always within 8 weeks. They often begin with insomnia, restlessness and perplexity, later progressing to suspiciousness and marked confusion with psychotic symptoms. These symptoms often fluctuate dramatically in their nature and intensity over a short space of time. There is some debate as to whether the puerperal psychoses represent a separate disease entity, a mood disorder with psychotic features, a schizophrenic episode, an organic psychosis or a combination of the aforementioned. In 80% of cases, the clinical presentation resembles a mood disorder (depression or mania) with delusions and hallucinations. Even when typical schizophrenic symptoms are present, patients often have associated mood symptoms.

## Epidemiology

Puerperal psychosis develops in about two in 1000 childbirths.

## Aetiology

The evidence seems to indicate that puerperal psychosis is most closely related to bipolar affective disorder (possibly depression). The relatives of patients with puerperal psychosis have a similar incidence of mood disorders as the relatives of patients with mood disorders. Patients with puerperal psychosis are also more likely to have a past psychiatric history of a mood disorder or have a family history of mental illness. Psychosocial factors seem less important, unlike in postnatal depression. Occasionally, a puerperal psychosis may be due to an obstetric complication (e.g. pre-eclampsia, puerperal infection) or medication. Figure 20.2 summarizes the risk factors for puerperal psychosis.

## Management

As with postnatal depression, the assessment of risk of infanticide and suicide on mental state examination is crucial. Concerning symptoms include:

| Risk factors for puerperal psychosis |
| --- |
| Previous puerperal psychosis |
| History of mood disorder |
| Family history of psychotic illness or mood disorder |
| Primiparous mother |
| Delivery associated with caesarean section or perinatal death |

Fig. 20.2 Risk factors for puerperal psychosis.

- Thoughts of self-harm or harming the baby.
- Severe depressive delusions (e.g. belief that the baby is, or should be, dead).
- Command hallucinations instructing the mother to harm herself or her baby.

Hospitalization is invariably necessary, with joint admissions to a mother-and-baby unit being indicated when the mother is able to look after her infant with some supervision; detention under mental health legislation may be necessary. The pharmacological treatment is the same as for other psychotic episodes, with antipsychotics, antidepressants and lithium, depending on the clinical presentation. Benzodiazepines may be needed in cases of severe behavioural disturbance. All psychotropic drugs should be used with caution in breast-feeding mothers (see Fig. 20.1); it is often advisable to bottle-feed. ECT is particularly effective in severe or treatment-resistant cases, irrespective of the clinical presentation.

Psychosocial interventions are similar to those for other psychotic episodes but also include providing support for the father.

## Prognosis

Most cases of puerperal psychosis will have recovered by 3 months – 75% within 6 weeks. There is about a 30% chance of experiencing a recurrence after future childbirths. Women who have had both puerperal and non-puerperal depressive or manic episodes (i.e. have an established mood disorder) have a 50–85% chance of future puerperal episodes.

The prevalence of postnatal blues, postnatal depression and puerperal psychosis is inversely related to their severity:
- Postnatal blues develops after one in two childbirths.
- Postnatal depression develops after one in eight childbirths.
- Puerperal psychosis develops after about one in 500 childbirths.

- What types of psychiatric symptoms occur in the premenstruum, pregnancy, the puerperium and the menopause?
- What types of symptoms occur in PMS and where do they occur in the menstrual cycle?
- What is the risk of mental illness following miscarriage and termination of pregnancy?
- What is the difference between pseudocyesis and couvade syndrome?
- What are the symptoms and management of postnatal blues?
- How does the aetiology of postnatal depression differ from the aetiology of postnatal blues and puerperal psychosis?
- How would you manage a woman with postnatal depression who wanted to continue breast-feeding?
- What factors on mental state examination would concern you when assessing risk in a woman with puerperal psychosis?
- How is puerperal psychosis related to bipolar affective disorder (with reference to clinical features and aetiology)?

## Suggested further reading

Burt V K, Stein K 2002 Epidemiology of depression throughout the female life cycle. Journal of Clinical Psychiatry 63(Suppl. 7): 9–15

Connolly M 2001 Premenstrual syndrome: an update on definitions, diagnosis and management. Advances in Psychiatric Treatment 7: 469–477

Cooper P J, Murray L 1998 Fortnightly review: postnatal depression. British Medical Journal 316(7148): 1884–1886

Misri S, Kostaras X 2000 Reproductive psychiatry: an overview. URL: http://www.medscape.com/viewprogram/138

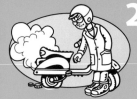

# 21. The Sleep Disorders

Sleeping is intimately related to mental health. Not only can psychiatric illnesses such as depression and schizophrenia disturb the quantity and quality of sleep, but certain psychiatric drugs can also have the same effect. Furthermore, persistent primary sleep disturbances, which are common, can result in significant psychological consequences in an otherwise mentally healthy individual.

## Definitions and classification

Sleep is divided into five distinct stages as measured by polysomnography (see later), which includes four stages of non-rapid eye movement (stages 1, 2, 3 and 4) and a rapid eye movement stage (REM). Figure 21.1 summarizes the key characteristics of the stages of sleep.

The DSM-IV organizes the sleep disorders into four sections according to their causes:
1. Primary sleep disorders.
2. Sleep disorders secondary to another mental illness.
3. Sleep disorders secondary to another medical condition.
4. Sleep disorders secondary to the use of a substance.

This chapter will focus principally on primary sleep disorders, which by definition are not caused by another medical condition (e.g. arthritis) or mental illness (e.g. depression) and do not occur secondary to the use of a substance (e.g. alcohol). These disorders are presumed to arise from some defect of an individual's endogenous sleeping mechanism (mainly hypothalamus) coupled with unhelpful learned behaviours (e.g. worrying about not sleeping).

The primary sleep disorders, in turn, are divided into the *dyssomnias* and the *parasomnias*:
1. The dyssomnias are characterized by abnormalities in the amount, quality or timing of sleep. They include primary insomnia, primary hypersomnia, narcolepsy, circadian rhythm sleep disorders and breathing-related sleep disorders.

2. The parasomnias are characterized by abnormal episodes that occur during sleep or sleep–wake transitions. They include nightmares, night terrors and sleepwalking.

## Insomnia

Insomnia describes sleep of insufficient quantity or poor quality due to:
- Difficulty in falling asleep.
- Frequent awakening during the course of sleep.
- Early morning awakening with subsequent difficulty getting back to sleep.
- Sleep that is not refreshing despite being adequate in length.

In addition to daytime tiredness, persistent insomnia can have significant effects on mood, behaviour and performance. Some researchers have suggested that insomnia may play a contributing or even causal role in some cases of depression. It has been shown that insomnia can also lead to an impairment of health-related quality of life similar to congestive cardiac failure or depression.

*Primary insomnia* is diagnosed when patients present with insomnia for at least a month not attributable to a medical condition, psychiatric disorder, use of a substance or other dyssomnia (e.g. circadian rhythm sleep disorder) or parasomnia.

The numerous causes of insomnia as summarized in Figure 21.2 include primary sleep disorders, medical and psychiatric illness and substance use.

### Assessment of insomnia

The assessment of insomnia involves excluding a medical, psychiatric or substance-related cause of insomnia. Many cases of primary insomnia are related to poor sleep hygiene (see Fig. 21.3). Therefore it is essential to enquire about sleeping times, daytime sleeping, drinking of coffee, erratic sleeping hours, etc. It is also useful to obtain collateral information from the patient's sleeping partner regarding sleeping patterns, snoring and movements during the night.

The following questions might be helpful in eliciting the key symptoms of insomnia:

| Stage of sleep | Duration spent in this phase during night | Characteristics and electroencephalogram (EEG) findings |
| --- | --- | --- |
| Stage 1 | 5% | • Transition from wakefulness to sleep<br>**EEG: theta waves**<br> 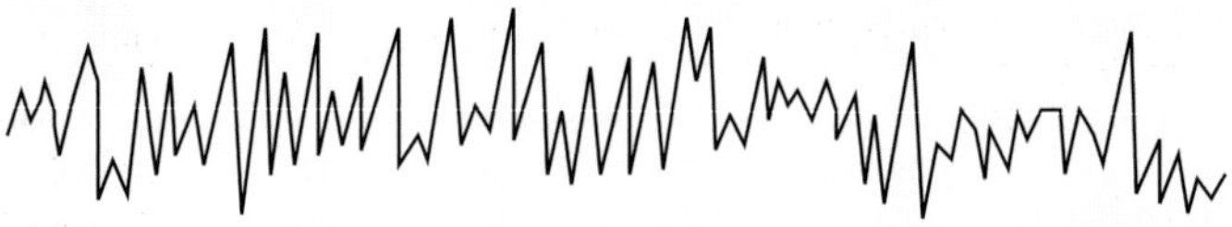<br>Theta waves: low amplitude, spike-like waves, 4–7Hz |
| Stage 2 | 45% | **EEG: sleep spindles and K-complexes** 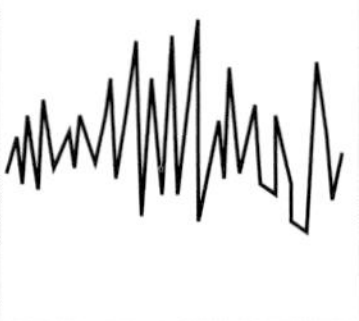<br><br>Sleep spindles: short rhythmic waveform clusters of 12–14Hz 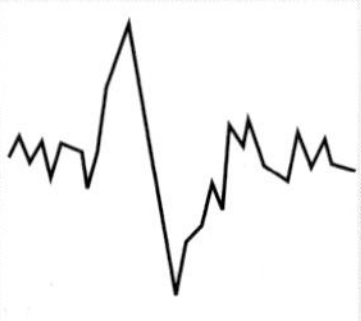  K-complex: sharp negative wave followed by a slower positive component |
| Stage 3 and 4 (Slow wave sleep) | 25% | • Deep sleep<br>• Unusual arousal characteristics: disorientation, sleep terrors, sleepwalking<br>• Occur in first third to half of night<br>**EEG: delta waves**<br>*Stage 3 – delta waves <50%*<br>*Stage 4 – delta waves >50%*<br> 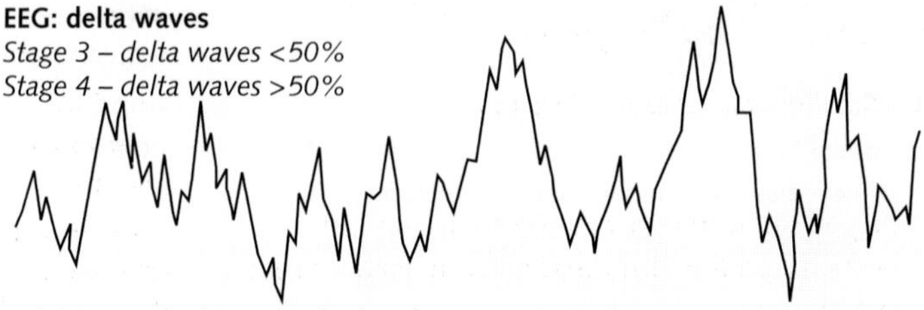<br>Delta waves: high amplitude, low frequency (<4Hz) |
| REM | 25% | • Occurs cyclically through the night, every 90 minutes alternating with non-REM sleep<br>• Each episode increases in duration – most episodes occur in last third of night<br>• Features penile erection, skeletal muscle paralysis, and surreal dreaming (including nightmares)<br>**EEG: low amplitude, high frequency, with saw-tooth waves**<br> 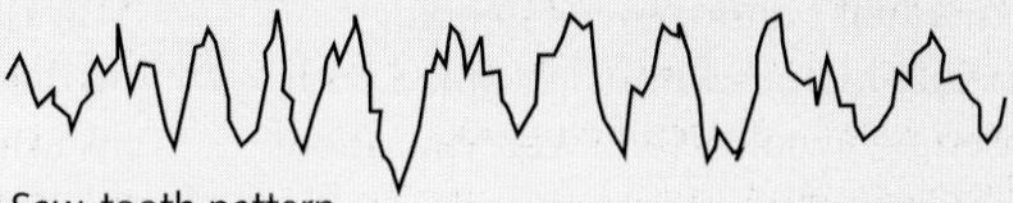<br>Saw-tooth pattern |

**Fig. 21.1** Stages of sleep.

• Do you fall asleep quickly or do you find yourself tossing and turning for some time before dropping off?

• Do you wake up repeatedly in the night or can you sleep through once you have managed to get to sleep?

| Common causes of insomnia |
| --- |

**Primary sleep disorders**
- Dyssomnias
  a. Primary insomnia
  b. Circadian rhythm sleep disorders (jet-lag, shift-work)
  c. Breathing-related sleep disorders (sleep apnoea syndromes)
- Parasomnias (all)

**Psychiatric**
- Anxiety
- Depression
- Mania
- Schizophrenia

**Medical**
- Painful conditions (malignancies, arthritis, reflux disease)
- Cardiorespiratory discomfort (dyspnoea, coughing, palpitations)
- Nocturia (prostatism, urinary tract infections)
- Metabolic or endocrine conditions (thyroid disease, renal or liver failure)
- Central nervous system lesion (especially brainstem and hypothalamus)

**Substances**
- Caffeine and other stimulants
- Alcohol
- Prescribed drugs (e.g. SSRIs, some antipsychotics)
- Substance withdrawal syndrome

**Fig. 21.2** Common causes of insomnia.

| Correct sleep hygiene |
| --- |

- Avoid sleeping during the day
- Exercise during the day and maintain a healthy diet
- Eliminate the use of stimulants (e.g. caffeine, nicotine, alcohol), especially around bedtime
- Condition the brain by only using the bed for sleeping and sex – not for reading, watching TV, etc.
- Go to bed and awaken at the same time each day
- Avoid stimulating activities before bedtime (e.g. television, games). Instead, engage in relaxation techniques or reading
- Try having a hot bath or drinking a cup of warm milk near bedtime
- Avoid large meals near bedtime
- Ensure that the bed is comfortable and that the bedroom is quiet
- Do not lie in bed awake for longer than 15 minutes. Get up and do another relaxing activity and try sleeping later

**Fig. 21.3** Correct sleep hygiene.

- Do you sometimes awaken too early in the morning and then find that you are unable to get back to sleep?
- Is your sleep refreshing or do you still feel tired in the morning?

In treatment-resistant cases it might be necessary to refer the patient to a sleep specialist for further investigation. *Polysomnography* is the simultaneous process of monitoring multiple electrophysiological parameters during sleep. Tests include the electroencephalogram (EEG), electrocardiogram (ECG), electromyogram, electrooculogram (eye movement), blood oxygen saturation, chest and abdominal excursion, mouth and nose air entry rates and the loudness of snoring.

## Management of primary insomnia
It follows that the most important aspect of management is providing education about correct sleep hygiene. Sleep hygiene, which is described in Figure 21.3, includes a number of non-specific, non-pharmacological measures that should lead to an improvement in sleep.

There is a limited role for medication in the treatment of primary insomnia. Insomnia associated with depression may be helped by an antidepressant with sedative properties (e.g. mirtazapine, trazodone, amitriptyline). Hypnotics may help with sleep in the short term, but the development of tolerance to their effects (usually within 2 weeks), possible dependence and their propensity to cause rebound insomnia limit their use. Therefore, they should only be prescribed on a time-limited basis, ideally for use on alternate or occasional nights rather than every night. Short-acting benzodiazepines (e.g. temazepam) are preferred, as they do not leave patients feeling drowsy the next day and do not accumulate with repeated doses. The related short-acting compounds: zopiclone, zolpidem and zaleplon, which act on receptors similar to the benzodiazepines, are also very effective in the short term. Note, however, that they are also associated with the rapid development of tolerance and possible dependence.

## Hypersomnia and narcolepsy
Hypersomnia describes excessive sleepiness that manifests as either a prolonged period of sleep or sleep episodes that occur during normal waking hours.

*Primary hypersomnia* is diagnosed when patients present with hypersomnia for at least a month not attributable to a medical condition, psychiatric

133

There is a considerable inter-individual variation in normal sleep duration. Some individuals, termed 'short sleepers', require less sleep than average. They fall asleep quickly and do not suffer from intermittent awakening or daytime fatigue. Some of them may attempt to prolong their sleeping time, which may resemble a primary insomnia.

disorder, use of a substance or other dyssomnia (especially narcolepsy and sleep apnoea) or parasomnia.

*Narcolepsy* is seen as a neurological condition, mainly due to an abnormality of the REM-inhibiting mechanism and is characterized by a tetrad of:

1. Irresistible attacks of refreshing sleep that may occur at inappropriate times (e.g. driving).
2. Cataplexy (sudden, bilateral loss of muscle tone usually precipitated by intense emotion leading to collapse, and lasting for seconds to minutes).
3. Hypnagogic or hypnopompic hallucinations (see p. 23).
4. Sleep paralysis at the beginning or end of sleep episodes.

Patients usually have 2–6 episodes of sleep per day which usually last 10–20 minutes. Hypnagogic/hypnopompic hallucinations and the paralysis of voluntary muscles occur as a result of elements of REM sleep intruding into the transition between sleep and wakefulness. All four symptoms occur in less than 50% of cases and the diagnosis is usually made with evidence of sleep attacks and cataplexy. Other features may include persistent tiredness (narcoleptics often experience broken sleep) and problems with memory and concentration.

The numerous causes of hypersomnia as summarized in Figure 21.4 include primary sleep disorders, medical and psychiatric illness, substance use and sleep deprivation.

The *treatment* of primary hypersomnia is usually with stimulants such as dexamphetamine and methylphenidate. The treatment of narcolepsy includes taking forced naps at regular times. In some cases, stimulants are needed to reduce daytime sleepiness; tricyclic antidepressants increase muscle tone and may help to control cataplexy and sleep paralysis.

### Common causes of hypersomnia

**Primary sleep disorders**
- Dyssomnias
  a. Primary hypersomnia
  b. Narcolepsy
  c. Breathing-related sleep disorders (sleep apnoea syndromes)
  d. Circadian rhythm sleep disorders (jet-lag, shift-work)
- Parasomnias (all)
Psychiatric
- Depression with atypical features

**Medical**
- Encephalitis and meningitis
- Stroke, head injury, space occupying lesion
- Degenerative neurological conditions
- Toxic, metabolic or endocrine abnormalities
- Kleine–Levin syndrome

**Substances**
- Alcohol
- Prescribed drugs (e.g. antipsychotics, benzodiazepines, tricyclic antidepressants)
- Substance withdrawal syndrome

**Secondary to insomnia or sleep deprivation**

**Fig. 21.4** Common causes of hypersomnia.

Insomnia is a common complaint in depression; however, only early morning awakening is part of the *somatic syndrome* (see p. 4) of depression. A fifth of depressed patients may experience hypersomnia. Increased appetite or weight gain and hypersomnia may be referred to as atypical depressive features.

## Circadian rhythm sleep disorders

Circadian rhythm sleep disorder (sleep–wake schedule disorder) is characterized by a lack of synchrony between an individual's endogenous circadian rhythm for sleep and that demanded by their environment, resulting in their being tired when they should be awake (hypersomnia) and being awake when they should be sleeping (insomnia). This disorder results from either a malfunction of the internal 'biological clock' that regulates sleep or from an unnatural environmental change (e.g. jet lag, night-shift work). Individuals with *delayed sleep phase syndrome (DSPS)*, have a normal length of sleep, but the timing of sleep and wakefulness is set later than other individuals from the same environment. DSPS often occurs in adolescents when a pattern of going to bed late is established (late-night social activities combined with caffeine, nicotine, alcohol), which resets the biological clock to a later time. Awakening at a time to meet daily commitments becomes excruciatingly difficult and daytime drowsiness ensues.

## Breathing-related sleep disorders

These disorders feature a repeated disruption of sleep due to abnormalities of ventilation during sleep. This results in unrefreshing sleep and excessive sleepiness during the day. *Obstructive sleep apnoea syndrome*, the most common breathing-related sleep disorder, is characterized by obstruction of the upper airways during sleep, in spite of an adequate respiratory effort. Typically, an individual will have noisy breathing during sleep with loud snoring interspersed with apnoeic episodes lasting from 20 to 90 seconds, sometimes associated with cyanosis. It is not an uncommon condition, affecting 4% of middle-aged men, 2% of adult women and 1% of children. The prevalence is much higher in obese, elderly or hypertensive individuals and is also prominent in some forms of mental retardation, e.g. Down's syndrome. This illness has significant cardiovascular and neuropsychiatric morbidity and should be actively excluded when an at-risk patient presents with hypersomnia, impairment of concentration and memory or other psychiatric symptoms. Collateral history from a bed-partner, who is often aware of the sleeping difficulties, can be extremely useful in this regard.

Many primary sleep problems often present with psychiatric symptoms that are misdiagnosed as primary psychiatric illnesses and treated symptomatically. For example, depression is one of the conditions for which patients are sometimes treated before their obstructive sleep apnoea syndrome is correctly diagnosed.

## Sleep terrors (night terrors)

Sleep terrors are episodes that feature an individual (usually a child) abruptly waking from sleep, usually with a scream, appearing to be in a state of extreme terror and panic. These episodes are associated with:

- Autonomic arousal, e.g. tachycardia, dilated pupils, sweating and rapid breathing.
- A relative unresponsiveness to the efforts of others to comfort the person, who appears confused and disorientated.

Upon full awakening, there is amnesia for the episode and no recall of any dream or nightmare. Sleep terrors last from 1 to 10 minutes, and usually occur during slow wave sleep (stage 3 and 4) and are therefore predominant in the first third of the night. Sleep terrors are seen in up to 6% of children aged 4–12 and usually resolve by adolescence. Sleepwalking and sleep terrors seem to be related conditions as they share clinical and aetiological similarities. Sleep terrors should be distinguished from nightmares and epileptic seizures, although seizures seldom occur during sleep.

## Nightmares

Between 10% and 50% of children aged 3–5 experience repeated nightmares, although they occur occasionally in up to 50% of adults. Nightmares are characterized by an individual waking from sleep due to an intensely frightening dream involving threats to survival, security or self-esteem. Nightmares are distinguished from sleep terrors by the observation that not only is the individual alert and orientated immediately after awakening but is also able to recall the dream in vivid detail. Furthermore, nightmares tend to occur during the second half of the night because they arise almost exclusively during REM sleep, which tends to be longer and have more intense, surreal dreaming during the latter part of the night.

## Sleepwalking (somnambulism)

Sleepwalking is characterized by an unusual state of consciousness in which complex motor behaviour, including walking around, occurs during sleep. While sleepwalking, the individual has a blank staring face and is relatively unresponsive to the communicative efforts of others and is difficult to awaken. When sleepwalkers do wake up, either during an episode or the following morning, they have no recollection of the event ever having occurred and have no impairment of cognition or behaviour, although they may have an initial brief period of disorientation subsequent to waking up from a sleepwalking episode. Sleepwalking usually occurs during slow wave sleep (stage 3 and 4) and is therefore predominant in the first third of the night. The peak prevalence of sleepwalking occurs at the age of 12, with an onset between the age of 4 and 8 years.

About 2–3% of children and about 0.5% of adults have regular episodes. Sleepwalking runs in families with 80% of sleepwalkers having a positive family history for sleepwalking or sleep terrors.

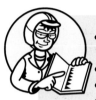

- What are the differences between slow wave (stages 3 and 4) and REM sleep and what parasomnias are they associated with?
- What are the three main causes of secondary sleep disorders?
- What non-pharmacological strategies may be used to treat primary insomnia?
- What is the role of the benzodiazepines in treating primary insomnia?
- What are the four characteristic symptoms of narcolepsy?
- How do circadian rhythm sleep disorders cause hypersomnia?
- Name four risk factors for obstructive sleep apnoea syndrome.
- How do you distinguish between nightmares and night terrors (sleep terrors)?

## Suggested further reading

Stores G 2003 Misdiagnosing sleep disorders as primary psychiatric conditions. Advances in Psychiatric Treatment 9: 69–77

Doghramji K 2000 Sleepless in America: diagnosing and treating insomnia. URL: http://www.medscape.com/viewprogram/347

Doghramji K 1999 Clinical frontiers in the sleep/psychiatry interface. URL: http://www.medscape.com/viewprogram/689

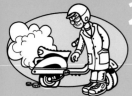

# 22. The Psychosexual Disorders

Healthy sexual functioning requires a healthy body and, perhaps more importantly, a healthy mind and relationship. Physical or psychological problems or, as is often the case, a combination of the two can cause a wide variety of sexual problems. Mental health workers may be consulted about sexual problems that are largely due to intrapsychic or inter-personal conflicts (not predominantly due to a biological problem) – i.e. psychosexual problems.

The psychosexual disorders can be classified into three groups:
- Sexual dysfunction.
- Disorders of sexual preference (paraphilias).
- Gender identity disorders.

Women have a large inter-individual variability in the type, and duration, of stimulation that results in orgasm. The diagnosis of female orgasmic disorder should only be made if the ability to achieve orgasm is less than would be reasonably expected for a woman's age, sexual experience and quality of sexual activity – and then only if the orgasmic dysfunction results in marked distress or relationship difficulties.

## Sexual dysfunction

### Clinical features

Following the original description by Masters and Johnson, the DSM-IV describes the sequence of psychological and physiological responses to sexual stimulation in a four-phase sexual response cycle, which is summarized in Figure 22.1.

*Sexual dysfunctions* describe abnormalities of the sexual response cycle or pain associated with sexual intercourse that lead to difficulties in participating in sexual relationships. Although this chapter is focused on psychosexual or psychogenic sexual dysfunction, the sexual response cycle consists of both psychological and biological processes and it is rarely possible to identify cases with a purely organic or purely psychogenic aetiology. Nevertheless, both the ICD-10 and the DSM-IV stipulate that a sexual dysfunction disorder should only be diagnosed when there is a suspected psychogenic component to the problem, i.e. it should not be due exclusively to a medical condition or use of a substance. Figure 22.2 summarizes the sexual dysfunction disorders.

### Epidemiology

A comprehensive survey was conducted in the USA on a representative sample of 3159 people between the ages of 18 and 59. The findings indicate that sexual dysfunction is very common with a prevalence of about 43% in women and 31% in men. The reported frequency of specific sexual dysfunction is shown in Figure 22.3. Further findings from the same study include:
- The prevalence of sexual problems in women tends to decrease with increasing age except for those who report trouble lubricating.
- Men, in contrast, have an increased prevalence of erectile problems and lack of interest in sex with increasing age.
- Sexual dysfunction is more likely among people with poor physical and emotional health.
- Sexual dysfunction is highly associated with negative experiences in sexual relationships.
- Married individuals and those with high educational attainment are at a lower risk of experiencing sexual dysfunction.

### Aetiology

There are many, often interrelated, psychosocial factors that may result in psychogenic sexual dysfunction:
- Ambivalent attitude about sex or intimacy (anxiety, fear, guilt, shame).
- History of rape or childhood sexual abuse.
- Fears of consequences of sex, e.g. impregnation, sexually transmitted diseases.

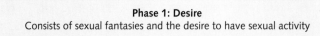

---

**Phase 1: Desire**
Consists of sexual fantasies and the desire to have sexual activity

↓

**Phase 2: Excitement**
Consists of the subjective sense of sexual pleasure and the accompanying physiological changes (e.g. erection in the man; vaginal lubrication in the woman)

↓

**Phase 3: Orgasm**
Consists of the peaking of sexual pleasure, release of sexual tension and rhythmic contraction of the perineal muscles and pelvic reproductive organs (men: sensation of ejaculatory inevitably followed by ejaculation; women: contractions of outer third of vagina)

↓

**Phase 4: Resolution**
Consists of a sense of muscular relaxation and general well being. Men are refractory to further erection and orgasm for a period of time. Women may be able to have multiple orgasms.

**Fig. 22.1** The DSM-IV's four-phase sexual response cycle.

| Sexual dysfunction disorders | | |
|---|---|---|
| **Phase of cycle** | **Dysfunction*** | **Description** |
| Desire | Lack or loss of sexual desire [Hypoactive sexual desire disorder] | Loss of desire to have or fantasize about sex – not due to other sexual dysfunction (e.g. erectile dysfunction, dyspareunia) |
| | Sexual aversion and lack of sexual enjoyment [Sexual aversion disorder] | Avoidance of sex due to negative feelings (fear, anxiety, repulsion), or lack of enjoyment |
| Excitement | Failure of genital response [Male erectile disorder; Female sexual arousal disorder] | Inability to attain or maintain sexual intercourse due to an inadequate erection in men, or poor lubrication–swelling response in women |
| Orgasm | Orgasmic dysfunction [Male/female orgasmic disorder] | Recurrent absence or delay of orgasm or ejaculation despite adequate sexual stimulation |
| | Premature ejaculation [Premature ejaculation] | Recurrent ejaculation with minimal sexual stimulation before the man wishes |
| Sexual pain | Nonorganic dyspareunia [Dyspareunia not due to a general medical condition] | Genital pain during sex in men or women – not due to other sexual dysfunction (e.g. poor lubrication–swelling response, vaginismus) or medical condition (e.g. atrophic vaginitis) |
| | Vaginismus [Vaginismus not due to a general medical condition] | Recurrent, involuntary spasm of the muscles that surround the outer third of the vagina, causing occlusion of the vaginal opening |

*The DSM-IV terms are in parentheses; the ICD-10 terms are not

**Fig. 22.2** Sexual dysfunction disorders.

| Reported frequency of sexual dysfunction in Americans aged 18-59 years | | |
|---|---|---|
| Men | Premature ejaculation | 31% |
| | Lack of sexual interest | 15% |
| | Erectile difficulties | 10% |
| | Unable to achieve orgasm | 10% |
| Women | Lack of sexual interest | 32% |
| | Unable to achieve orgasm | 26% |
| | Trouble lubricating | 21% |
| | Dyspareunia | 16% |

**Fig. 22.3** Reported frequency of sexual dysfunction in Americans aged 18–59 years. (Data from Laumann EO et al 1999 Sexual Dysfunction in the United States: prevalence and predictors. JAMA 281: 537–544)

- A poor or deteriorating relationship. This includes feeling undesirable or finding the partner undesirable; lack of trust; feelings of resentment or hostility, lack of respect, fear of rejection, etc.
- Anxiety about sexual performance or physical attractiveness.
- Fatigue, stress or difficult psychosocial circumstances.

Frequently, there is more than one psychosocial problem that can affect more than one of the phases of the sexual response cycle. For example, the belief that sex is inherently sinful, in the context of an abusive relationship may lead to a lack of desire, a poor lubrication–swelling response and difficulty in reaching orgasm.

## Differential diagnosis

Other causes of sexual dysfunction should be excluded when assessing a patient with sexual dysfunction. These include:

- Medical conditions, e.g. diabetes mellitus, vascular disease, vaginitis, endometriosis, trauma or radical surgery (pelvic fractures, spinal cord injuries, prostatectomy), multiple sclerosis, thyroid disease, hyperprolactinaemia, etc.
- Prescribed or illicit drugs. See Figure 22.4.
- Psychiatric illness: mental disorders such as depression, anxiety and alcohol dependence are frequently associated with sexual dysfunction.

In addition, psychiatric medication often results in sexual dysfunction as a side-effect. However, sexual functioning frequently improves as the patient's mental illness (e.g. depression) improves, even though the medication (e.g. antidepressants) may have adverse sexual effects.

 The finding that patients have a clear biological component to their sexual dysfunction does not rule out a psychogenic sexual dysfunction, as the two are often interrelated. For example, a 55-year-old man with diabetes and advanced atherosclerosis notices a weakened erection; he subsequently becomes anxious during sex, fearing that he is losing his virility. This leads to a complete loss of his erectile potency.

## Assessment considerations

- The wide differential diagnosis requires a comprehensive history including medical, psychiatric, sexual and relationship histories as well as current medication and recreational substance use.

**Prescribed and recreational drugs associated with sexual dysfunction**

**Psychiatric drugs**
- Antidepressants (tricyclics, SSRIs and MAOIs)
- Antipsychotics (especially typical antipsychotics)
  - Benzodiazepines
  - Lithium

**Recreational drugs**
- Alcohol
- Amfetamines
- Cannabis
- Cocaine
- Opiates

**Medical drugs**
- Anticonvulsants
- Antihistamines
- Antihypertensives (including beta-blockers)
- Digoxin
- Diuretics

**Fig. 22.4** Prescribed and recreational drugs associated with sexual dysfunction.

- In addition to a thorough physical examination including genitalia, the investigation of dyspareunia or vaginismus in women requires specialist gynaecological examination (e.g. endometriosis, atrophic vaginitis).
- In addition to indicated blood tests (e.g. thyroid functions, fasting glucose, liver and renal functions, prolactin, testosterone, sex hormone binding globulin), special investigations are performed to exclude medical causes of sexual dysfunction, e.g. monitoring of nocturnal penile tumescence (excludes organic causes of impotence if able to have erection during REM sleep) and monitoring penile blood flow (internal pudendal artery) with Doppler ultrasonography.

## Management considerations

- Many patients may need no more than reassurance, advice and sex education. Furthermore, patients who have significant relationship difficulties may be advised to engage in relationship counselling (e.g. Relate) or marital therapy before attempting specific treatment for sexual dysfunction.
- Some couples with minor problems benefit from self-help instruction manuals (bibliotherapy) and videotapes, particularly those with no major relationship difficulties.
- Urology clinics deal mainly with organic sexual dysfunction, particularly erectile problems.
- Sexual dysfunction clinics have multidisciplinary teams that focus on both psychological and physical aspects of sexual dysfunction and are best equipped to deal with cases that do not respond to non-specific measures.
- Some couples benefit from sex therapy, in which partners are treated together and are taught to communicate freely about sex, in addition to receiving education about sexual anatomy and the physiology of the sexual response cycle. They also take part in graded assignments, beginning with caressing of their partner's body, without genital contact, for their own and then their partner's pleasure (Sensate Focus: Masters & Johnson 1970). These behavioural tasks progress through a number of stages with increasing sexual intimacy, with the focus remaining on pleasurable physical contact as opposed to the monitoring of sexual arousal or the preoccupation with achieving orgasm. Couples suitable for sex therapy include those with a significant psychological component to their problem, those with reasonable motivation and those with a reasonably harmonious relationship.
- Figure 22.5 summarizes some of the specific exercises often used in the context of sex therapy that may be helpful with particular problems.
- Biological treatments may be very effective, especially for erectile problems (e.g. oral sildenafil (Viagra®), intracavernosal injections (prostaglandin E1), vacuum devices, prosthetic implants and surgery for venous leakage). Testosterone may increase sexual drive in patients with low levels. SSRIs and tricyclic antidepressants may delay ejaculation, but this is rarely a long-term solution.

## Prognosis

Vaginismus has an excellent prognosis. Premature ejaculation and psychogenic erectile dysfunction also respond fairly well to treatment. Problems associated with poor sexual desire, especially in men, seem more resistant to treatment.

| Specific exercises useful in sexual dysfunction | |
|---|---|
| **Sexual dysfunction** | **Exercise** |
| Female orgasmic disorder | Exercises in sexual fantasy and masturbation, sometimes with a vibrator |
| Premature ejaculation | Squeeze technique: woman squeezes the glans of her partner's penis for a few seconds when he feels that he is about to ejaculate |
| | Start-stop method: stimulation is halted and arousal is allowed to subside when the man feels that ejaculation is imminent. The process is then repeated |
| | Quiet vagina: man keeps penis motionless in vagina for increasing periods before ejaculating |
| Vaginismus | Desensitization, first by finger insertion followed by dilators of increasing size |

**Fig. 22.5** Specific exercises useful in sexual dysfunction.

## Disorders of sexual preference (paraphilias)

The DSM-IV describes the essential features of a paraphilia as recurrent, intensely sexually arousing fantasies, sexual urges or behaviours involving: (1) non-human objects; (2) the suffering or humiliation of oneself or one's partner; or (3) children or other non-consenting individuals. It is useful to divide the paraphilias into two groups:

1. Abnormalities of the *object* of sexual interest, e.g. paedophilia, fetishism, transvestic fetishism.
2. Abnormalities of the *sexual act*, e.g. exhibitionism, voyeurism, sexual sadism, sexual masochism.

Figure 22.6 summarizes the specific paraphilias.

The paraphilias are mainly confined to men (with the exception of sexual masochism) and usually begin in late adolescence or early adulthood and tend to be chronic. Paedophilia and exhibitionism are frequently seen in a forensic setting and account for the majority of sexual offenders referred for a psychiatric opinion.

The aetiology is unknown, but there is often an impaired capacity for affectionate sexual activity and paraphilics frequently have diagnosable personality disorders.

Treatment options include behaviour therapy, e.g. covert sensitization, where patients attempt to pair paraphilic thoughts with humiliating consequences; and aversion therapy which involves pairing paraphilic thoughts with a noxious stimulus such as an unpleasant odour or taste. Individual psychodynamic and group therapies are also used. Cognitive-behavioural therapy programmes and anti-androgens (e.g. cyproterone acetate) have shown some efficacy in the treatment of some paedophiles and exhibitionists; however, there is little evidence that any treatment is consistently effective in either of these conditions.

Paraphilias associated with a young age of onset, a high frequency of acts, no remorse about acts and a lack of motivation for change have a particularly poor prognosis.

| The paraphilias | |
|---|---|
| **Abnormalities of the object of sexual interest** | |
| Paedophilia | Sexual fantasies, urges or behaviours involving prepubertal children |
| Fetishism | Sexual fantasies, urges or behaviours involving inanimate objects or parts of the body that are not directly erogenous |
| Transvestic fetishism | Sexual fantasies, urges or behaviours involving cross-dressing (wearing of clothes of the opposite sex). Rare in women |
| Zoophilia (bestiality) | Sexual fantasies, urges or behaviours involving animals |
| Necrophilia | Sexual fantasies, urges or behaviours involving corpses |
| **Abnormalities of the sexual act** | |
| Exhibitionism | Sexual fantasies, urges or behaviours involving the exposure of genitals to unsuspecting strangers |
| Voyeurism | Sexual fantasies, urges or behaviours involving the act of observing unsuspecting people engaging in sexual activity or undressing |
| Sexual sadism | Sexual fantasies, urges or behaviours involving the infliction of acts of physical or psychological suffering or humiliation on others |
| Sexual masochism | Sexual fantasies, urges or behaviours involving the infliction of acts of humiliation or suffering on oneself |

**Fig. 22.6** The paraphilias.

## Gender identity disorders

*Gender identity* describes an individual's inner sense of being male or female. This usually corresponds to an individual's *sexual identity*, which comprises all an individual's biological and anatomic sexual characteristics, i.e. external genitalia, internal genitalia, chromosomes, sex hormones and secondary sex characteristics. *Sexual orientation* describes the preferred gender of an individual's sexual desires, i.e. heterosexual (opposite sex), homosexual (same sex) and bisexual (both sexes).

An individual whose gender identity does not correspond to his or her sexual identity has a *gender identity disorder*. This is a DSM-IV term; the ICD-10 term for the same disorder is *transsexualism*. Gender identity disorder or transsexualism is characterized by:

- A desire to live and be accepted as a member of the opposite sex (may include cross-dressing and attempts at passing as the opposite sex).
- A strong sense of discomfort with, or inappropriateness of, one's own anatomic sex (may include attempts to minimize or remove one's primary and secondary sexual characteristics, e.g. hormone therapy, surgery).

Gender identity disorder in children may manifest as a strong desire to participate in the typical games that are played by the opposite sex, cross-sex roles in make-believe play and a preference for playmates of the opposite sex.

At clinic centres the male-to-female ratio is about 3:1. The cause of this condition is unknown. There is no convincing evidence of abnormalities in genetic make-up, upbringing or endocrine function. However, a minority of men with transvestic fetishism may progress to transsexualism after many years, coinciding with diminishing sexual arousal from cross-dressing.

The treatment of gender identity disorder requires specialist care. Patients who are committed to gender change may be helped with hormones and surgery, usually after they have completed a 'real life test', which involves living as the opposite sex for at least a year. The success of gender reassignment surgery in terms of long-term outcome is not conclusive.

Do not confuse transsexualism with transvestic fetishism. In transsexualism, individuals cross-dress in an attempt to live and be accepted as a member of the opposite sex; whereas in transvestic fetishism, individuals are sexually aroused by cross-dressing, but are content with their gender identity. Note that in a small minority of cases, transvestic fetishism may progress to transsexualism

- How is sexual dysfunction classified in relation to the four-phase sexual response cycle?
- What are the three most common sexual dysfunctions in men and women respectively?
- How does age, physical and relationship health and educational achievement affect sexual functioning?
- How may antidepressants worsen and improve sexual functioning?
- What are the principles of sex therapy and which type of couples are most suitable?
- What three techniques may be useful in treating premature ejaculation?
- What biological treatments may be very effective in erectile dysfunction?
- Which sexual dysfunctions have the best prognosis?
- Which two paraphilias are most often seen in forensic settings and how do they differ in terms of their classification?
- Which interventions have shown limited efficacy in the treatment of paraphilias?
- How does transsexualism differ from transvestic fetishism and how may they be associated?

## Suggested further reading

Baldwin D, Mayers A 2003 Sexual side-effects of antidepressant and antipsychotic drugs. Advances in Psychiatric Treatment 9: 202–210

Di Ceglie D 2000 Gender identity disorder in young people. Advances in Psychiatric Treatment 6: 458–466

Hawton K 1995 Treatment of sexual dysfunctions by sex therapy and other approaches. British Journal of Psychiatry 167: 307–314

Padma-Nathan H 2001 Challenges and solutions in the treatment of erectile dysfunction. URL: http://www.medscape.com/viewprogram/603

Phanjoo A L 2000 Sexual dysfunction in old age. Advances in Psychiatric Treatment 6: 270–277

# 23. Child and Adolescent Psychiatry

Children are often not able to verbalize any psychological symptoms they might have in explicit terms. In fact 'the problem' is usually brought to the psychiatrist's attention by someone else, e.g. parent, schoolteacher, paediatrician. Therefore the presenting problem is invariably a complaint about the child's abnormal behaviour or performance rather than their psychological symptoms. Inevitably, this means that the clinician is presented with a non-specific presentation (e.g. 'being disruptive in the classroom').

Furthermore, problems need to be seen in the context of a child's developmental stage; for example, 'temper tantrums' are normal for a 2-year-old child, but should have subsided by age 5.

## Considerations in the assessment of children

- Parents or carers usually accompany children and young adolescents. It is often useful to first interview them, with or without the child present, to obtain a full description of the current concerns as well as complete psychiatric, neurodevelopmental, educational and medical history. An indirect evaluation of the parents' personalities, marital relationship and style of parenting often creates another perspective from which to understand the context of the 'presenting complaint'.
- An interview with the child usually follows. The explicit information gathered from this interview will depend on the age of the child. Younger children may not be able to articulate their inner experiences; therefore, it is often necessary to observe them in play situations.
- The obtaining of collateral information is extremely important in fully understanding the development of the presenting problem and the child's premorbid functioning. It includes obtaining academic, educational or psychological reports as well as discussions with teachers and any other involved agencies.
- Further information can be obtained from structured and semi-structured interviews (e.g.

Kiddie Schedule for Affective Disorders and Schizophrenia (K-SADS-P); Diagnostic Interview Schedule for Children (NIMH-DISC-IV)), and parent/teacher rating scales.

## Classification

The ICD-10 groups the psychiatric disorders in children and adolescents into four broad categories:
1. Mental retardation (learning disability).
2. Developmental disorders (specific and pervasive).
3. Acquired disorders with onset usually in childhood or adolescence.
4. Acquired 'adult' disorders with onset in childhood or adolescence.

Figure 23.1 provides an overview of the conceptual framework for the disorders of childhood and adolescence.

## Mental retardation (learning disability)

### Definition and diagnosis
Mental retardation is the umbrella term used to describe a group of individuals who have suffered an interruption in the normal development of the brain, from any possible cause, that leads to *subaverage intellectual functioning* and thus an *impaired ability to adapt* to the normal demands of daily living. Mental retardation usually presents in early childhood and is a lifelong condition.

Intellectual functioning is usually defined by the intelligence quotient (IQ), which is assessed by standardized intelligence tests (e.g. Wechsler Intelligence Scales for Children). An IQ of 70 or below, which is about two standard deviations below the mean, is said to represent subaverage intellectual functioning.

Adaptive functioning is a measure of how patients cope with tasks of living such as communication, self-care, social skills, and academic and vocational

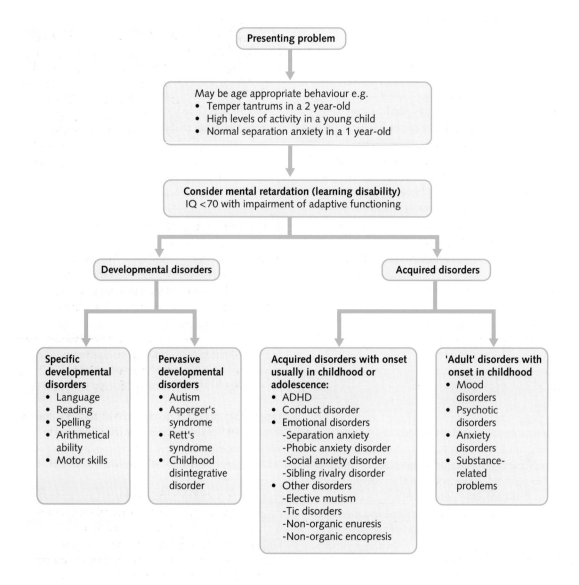

**Fig. 23.1** Conceptual framework for the disorders of childhood and adolescence.

skills. This is assessed by a thorough developmental, psychiatric and medical history from the patient's parents in addition to reports from teachers and other care providers. Standardized scales measuring adaptive functioning should be used whenever possible (e.g. Vinelands Adaptive Behaviour Scale).

It is important to remember the limitations of using standardized testing instruments and scales. Differences in sociocultural background and native language as well as sensory, motor or communication handicaps may lead to patients obtaining falsely low IQ scores. Therefore, patients obtaining IQ scores lower than 70 should not be diagnosed as having mental retardation if there is no

Whereas dementia describes a loss of cognitive ability already acquired, mental retardation usually describes the failure to develop a normal level of cognitive functioning in the first place. Note that individuals with mental retardation due to Down's syndrome are at very high risk for developing Alzheimer's disease in later life.

146

evidence of significant impairments in adaptive functioning.

## Classification and clinical features

The ICD-10 specifies mental retardation as mild, moderate, severe and profound according to the degree of intellectual and adaptive impairment. Figure 23.2 summarizes the clinical features of the degrees of mental retardation. In addition to the impairment of adaptive functioning, patients may have clinical features associated with the specific cause of their mental retardation (e.g. Down's syndrome: epicanthic folds with oblique palpebral fissures, broad hands with single transverse palmar crease, flattened occiput, cardiac septal defects). Other features associated with mental retardation include aggression, self-injurious behaviours, repetitive stereotypical motor movements and poor impulse control.

Many clinicians in the UK prefer the term *learning disability* to the term *mental retardation*, which is used in both the ICD-10 and DSM-IV; others prefer the term *mental handicap*. The varying use of these terms probably does more to confuse than to prevent the unfortunate stigmatization of these patients. For examination purposes, the term *learning disability* is probably more politically correct.

## Epidemiology and aetiology

- The prevalence of mental retardation in the general population is about 1–2%.
- The male-to-female ratio is approximately 1.5:1.
- 85% of cases are mild (see Fig. 23.2).

In 30–40% of cases of mental retardation no clear aetiology can be determined and patients with mild mental retardation may represent the lower end of a normal distribution curve for intellectual functioning. Specific causes, however, are likely to be found in patients with severe or profound mental retardation. Remember that mental retardation is a descriptive term and should still be used regardless of whether patients have a specific psychiatric or physical cause for their intellectual impairment or not (e.g. autism, Down's syndrome). Figure 23.3 lists the potential identifiable causes of mental retardation.

The DSM-IV uses a multi-axial diagnostic system that separates Axis I conditions (major mental illnesses, e.g. psychotic and mood disorders), Axis II conditions (personality disorders and mental retardation) and Axis III conditions (general medical conditions) so that all three areas potentially requiring clinical attention are considered.

## Management and prognosis

Prevention of mental retardation includes:

- Improved perinatal and child healthcare.
- Early detection of metabolic abnormalities, which, if left untreated, can lead to mental retardation (e.g. neonatal hypothyroidism, phenylketonuria).
- Genetic counselling, amniocentesis and chorionic villus sampling with the option of therapeutic abortion in pregnant women over the age of 35 or those with a family history of genetic disorders.

Intellectual functioning does not improve in most cases of mental retardation. However, adaptive functioning may improve with:

- Comprehensive educational and vocational programmes.
- Family education and support.
- Behaviour therapy for behavioural difficulties (aggressive and destructive behaviours).
- In some cases, medication may be helpful in managing aggressive and destructive behaviour (antipsychotics, benzodiazepines, lithium, carbamazepine).
- Appropriate residential placement.
- Treatment of co-morbid psychiatric and medical conditions.

The prevalence of other psychiatric disorders (e.g. schizophrenia, depression) is 3–4 times higher in patients with mental retardation than in the general population. Therefore, it is important to exclude these whenever there is a change in a patient's behaviour pattern.

| Degrees of mental retardation (learning disability) | | |
|---|---|---|
| Degree of mental retardation | Intelligence quotient (IQ) range | Adaptive functioning |
| Mild (85% of cases) | 50–69 | Often only identified at a later age<br>Delayed, but usually adequate use of language and self-care<br>Difficulties in academic work (reading and writing) but greatly helped by educational programmes<br>Usually capable of unskilled or semi-skilled manual labour<br>May be able to live independently |
| Moderate (10% of cases) | 35–49 | Language and comprehension limited<br>Self-care and motor skills retarded, may need supervision<br>May be able to do simple practical work with supervision<br>Completely independent living rarely achieved, usually settle in supervised accommodation |
| Severe (3–4% of cases) | 20–34 | Marked degree of motor impairment<br>Little or no speech during early childhood; may learn to talk in school-age period<br>Capable of only elementary self-care skills<br>May be able to perform simple tasks under close supervision<br>Usually settle in group homes, family settings |
| Profound (1–2% of cases) | <20 | Severely limited in ability to understand or comply with requests or instructions<br>Often severe motor impairment with restricted mobility and incontinence<br>Little or no self-care<br>Usually require residential care |

**Fig. 23.2** Degrees of mental retardation (learning disability).

# Developmental disorders

The developmental disorders are a heterogeneous group of disorders whose defining characteristic is an inherent impairment in the development of the brain resulting in an impaired acquisition of (or loss of, in the case of the pervasive developmental disorders) expected cognitive, motor, social or adaptive skills. The onset of these disorders is usually in infancy or early childhood and they tend to follow a chronic, steady course (see Fig. 23.1)

## Specific developmental disorders

These disorders are marked by the disturbed acquisition of a *specific* cognitive or motor function during a child's development, e.g. language, reading, spelling, arithmetical ability, and motor skills. Other areas of cognitive functioning are average or even above average; therefore, a child may have a specific reading disorder (developmental dyslexia) but be of normal intelligence and have no problem with

writing or mathematics. These disorders are not simply the consequence of a lack of opportunity to learn, sensory impairment or neurological disease but are thought to arise from some specific biological abnormality in cognitive processing. Compared with mental retardation, patients have less difficulty with overall social and personal functioning, although the consequences of the delay (e.g. school problems, teasing) might lead to emotional or behavioural problems.

## Pervasive developmental disorders

The pervasive developmental disorders are characterized by:

- Severe impairments in social interactions and communication skills.
- Restricted, stereotyped interests and behaviours.

These behavioural abnormalities pervade all areas of these patients' functioning and are usually evident within the first few years of life. Although they are often associated with mental retardation, this is not

| Causes of mental retardation (learning disability) | |
| --- | --- |
| Genetic | Chromosomal: Down's syndrome, fragile X syndrome, Prader–Willi syndrome<br>Other: phenylketonuria, neurofibromatosis, tuberous sclerosis, Lesch–Nyhan syndrome, Tay–Sachs disease, other enzyme deficiency diseases |
| Prenatal | Congenital infections (TORCH infections): toxoplasmosis, rubella, cytomegalovirus, herpes simples and zoster (chicken pox), also syphilis and acquired immune deficiency syndrome (AIDS)<br>Substance use during pregnancy (including alcohol: fetal alcohol syndrome) or prescribed drugs with teratogenic effects<br>Complications of pregnancy: pre-eclampsia, intrauterine growth retardation, antepartum haemorrhage |
| Perinatal | Birth trauma (intracranial haemorrhage) and hypoxia<br>Prematurity: intraventricular haemorrhage, hyperbilirubinaemia (kernicterus)<br>Infections |
| Environmental | Poor, socioculturally deprived children<br>Neglect, malnutrition, poor linguistic and social stimulation<br>Abuse |
| Psychiatric conditions | Pervasive developmental disorders (e.g. autism, Rett's syndrome) |
| Medical conditions in childhood | Infections: meningitis, encephalitis<br>Head injury<br>Toxins (e.g. lead) |

**Fig. 23.3** Causes of mental retardation (learning disability).

essential for the diagnosis, the emphasis being on deviant *behaviour* irrespective of intellectual functioning. The pervasive developmental disorders include autism, Asperger's syndrome, Rett's syndrome and childhood disintegrative disorder.

## Autism (childhood autism, autistic disorder)
### Diagnosis and clinical features
The three characteristic features of autism manifest within the first 3 years of life and include:

1. *Impairment in social interaction* as evidenced by the poor use of non-verbal behaviours (e.g. eye contact, facial expression, gestures) and a failure to develop and share in the enjoyment of peer relationships.
2. *Impairment in communication* as evidenced by poor development of spoken language; extreme difficulty in initiating or sustaining conversation; repetitive use of idiosyncratic language and lack of imitative or make-believe play.
3. *Restricted, stereotyped interests and behaviours* as evidenced by intense preoccupations with interests such as dates, phone numbers and timetables; inflexible adherence to routines and rituals; repetitive, stereotyped motor movements such as clapping, rocking or twisting and an

unusual interest in parts of hard or moving objects.

In addition to these diagnostic features, patients may also exhibit behavioural problems such as aggressiveness, impulsivity and self-injurious behaviour. Although autistic children can be of normal intelligence, 75% have significant mental retardation. Epilepsy may develop in about 25–30% of cases.

### Epidemiology and aetiology
- The prevalence of autism in the general population is about 0.05% (5 cases per 10 000 people).
- The male-to-female ratio is approximately 3–5:1, but girls are more seriously affected.
- The exact cause of autism has not been clarified but genetic, prenatal, perinatal and immunological factors have been implicated. Phenylketonuria, tuberous sclerosis and congenital rubella are associated conditions. Notwithstanding the turbulent speculation in the mass media, there is no good evidence that indicates that the MMR vaccine (mumps, measles, rubella) results in autism.

### Management and prognosis

- Prognosis is poor: only 1–2% achieve full independence; 20–30% achieve partial independence.
- Autistic children with IQs above 70 and those who have good language development by age 5–7 have the best prognosis.
- Prognosis is improved if the home environment is supportive – family education and support are crucial.
- Treatment approach is similar to mental retardation.

### Asperger's syndrome

Asperger's syndrome is similar to autism in that there is impairment in social interaction coupled with restricted, stereotyped interests and behaviours. However, there are no significant abnormalities in language acquisition and ability, or in cognitive development and intelligence. Asperger's syndrome is far more prevalent in boys, and schizoid and anankastic personality traits are common (see p. 77). Many authors conceptualize Asperger's syndrome as a disorder on the so-called *autistic spectrum*.

### Rett's syndrome (disorder)

Rett's syndrome, which has almost only been seen in girls, is initially characterized by an apparently normal antenatal development with a normal head circumference at birth, followed by an apparently normal psychomotor development in the first 5 months after birth. From 6 months to 2 years of age, a progressive and destructive encephalopathy results in a deceleration of head growth; loss or lack of development of language and loss of purposeful hand movements and fine motor skills, with subsequent development of stereotyped hand movements (e.g. midline hand-wringing). After a decade, most girls are bound to a wheelchair with incontinence, muscle wasting and rigidity and almost no language ability.

### Childhood disintegrative disorder (Heller's syndrome)

This disorder, which is more common in boys, is characterized by about 2 years of normal development, followed by a loss of previously acquired skills (language, social and adaptive skills, play, bowel and bladder control and motor skills) before age 10. It is also associated with an autism-like impairment of social interaction as well as repetitive, stereotyped interests and mannerisms. Thus, after

the deterioration, these children may resemble autistic children.

## Acquired disorders

The *acquired disorders* of childhood are illnesses 'superimposed' on a relatively normally developing child, implying that if the illness were 'removed', a more or less normally developed child would remain. They tend to follow a fluctuating course and are often amenable to treatment. Acquired disorders can further be divided into those disorders developing specifically in childhood and the 'adult' psychiatric disorders that have their onset in childhood (see Fig. 23.1).

## Acquired disorders with onset usually in childhood or adolescence

### Attention-deficit/hyperactivity disorder – DSM-IV (ICD-10: Hyperkinetic disorder)

*Diagnosis and clinical features* Attention-deficit/hyperactivity disorder (ADHD) usually has its onset before the age of 6 or 7 and is characterized by: (1) *impaired attention*; or (2) *hyperactivity or impulsivity*:

1. Impaired attention ability includes difficulty sustaining attention in work or play tasks; not listening when being spoken to; being highly distractible – moving from one activity to another; reluctance to engage in activities that require a sustained mental effort (e.g. schoolwork) and being forgetful or regularly losing things.
2. Hyperactivity includes restlessness; incessant fidgeting; running and jumping around in inappropriate situations; excessive talkativeness or noisiness and difficulty engaging in quiet activities. Impulsivity includes difficulty awaiting turn, interrupting others' conversations or games and prematurely blurting out answers to questions.

These symptoms should be evident in more than one situation, e.g. at school and at home, and should have been present for at least 6 months.

It is important to distinguish ADHD from:

- Age-appropriate behaviours in young active children. ADHD is usually not recognized until the child has started school because of the normal variation of behaviours in preschool children.

However, ADHD is diagnosed and treated in clear cases in young children.

- Children placed in academic settings inappropriate to their intellectual ability. This includes children with learning disabilities and highly intelligent children in an under-stimulating environment.
- Other mental illnesses (e.g. pervasive developmental disorders, depression, etc.).

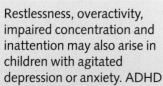

Restlessness, overactivity, impaired concentration and inattention may also arise in children with agitated depression or anxiety. ADHD should not be diagnosed in these cases unless there is clear evidence that these symptoms were present before, or persist after the resolution of, the depression or anxiety.

### Epidemiology and aetiology

- The prevalence of ADHD in the USA is 3–7% in school-age children. It is about 1% in the UK, probably due to the narrower diagnostic criteria in the ICD-10, where it is termed *hyperkinetic disorder*.
- The male-to-female ratio is approximately 3–9:1.
- The cause of ADHD is not known. Genetic factors, brain damage, dietary factors and psychosocial factors (prolonged emotional deprivation) have all been implicated.

### Management and prognosis

- Pharmacological: central nervous system stimulants such as methylphenidate (Ritalin®) and dexamfetamine have been shown to be highly effective in up to three-quarters of children, improving ability to sustain attention and academic efficiency. Antidepressants (e.g. imipramine, desipramine), clonidine and some antipsychotics are second line options.
- Psychotherapy: behaviour modification in a structured environment, family education and support (parental permissiveness is not helpful).
- Improvement usually occurs with development and remission of symptoms usually occurs between the ages of 12 and 20 although 15%

of patients have symptoms persisting into adulthood.

- Unstable family dynamics and coexisting conduct disorder are associated with a worse prognosis.

A particular concern with the use of stimulants such as methylphenidate (Ritalin®) is that they cause growth suppression with prolonged use. They are therefore prescribed in specialist settings where growth and weight can be monitored. Drug-free periods (drug holidays) usually allow children to make up the growth.

### Conduct disorder

The onset of conduct disorder is usually before the age of 18. Most affected boys meet the criteria by age 10–12 years and most affected girls by age 14–16 years. The disorder is characterized by a repetitive and persistent pattern of:

- Aggression to people and animals.
- Destruction of property (including fire-setting).
- Deceitfulness or theft.
- Major violations of age-appropriate societal expectations or rules (e.g. truancy, staying out at night, running away from home).

Aetiological factors include genetic factors, parental psychopathology (mental illness, substance abuse, antisocial personality traits), child abuse and neglect, poor socioeconomic status and educational impairment. Prevalence estimates vary from 5 to 15% of adolescent boys and from 2 to 10% of adolescent girls. More boys than girls are affected with a male-to-female ratio of approximately 3–12:1. Many adolescents improve by adulthood; however, a substantial proportion goes on to develop antisocial personality disorder and substance-related problems, especially those children with an early age of onset of symptoms. Management strategies include behaviour, cognitive, family and group therapy.

Oppositional defiant disorder describes a persistent pattern of negativistic, defiant, hostile and disruptive behaviour *in the absence* of behaviour that violates the law or the basic rights of others as occurs in conduct disorder (e.g. theft, cruelty, bullying, assault). Children with this disorder deliberately defy requests or rules, are angry and resentful and annoy others on purpose.

The risk of developing conduct disorder is increased in children with a biological or adoptive parent with antisocial personality disorder or a sibling with conduct disorder.

### Emotional disorders

The emotional disorders in childhood are marked by depression or anxiety and often seem to be exaggerations of normal developmental trends rather than discrete illnesses in themselves. They seldom persist into adult life and tend to have a good prognosis. The treatment of these disorders is focused on behavioural and family therapy. They include:

- Separation anxiety disorder: inappropriate and excessive anxiety about separation from those to whom the child is attached. Normal separation anxiety occurs in well-adjusted children from 6 months to 2 years. This disorder is only diagnosed when the anxiety is of such a severity that it is markedly different from other children of a similar age or when it persists beyond the usual age period.
- Phobic anxiety disorder: a *developmental phase* specific fear or phobia (e.g. fear of animals in preschool children) that features a degree of anxiety that is clinically abnormal. Note that non-developmental phobias (e.g. agoraphobia) do not fall under this category but fall under the adult phobia category (see Ch. 5).
- Social anxiety disorder: a persistent and recurrent fear or avoidance of strangers. Normal stranger anxiety occurs in well-adjusted children from 8 months to 1 year. This disorder is only diagnosed when the anxiety is of such a severity that it is markedly different from other children of a similar age or when it persists beyond the usual age period.
- Sibling rivalry disorder: abnormal levels of sibling rivalry or jealousy following the birth of a younger sibling. Some emotional disturbance or jealousy is

normal after the birth of a sibling. This disorder is diagnosed when the disturbance is excessive or persistent.

School refusal is the refusal to go to school because of anxiety in spite of parental pressure. It may be caused by separation anxiety (younger children) or be a symptom of another mental illness such as depression, adjustment disorder (change from junior to secondary school) or social phobia. Truancy, on the other hand, is an absence from school by choice and is associated with conduct disorder, poor academic performance, family history of antisocial behaviour and large family size.

## Other disorders with onset usually in childhood or adolescence
### Elective mutism (selective mutism)

Elective mutism is a condition characterized by a marked selectivity in speaking depending on the specific social situation. The child will typically speak normally in certain situations (e.g. at home), but is mute in others (e.g. at school). These children have adequately developed language comprehension and ability, although a minority may have speech delay or articulation problems. It usually presents before the age of 5, is slightly more common in girls, and is associated with psychological stress, social anxiety and oppositional behaviour.

### Tic disorders

Tics are sudden, involuntary, rapid, recurrent, non-rhythmic motor movements or vocalizations that are experienced as irresistible. They are divided into:

- Simple motor tics: eye-blinking, neck-jerking, facial grimacing.
- Simple vocal tics: grunting, coughing, barking, sniffing.
- Complex motor tics: jumping, touching or hitting oneself, echopraxia (see p. 27), copropraxia (use of obscene gestures).
- Complex vocal tics: senseless repetition of words, coprolalia (use of obscene words or phrases), palilalia, echolalia (see p. 26).

*Gilles de la Tourette's syndrome* is characterized by the presence of *both* multiple motor tics and one or more vocal tics for more than 1 year. The motor tics usually present by age 7 years, although tics can present as early as 2 years of age. Obsessions and compulsions (OCD) and attention difficulties and impulsivity (ADHD) are associated conditions that may require treatment (see p. 47). Pharmacotherapy is the most effective treatment for tics but behaviour therapy may reduce the stress that aggravates them. Dopamine antagonists such as haloperidol, pimozide and sulpiride, as well as atypical antipsychotics, are most commonly used, but side-effects are a concern. SSRIs and clomipramine may be useful in treating associated obsessions and compulsions.

Other tic disorders include *transient tic disorder* (motor and/or vocal tics lasting no longer than 12 months), and *chronic motor or vocal tic disorder* (either motor or vocal tics, but not both).

Tics may be aggravated by anxiety, stressful situations or stimulants, e.g. caffeine, methylphenidate and amfetamines. In contrast, sleep, relaxation or concentration on absorbing activities reduces their frequency.

## Non-organic enuresis

This condition is characterized by the involuntary voiding of urine into the bed or clothes in children who, according to their mental age, should have established consistent bladder control (therefore ordinarily not diagnosed before the age of 5). It may occur day or night and is not directly caused by any medical condition (e.g. seizures, diabetes, urinary tract infection, structural abnormalities of the urinary tract) or use of a substance (e.g. diuretic). Two types of enuresis have been described: *primary enuresis* means that urinary continence has never been established and *secondary enuresis* means that continence has been achieved in the past.

*Prevalence* 5–10% of 5-year-olds; 3–5% of 10-year-olds, 1% of adolescents over age 15.

*Male-to-female ratio* 1:1 in 5-year-olds; 2:1 in adolescents.

*Aetiology* Genetic factors, developmental delays, psychosocial stressors (moving house, birth of a sibling, start or change of school, divorce, bereavement), inadequate toilet training.

### Treatment

- Exclude a physical problem (e.g. urinary tract infection).
- Parental education about appropriate toilet training (especially in primary enuresis).
- Behaviour therapy (pad and buzzer apparatus, star chart, bladder training).
- Pharmacotherapy as a last resort: imipramine (Tofranil®), nasal desmopressin.

*Prognosis* Most cases resolve by adolescence.

About 75% of children with non-organic enuresis have a first-degree biological relative who has had the same problem.

## Non-organic encopresis

This condition is characterized by the deposition of normal faeces (i.e. not diarrhoea) in inappropriate places, in children who, according to their mental age, should have established consistent bowel control (therefore ordinarily not diagnosed before the age of 4). It may be due to unsuccessful toilet training where bowel control has never been achieved (primary encopresis), or may occur after a period of normal bowel control (secondary encopresis). Encopresis may result from a developmental delay, coercive or punitive potty training, emotional, physical or sexual abuse, a disturbed parent–child relationship, marital conflict or feature as a symptom of another psychiatric disturbance (e.g. autism). About 1% of 5-year-olds have the condition and it is more common in males. Management includes ruling out an organic cause (constipation with overflow incontinence, anal fissure, gastrointestinal infection), assessing and treating disturbed family dynamics (ruling out child abuse), parental guidance regarding toilet training and behaviour therapy (e.g. star chart). Stool softeners may be used for constipation. The prognosis is good with 90% of cases improving within a year.

## 'Adult' disorders with onset in childhood

All psychiatric disorders that usually present in adulthood can also develop in childhood (e.g. mood disorders, psychotic disorders, anxiety disorders, substance-related problems). The diagnostic criteria are essentially the same as for adults (see relevant chapters).

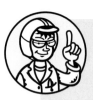

Depression in childhood may present with irritable rather than depressed mood and with failure to make expected weight gains rather than weight loss.

## Child abuse

Child abuse includes the overlapping concepts of physical (non-accidental injury), sexual and emotional abuse as well as neglect or deprivation of the child. Figure 23.4 lists the risk factors associated with child abuse.

In addition to the physical manifestations of abuse, children who have been abused may present with failure to thrive and symptoms of depression, anxiety, aggression, precocious sexual behaviour, post-traumatic stress disorder and suicidal behaviour. They are also at an increased risk for the development of a substantial range of psychiatric problems in later life. It is often difficult making the diagnosis, so a high index of suspicion is needed. Remember that the child's safety is always the main priority and healthcare professionals should have a low threshold for informing social services when their suspicions are raised.

- How are psychiatric disorders in children classified?
- What are the two essential characteristics of mental retardation (learning disability)?
- How is mental retardation classified?
- What prenatal factors are associated with mental retardation?
- What environmental and physical conditions should you exclude before diagnosing a child with a specific reading disorder?
- What are the three main characteristics of autism?
- What is the difference between Rett's syndrome and childhood disintegrative disorder?
- What common conditions should attention-deficit/hyperactivity disorder (ADHD) be distinguished from?
- What is the pharmacological treatment of ADHD? What concerns are there with this treatment?
- How does conduct disorder differ from oppositional defiant disorder?
- What are the causes of school refusal and how does it differ from truancy?
- What types of tics occur in Gilles de la Tourette's syndrome, and with what other conditions is it associated?
- What is the treatment of non-organic enuresis?
- How may depression present in children?
- What are the risk factors for child abuse?

| Risk factors for child abuse | |
| --- | --- |
| **Parent/environmental factors** | **Child factors** |
| Parents who were abused | Low birth weight or prematurity |
| Parental substance abuse | Early maternal separation |
| Parental mental illness | Unwanted child |
| (mental retardation, depression, | Mental retardation or physical disability |
| schizophrenia, personality | Challenging behaviour |
| disorders) | Hyperactivity |
| Step-parent | Excessive crying |
| Young, immature parents | |
| Parental criminality | |
| Poor socioeconomic status and | |
| overcrowding | |

**Fig. 23.4** Risk factors for child abuse.

## Suggested further reading

Coghill D 2003 Current issues in child and adolescent psychopharmacology. Part 1: Attention-deficit hyperactivity and affective disorders. Advances in Psychiatric Treatment 9: 86–94

Coghill D 2003 Current issues in child and adolescent psychopharmacology. Part 2: Anxiety and obsessive-compulsive disorders, autism, Tourette's and schizophrenia. Advances in Psychiatric Treatment 9: 289–299

Fitzgerald M, Corvin A 2001 Diagnosis and differential diagnosis of Asperger syndrome. Advances in Psychiatric Treatment 7: 310–318

Kramer T, Garralda M E 2000 Child and adolescent mental health problems in primary care. Advances in Psychiatric Treatment 6: 287–294

Scott S 2002 Classification of psychiatric disorders in childhood and adolescence: building castles in the sand? Advances in Psychiatric Treatment 8: 205–213

Patients arbitrarily come under the care of old-age psychiatrists at the age of 65 years, as it is the average age of retirement. The number of people over the age of 65 has more than doubled since the 1930s and now accounts for approximately 16% of the British population. As life expectancy continues to increase, this percentage is likely to rise. Between 1995 and 2025 the number of people aged 80 and over should increase by nearly a half and the number of people aged 90 and over is set to double.

## Mental illness in the elderly

### The psychosocial consequences of ageing

Not only is ageing associated with a decline in physical health but also psychological and social changes. The psychological changes with ageing include a decline in intellectual functioning as evidenced by:

- Mental slowing: there is slowing of the speed of processing of new information and an increase in reaction times. There tends to be no impairment of well-rehearsed (e.g. verbal comprehension) and knowledge-based skills.
- Impaired long-term remote memory, although memory for events of personal significance remains intact. There tends to be no impairment of short-term memory (as measured by digit span).

Important social challenges include: coming to terms with retirement; income reduction; living alone or being separated from family; death of spouse, siblings and peers; and coping with deteriorating physical health and mobility.

### Epidemiology of mental illness in the elderly

The prevalence of all mental illness tends to increase with age and is about 25–30% in people over the age of 65. The prevalence of mental illness tends to be higher in residential homes. Figure 24.1 summarizes the prevalence of the individual psychiatric disorders in the elderly.

## Depressive disorders

Depression in the elderly presents similarly to that in younger people, although certain features seem more prevalent:

- Severe psychomotor agitation or retardation.
- Apparent cognitive impairment (depressive pseudodementia).
- Poor concentration.
- Generalized anxiety.
- Excessive concerns about physical health (hypochondriasis).
- When psychotic, the elderly may have hypochondriacal delusions, delusions of poverty and nihilistic delusions (see p. 25).

Depression is often underdiagnosed in the elderly, so a high index of suspicion is needed. This is important considering that the elderly are at a high risk for completed suicide, even though the prevalence of parasuicide in this group is lower than in adults.

The principles of treatment are the same as for adults, although medication should be introduced cautiously as the elderly have an increased risk of developing adverse side-effects and generally need lower doses; postural hypotension is a particular problem with tricyclic antidepressants. Electroconvulsive therapy (ECT) is a very effective treatment for depression in this population group and should be considered for severe depression, suicidal ideation, severe psychomotor retardation, failure to respond to or tolerate medication, and previous good response to ECT. Lithium augmentation may be used in treatment-resistant cases, although the dose is generally half that used in adults. Patients in this age group often need lifelong antidepressant treatment to reduce the chance of relapse. Psychosocial intervention in the form of social support and possibly cognitive-behavioural therapy are also important.

Poor prognostic factors include co-morbid physical illness, late detection of illness and poor compliance with antidepressant medication. Elderly depressed patients have a higher mortality than the non-depressed do, even when physical illness is taken into account.

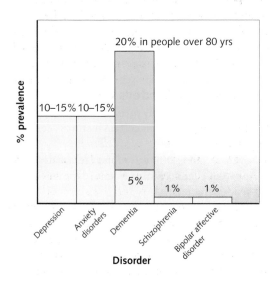

**Fig. 24.1** Prevalence of mental illness in people over the age of 65.

Cotard's syndrome describes the presence of nihilistic and hypochondriacal delusions as part of a depressive psychosis and is typically seen in the elderly.

## Mania

Unlike depression, the incidence of bipolar affective disorder does not increase with age, although late onset cases seem to be less influenced by genetic factors (fewer of these patients have positive family histories for mood disorders). In a fifth of cases, mania is precipitated by an acute medical condition, e.g. stroke or myocardial infarction. The presentation and treatment is similar to that of adults.

## Dementia and delirium

See Chapters 9 and 16.

## Late-onset schizophrenia (late paraphrenia)

Old-age psychiatrists in the UK used the term *late-onset schizophrenia* or *late paraphrenia* to denote a group of patients who develop psychotic symptoms late in life, usually over the age of 60. Late-onset schizophrenia is characterized predominantly by delusional thinking, usually of a persecutory or grandiose nature. These delusions tend not to be as fantastic as they sometimes are in earlier onset schizophrenia, e.g. rather than believing that secret agents are monitoring them by satellite, paraphrenics will assert that the neighbours have been poisoning their water supply. Hallucinations may occur but disorganized thinking, inappropriate affect and catatonic features almost never feature.

The aetiology of late-onset schizophrenia seems different to early-onset schizophrenia especially as regards genetic loading: the risk of schizophrenia in first-degree relatives is highest for a young schizophrenic, intermediate for a paraphrenic and lowest for an unaffected person in the general population. Also, late-onset schizophrenia is far more common in women than men – unlike early-onset schizophrenia, which has a closer sex ratio. Sensory deprivation, particularly hearing loss and social isolation, is also implicated in its aetiology.

The treatment is with antipsychotics but some work is needed in building up a therapeutic relationship as these patients are often difficult to engage and poor compliance is associated with a poor treatment response. Note that although late-onset schizophrenia does seem to be a distinct entity, it is not a term used by the ICD-10 or DSM-IV; here, these patients would be classified as having schizophrenia or delusional disorder.

Diogenes' syndrome or 'senile squalor' is the term used to describe an elderly recluse who lives in a state of perpetual filth and gross self-neglect, often with the hoarding of rubbish. This is purely a descriptive term and may occur in individuals with alcohol abuse, frontal lobe dysfunction, personality disorder and chronic psychotic illness. It may also occur at a younger age.

## Assessment considerations in the elderly

- Home assessments are a very important part of old age psychiatry. Patients can be assessed in their normal environment and collateral information can be obtained from family members. It is important to ascertain whether the patient can be managed at home (i.e. risk of harm to self and others; ability to carry out activities of daily living (ADL), drive and manage financial affairs, etc.), or whether additional community support or hospitalization is needed.

- Collateral information from the patient's general practitioner, family and neighbours is an important part of history taking.
- The mental state examination follows the same format as for adults, although extra consideration should be given to the assessment of cognitive functioning and it is advisable to always do a Mini-Mental State Examination (see Fig. 9.10, p. 62).
- A thorough physical examination is very important. Do not forget to assess hearing and vision as well as tremors and involuntary movements.
- Routine investigations in the newly diagnosed or hospitalized elderly include: full blood count, urea and electrolytes, liver function tests, thyroid function tests, calcium, glucose, serum proteins, mid-stream urine microscopy and culture, chest X-ray, ECG and CT scan when indicated. Remember that the chances of a physical illness causing or aggravating a mental deterioration are significant in the elderly.

## Treatment considerations in the elderly
### Physiological changes with ageing
There are a number of physiological changes that occur with ageing, which may affect the handling of certain drugs. Figure 24.2 describes the most important changes and their effects. The net result of these changes is that the tissue concentration of a drug may be increased by over 50%, especially in malnourished, dehydrated and debilitated patients. Therefore the adage, 'start low and go slow' applies especially to the use of psychotropic drugs in the elderly.

### Polypharmacy
The elderly receive almost a third of all prescriptions issued in the UK and 15% of these are for four drugs or more. This increases the risk of adverse reactions, drug interactions and poor compliance. The practice of prescribing psychotropic drugs for common symptoms such as insomnia and headache should be avoided as they may lead to further non-specific symptoms, e.g. confusion, drowsiness and light-headedness. Medication should not be a substitute for adequate social care, the lack of which often underlies many of these symptoms.

### Compliance
Compliance is often a problem with the elderly, especially with those who are visually impaired, confused, take numerous drugs and live alone. This may be improved by simplifying medication regimens, taking time to explain dosing schedules and labelling prescriptions clearly. Organizing supervision of medication taking by a relative, friend or community mental health nurse (CPN) may be necessary.

| Age-related changes in drug-handling and effects | |
|---|---|
| **Physiological change** | **Effect** |
| Reduction in renal clearance (glomerular filtration rate and tubular function) | Drugs excreted by filtration (e.g. lithium) need lower doses<br>Drug concentrations may rise rapidly with dehydration, heart failure, etc. |
| Decreased lean body mass and total body water and increased body fat | Volume of distribution increases for lipid-soluble drugs (most psychotropic drugs), and reduces for water soluble drugs (e.g. lithium) |
| Decreased plasma albumin | Reduced drug binding resulting in increased physiologically active unbound fraction |
| Reduced hepatic metabolism and first-pass metabolism | May increase the bioavailability and elimination of some drugs |
| Increased sensitivity to central nervous system drugs | Sedating drugs may result in drowsiness, confusion, falls and delirium<br>Sensitive to anticholinergic, postural hypotensive and parkinsonian effects of tricyclic antidepressants and conventional antipsychotics |
| Decreased total body mass | Lower doses of drugs needed (think in terms of 'mg/kg' as opposed to standard dose for all) |

**Fig. 24.2** Age-related changes in drug-handling and effects.

## Psychosocial interventions

Psychological treatment, such as supportive and cognitive behaviour therapy, has been applied with success in the elderly. Reality orientation and reminiscence therapies have been used to reduce confusion and stimulate remote memories in patients with dementia. Practical psychosocial interventions such as memory aids (e.g. notebooks, calendars) and assistance with mobility and daily activities by a support worker should not be underestimated. Activities of daily living (ADL) scales, which assess skills such as washing, dressing, eating, shopping, etc., give carers an indication of patients' strengths and weaknesses and enable them to tailor a package that caters specifically for these.

- What are the three most prevalent mental illnesses in people over the age of 65?
- What features are particularly prominent in depression in the elderly?
- What are the dangers of prescribing tricyclic antidepressants to the elderly considering age-related changes in physiology?
- How does late-onset schizophrenia differ from early-onset schizophrenia in terms of aetiology and clinical presentation?
- What is the role of home assessments in old age psychiatry?
- What factors should be considered before prescribing a benzodiazepine to an elderly patient on numerous cardiac drugs who lives alone?

## Suggested further reading

Bouman W P, Pinner G 2002 Use of atypical antipsychotic drugs in old age psychiatry. Advances in Psychiatric Treatment 8: 49–58

Cattell H 2000 Suicide in the elderly. Advances in Psychiatric Treatment 6: 102–108

Evans M, Mottram P 2000 Diagnosis of depression in elderly patients. Advances in Psychiatric Treatment 6: 49–56

British Journal of Psychiatry 2002 Old age psychiatry papers. British Journal of Psychiatry 180: 116–167

Forensic psychiatry, in its narrowest sense, is concerned with assessment and treatment of mentally ill offenders as well as the assessment of the dangerousness of individuals who may not yet have committed an offence. Certain patients may require treatment and rehabilitation in a secure environment, such as a special hospital, e.g. Broadmoor or Rampton Hospital, or regional secure unit.

## Mental illness and crime

The vast majority of patients suffering from a mental illness have never committed an offence, and most offences are not committed by people with a mental illness. However, there is a significantly higher prevalence of mental illness among prisoners than in the general population, with about a third of the male prisoners in England and Wales having a diagnosable mental disorder. Yet, this does not mean that mental illness causes people to offend. In fact, most evidence indicates that crime and mental illness are only weakly associated.

Certain mental disorders, however, have shown some association with both violent and non-violent crime and these are summarized in Figure 25.1.

- Note that the mental disorders associated with violent crime, that is personality disorders (especially psychopathy), alcohol and substance dependence and paranoid psychotic disorders, may have an additive effect to the risk of future violence when they occur in combination.
- Remember that delusions of jealousy (Othello's syndrome) are common with alcohol abuse and are linked to violent crime such as battering and homicide.

## Personality disorder and crime
### Psychopathy

The German clinician Koch first used the term 'psychopathy' in 1891. At that time it included all forms of personality disorder. However, the term was later used to describe individuals who exhibited antisocial behaviour. Unfortunately, the term 'psychopathic personality' and the related term 'psychopath' have been misused in both the medical and tabloid press. They were, for the most part, superseded by the term sociopathic personality disorder for a time and subsequently by the favoured, and currently used term, antisocial personality disorder (see Ch. 11).

Psychopathy is now narrowly defined by the Hare's Psychopathy Checklist – Revised (PCL–R) and is characterized, in part, by antisocial behaviour *and* emotional impairment such as the diminished capacity for guilt or remorse. Psychopathy is not synonymous with antisocial personality disorder as only a third of individuals diagnosed with antisocial personality disorder meet the criteria for psychopathy.

Note that the term 'psychopathic disorder' is a legal, not a psychiatric, term contained in the Mental Health Act (1983), which is defined as a persistent disorder or disability of the mind which results in abnormally aggressive or seriously irresponsible conduct. The act stipulates that individuals may be detained if it is deemed that treatment is likely to alleviate or prevent deterioration of this 'disorder'.

### Dangerous severe personality disorder (DSPD)

In February 1999, in the House of Commons, the English home secretary (Jack Straw) used the term 'dangerous severe personality disorder' (DSPD) to describe a group of '*individuals from whom the public at present are not properly protected, and who are restrained effectively neither by the criminal law, nor by the provisions of the Mental Health Act*'. This was coupled with a government consultation paper, which introduced proposals for tackling this problem in July 1999. In 2000, the government published its comprehensive White Paper on mental health law reform, which detailed legislation for a radically new mental health service for the assessment and

| Mental disorders associated with crime | |
| --- | --- |
| **Mental disorder** | **Associations with crime** |
| Personality disorder | Associated with violent crime, especially psychopathy (see text). Antisocial and borderline personality disorders are frequently diagnosed in forensic settings, often in association with co-morbid substance abuse |
| Alcohol and substance use | Alcohol leads to disinhibition and is strongly associated with violent crime. Alcohol intoxication may also lead to driving offences and public drunkenness. Drug intoxication is also associated with violent crime and offences may be committed to fund drug habits |
| Schizophrenia | There is conflicting evidence concerning schizophrenia and crime, but it appears as though schizophrenic patients commit more violent crimes than the general population. These crimes are associated with command hallucinations and paranoid delusions accompanied by strong affect. However, most offences committed by schizophrenics are minor and are manifestations of social incompetence |
| Mood disorders | Depression is associated with shoplifting and, in rare cases, homicide, or infanticide in postnatal depression. These cases are usually due to mood-congruent delusions (e.g. everyone would be better off dead) and are often followed by suicide. Offences by manic patients usually reflect financial irresponsibility or acts of aggression, which are usually not serious |
| Mental retardation | There is an association between mental retardation and sexual offences (especially indecent exposure), as well as arson |

**Fig. 25.1** Mental disorders associated with crime.

treatment of DSPD. This new legislation may permit the lifelong hospital detention of individuals facing no criminal charges, but who have been deemed to have a personality disorder that places them at risk of dangerous offending in the future.

You should be aware that a number of psychiatrists have expressed concern regarding the term DSPD and the proposals that have been presented for some of the following reasons:

- The definition of DSPD has not been adequately clarified. It is not a recognized psychiatric term and appears neither in the ICD-10 nor the DSM-IV. As it stands, there is little agreement among psychiatrists concerning the existing personality disorder categories.
- The concepts of risk, severity and dangerousness are fraught with complexity and are still subjects of debate in the psychiatric literature.
- There is currently no completely reliable violence risk prediction instrument, although tools like the Psychopathy Checklist – Revised (PCL–R) have shown some predictive value.
- A number of sadistically violent individuals suffer from other mental disorders, for example psychosis, and/or misuse substances; and most perpetrators of sexual violence do not have a personality disorder, or any other form of mental illness.

## Assessing dangerousness

The key principle in assessing dangerousness concerns an ethical conflict between protecting the community from a potentially violent offender and respecting the human rights of the individual in question. Despite much research on this very complex subject, the ability of experts to predict whether an individual will behave violently in the future is still not completely reliable. The approaches to the prediction of violence include:

- Unaided clinical risk assessment: assessment on an individual patient basis using unaided clinical judgement.
- Actuarial methods: time-consuming assessment using predetermined static actuarial or statistical variables, e.g. demographic factors.
- Structured clinical judgement: assessment utilizing both empirical actuarial knowledge and clinical expertise, e.g. Historical/Clinical/Risk Management 20-item (HCR-20) scale.

Figure 25.2 summarizes some of the factors that have been associated with the risk of violence.

A clinician confronted with an individual who poses a serious risk of violent behaviour may need to

| Factors associated with risk of violence | |
| --- | --- |
| Demographic factors | Male<br>Young age<br>Poor socioeconomic status<br>Poor social support<br>  • Relationship instability<br>  • Employment difficulties |
| History and background | Previous episodes of violence/convictions<br>  • Numerous serious offences<br>  • Young age at first violent offence<br>  • Sadistic, unprovoked or bizarre offences<br>  • Lack of remorse<br>Alcohol or substance misuse<br>Antisocial personality disorder; conduct disorder<br>Presence of a major psychiatric illness<br>Continued presence of precipitants of previous<br>  offences<br>Impulsivity/poor self-control<br>Poor compliance with psychiatric care or recent<br>  discontinuation of treatment<br>Drug use by father<br>History of parental fighting<br>Abuse in childhood |
| Mental state examination | Violence ideation<br>  • Violent fantasies<br>  • High degree of intent<br>  • Repeated threats<br>  • Presence of a victim<br>  • Planning of violence<br>  • Access to weapons<br>Paranoid beliefs/psychosis<br>  • Persecutory delusions/ideas<br>  • Delusions of external control<br>  • Delusions/ideas of jealousy (morbid jealousy)<br>  • Command auditory hallucinations<br>Irritability, hostility, psychomotor agitation<br>High psychopathy rating on PCL–R* |

*Psychopathy Checklist–Revised (PCL–R).

**Fig. 25.2** Factors associated with risk of violence.

discuss the case with colleagues, including social workers, psychiatrists and forensic specialists. Compulsory hospitalization may be required in serious cases. Clinicians may, and indeed have a duty to, breach confidentiality considerations to warn potential victims of serious threats that have been made, in consultation with the police.

 A past history of violent behaviour is the best predictor of future violent behaviour.

## Considerations in court proceedings

### Fitness to plead

Individuals with severe mental illness are not exempt from taking responsibility for their actions. However, defendants should be competent to stand trial and mount a defence against their charges. The term 'fitness to plead' is used in English law to describe this capacity. A jury determines this by assessing whether the charged can:

• Instruct counsel.
• Understand the nature of the charge.
• Challenge a juror.

- Follow the evidence brought before the court.
- Understand the difference between a plea of guilty and not guilty.

## Criminal responsibility

Before a defendant can be convicted, criminal responsibility needs to be determined. It should be determined whether, at the time of the offence, the person was able to control his own behaviour and choose whether to commit an unlawful act or not. Integral to this process is the concept of *mens rea* ('guilty intent' or 'guilty mind'), which means that the individual realized the nature of, and intended to commit, an unlawful act. A defendant may be deemed to be lacking *mens rea* due to:

- Their age. In England and Wales, children are only deemed legally responsible for their actions after the age of 14 years. Children under the age of 10 years are deemed incapable of criminal intent (*dolci incapax*). Children aged 10–14 years are not considered criminally responsible unless the prosecution can prove *mens rea*.
- By reason of insanity. In English law, legal insanity (not a psychiatric term) is defined in terms of the M'Naghten Rules, which state that: '*at the time of committing the act, the party accused was labouring under such a defect of reason, from disease of the mind, as to not know the nature and quality of the act he was doing, or, if he did know it, that he did not know what he was doing was wrong.*' If found 'not guilty by reason of insanity' an offender is usually detained in a hospital specified by the home secretary. Note that, in English law, legal insanity is a rare defence due to the alternative option of *diminished responsibility*.
- Diminished responsibility. In English law, a defence of diminished responsibility is only available in relation to charges for murder, and, if successful, will lead to the charged being found guilty only of manslaughter, which allows for flexible sentencing. It depends upon the presence of: '*an abnormality of mind (whether arising from a condition of arrested or retarded development of mind or any inherent causes or induced by disease or injury)*', as defined in Section 2 of the Homicide Act 1957. An 'abnormality of mind' is not a psychiatric term and is open to wide interpretation leading to successful defences such as 'emotional immaturity' and 'premenstrual tension'.
- Automatism. An act committed without presence of mind (e.g. during sleepwalking or epileptic seizure) may warrant this rare defence.

 Self-induced intoxication with alcohol or other drugs is not considered to be a defence to those crimes for which 'specific intent' need not be proved (e.g. rape, manslaughter, indecent assault). It may, however, indicate lack of intent in crimes for which 'specific intent' must be proved (e.g. murder, theft).

- What is the association between mental illness and crime?
- What psychiatric disorders are associated with violent crime?
- What is the difference between psychopathy, psychopathic disorder and antisocial personality disorder?
- How might the UK government's new mental health legislation proposals affect individuals deemed to have 'dangerous severe personality disorder' (DSPD)?
- What three methods have been used to predict violence?
- What factors on mental state examination are associated with a future risk of violence?
- Name four circumstances in which a person may be found to be lacking *mens rea*.

## Suggested further reading

Birmingham L 2003 The mental health of prisoners. Advances in Psychiatric Treatment 9: 191–199

Humphreys M 2000 Aspects of basic management of offenders with mental disorders. Advances in Psychiatric Treatment 6: 22–30

Rice M E, Harris G T, Quinsey V L 2002 The appraisal of violence risk. Current Opinion in Psychiatry 15(6): 559–589. Available from URL: http://www.medscape.com/viewarticle/444153

Snowden P 2001 Substance misuse and violence: the scope and limitations of forensic psychiatry's role. Advances in Psychiatric Treatment 7: 189–197

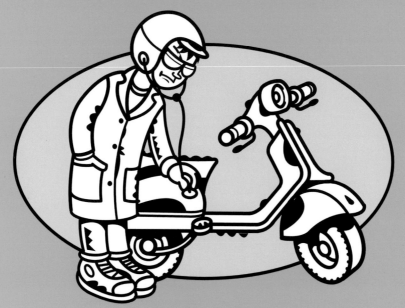

# ASSESSMENT, THERAPY AND SERVICE DELIVERY

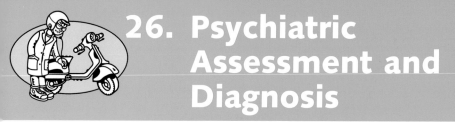

# 26. Psychiatric Assessment and Diagnosis

The psychiatric assessment is different from a medical or surgical assessment in that: (1) the history taking is longer and is aimed at understanding psychological problems that develop in patients, each with a unique background and social environment; and (2) a mental state examination is performed. Figure 26.1 provides an outline of the psychiatric assessment, which includes a psychiatric history, mental state examination, physical examination and formulation.

## Interview technique

- Whenever possible, patients should be interviewed in settings where privacy can be ensured – a patient who has just attempted suicide will be put more at ease in a quiet office than in an accident and emergency cubicle.
- Chairs should be at the same level and arranged at an angle, so that you are not sitting directly opposite the patient.
- Establishing rapport is an immediate priority and requires the display of genuineness, empathy and sensitivity by the interviewer.
- Notes may be taken during the interview; however, explain to patients that you will be doing so. Make sure that you still maintain good eye contact.
- Ensure that you and the patient are seated near the door. This allows an unobstructed exit for you or an agitated patient.
- Introduce yourself to the patient and ask them how they would like to be addressed. Explain how long the interview will last. In examination situations it may prove helpful to explain to patients that you may need to interrupt them due to time constraints.
- Keep track of, and ration, your time appropriately.
- Flexibility is essential, e.g. it may be helpful to put a very anxious patient at ease by talking about their background before zooming in on the presenting complaint.

Make use of both open and closed questions when appropriate:

*Closed questions* limit the scope of the response to one or two word answers. They are used to gain specific information, and can be used to control the length of the interview when patients are being over-inclusive. For example:

- Are you low in mood? (Yes or no answer)
- What time do you wake up in the morning? (Specific answer)

Note that closed questions can be used at the very beginning of the interview as they are easier to answer and help to put patients at ease, e.g. 'Do you live locally?'; 'Are you married?' – see 'identifying information' below.

*Open questions* encourage the patient to answer freely with a wide range of responses and should be used to elicit the presenting complaint, as well as feelings and attitudes. For example:

- How have you been feeling lately?
- What led you to feel this way?

All mental health workers need to work on being expert rapport-builders. Failure to establish rapport should be due to patient, not interviewer, factors, as the failure to establish rapport may be an important sign of mental illness. For example, patients with persecutory delusions may believe the interviewer is trying to harm them; or patients with paranoid personality traits may mistrust the interviewer's motives.

## Psychiatric history

The order in which you take the history is not as important as being systematic, making sure you cover all the essential subsections. A typical format for taking a psychiatric history is outlined in Figure 26.1 and will now follow in more detail.

### Identifying information
- Name.
- Age.

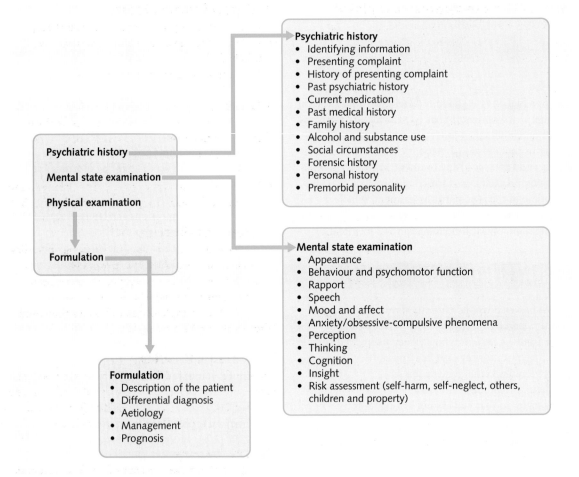

**Psychiatric history**
- Identifying information
- Presenting complaint
- History of presenting complaint
- Past psychiatric history
- Current medication
- Past medical history
- Family history
- Alcohol and substance use
- Social circumstances
- Forensic history
- Personal history
- Premorbid personality

Psychiatric history
Mental state examination
Physical examination
Formulation

**Mental state examination**
- Appearance
- Behaviour and psychomotor function
- Rapport
- Speech
- Mood and affect
- Anxiety/obsessive-compulsive phenomena
- Perception
- Thinking
- Cognition
- Insight
- Risk assessment (self-harm, self-neglect, others, children and property)

**Formulation**
- Description of the patient
- Differential diagnosis
- Aetiology
- Management
- Prognosis

**Fig. 26.1** Outline of the psychiatric assessment.

- Marital status and children.
- Occupation.
- Reason for the patient's presence in a psychiatric setting, e.g. referral to out-patient clinic by family doctor; or admitted to ward informally having presented at casualty.
- Legal status, i.e. if detained under mental health legislation.

For example:

*Mrs LM is a 32-year-old married housewife with two children aged 4 and 6 years, who was referred by her family doctor to a psychiatric out-patient clinic.*

## Presenting complaint

Open questions are used to elicit the presenting complaint. Whenever possible, record the main problems in the patient's own words, in one or two sentences, instead of using technical psychiatric terms, e.g.:

*Mrs LM complains of 'feeling as though I don't know who I am, like I'm living in an empty shell'.*

Patients frequently have more than one complaint, some of which may be related. It is helpful to organize multiple presenting complaints into groups of symptoms that are related, for instance, 'low mood', 'poor concentration' and 'lack of energy' are common features of depression, e.g.:

*Mrs LM complains firstly of 'low mood', 'difficulty sleeping' and 'poor self-esteem', and secondly of 'increased alcohol consumption' associated with withdrawal symptoms of 'shaking, sweating and jitteriness' in the morning.*

## History of presenting complaint

This section is concerned with eliciting the nature and development of each of the presenting complaints. The following headings may be helpful in structuring your questioning:

- Duration: when did the problems start?
- Development: how did the problems develop?
- Mode of onset: suddenly or over a period of time?
- Course: are symptoms constant, progressively worsening or intermittent?
- Severity: how much is the patient suffering? To what extent are symptoms affecting the patient's social and occupational functioning?
- Associated symptoms: certain complaints are associated with certain symptoms that should be enquired about if patients don't mention them spontaneously, e.g. when 'feeling low' is a presenting complaint, biological, cognitive, and psychotic features of depression as well as suicidal ideation should be asked about. Also, certain symptoms are common to many psychiatric conditions and these should be screened for, e.g. a primary complaint of insomnia may be a sign of depression, mania, psychosis or a primary sleep disorder.
- Precipitating factors: psychosocial stress frequently precipitates episodes of mental illness, e.g. bereavement, moving house, relationship difficulties.

As patients are not always forthcoming with all of their symptoms, it is wise to briefly screen all patients for the most common psychiatric disorders to ensure that you do not miss an important condition. Symptoms worth enquiring about include:

- Low mood (depression).
- Elevated mood and increased energy (hypomania and mania).
- Delusions and hallucinations (psychosis).
- Free-floating anxiety, panic attacks or phobias (anxiety disorders).
- Obsessions or compulsions (obsessive-compulsive disorder).
- Alcohol or substance abuse.

## Past psychiatric history

This is an extremely important section as it may provide clues to the patient's current diagnosis. It should include:

- Dates and duration of previous mental illness episodes.
- Details of previous treatments, including medication, psychotherapy, electroconvulsive therapy and hospitalizations.
- Details of previous contact with psychiatric services.
- Details of previous assessment or treatment under mental health legislation (e.g. Mental Health Act.)

## Current medication   + Psych. treatment

Note all the medication patients are using, including psychiatric, non-psychiatric and over-the-counter drugs. Also enquire how long patients have been on specific medication and whether it has been effective. Non-compliance as well as reactions and allergies should be recorded.

## Past medical history

Enquire about medical illnesses or surgical procedures. Past head injury or surgery, neurological conditions (e.g. epilepsy) and endocrine abnormalities (e.g. thyroid problems) are especially relevant to psychiatry.

## Family history

- Enquire about the presence of psychiatric illness (including suicide and substance abuse) in family members, remembering that genetic factors are implicated in the aetiology of many psychiatric conditions – a family tree may be useful to summarize information.
- Enquire whether parents are still alive and if not, causes of death. Also ask about significant physical illnesses in the family.
- Enquire about the quality of the patient's relationships with close family members.

## Alcohol and substance use

This section should never be overlooked, as alcohol/substance-related psychiatric conditions are not uncommon.

The CAGE questionnaire (see p. 72) is a useful tool to screen for alcohol dependence. If patients answer affirmatively to two or more questions, regard the screen as positive and go on to check if they meet the definitive criteria for the alcohol dependence syndrome (see p. 69). Try to elicit a patient's typical drinking day including daily intake of alcohol in units, type of alcohol used, time of first drink of the day and places where drinking occurs (e.g. at home alone or in a pub).

If illicit drugs have been or are being used, record the drug names, routes of administration (intravenous, inhaled, oral ingestion) and the years and frequency of use. Also enquire about possible dependence (see p. 66, Ch. 10).

## Social circumstances

This includes accommodation, social supports and relationships, employment and financial circumstances, and hobbies or leisure activities. This section is important in order to understand the social context in which the patient's problems developed.

## Forensic history

Enquire about the details and dates of previous offences and antisocial behaviour, including prosecutions, convictions and prison sentences. It is important to ask specifically about violent crime and the age of the patient's first violent offence.

## Personal history

The personal history consists of a brief description of the patient's life. Time constraints will not allow an exhaustive biographical account, but you should attempt to include significant events, perhaps under the following useful headings:

### Infancy and early childhood (until age 5)
- Pregnancy and birth complications (e.g. prematurity, fetal distress, caesarean section, etc.).
- Developmental milestones (age of crawling, walking, speaking, bladder and bowel control).
- Childhood illnesses.
- Unusually aggressive behaviour or impaired social interaction.

### Later childhood and adolescence (until completion of higher education)
- School record (academic performance, number and type of schools attended, age on leaving, and final qualifications).
- Relationships with parents, teachers and peers. History of physical, sexual or emotional abuse. Victim or perpetrator of bullying.
- Behavioural problems, including antisocial behaviour, drug use or truancy.
- Higher education and training.

### Occupational record
- Details of types and duration of jobs.

- Details of and reasons for unemployment and/or dismissal

### Relationship, marital and sexual history
- Puberty: significant early relationships and experiences as well as sexual orientation.
- Details and duration of significant relationships. Reasons for break-ups.
- Marriage/divorce details. Children.
- Ability to engage in satisfactory sexual relationships. Sexual dysfunction, fetishes or gender identity problems (enquire if problem is suspected).

Enquiring about a history of sexual abuse is important, especially in patients who exhibit personality traits suggestive of a personality disorder or in those who regularly self-harm. Tact and discretion are clearly essential; a useful question to screen for sexual abuse is: 'Have you ever had an unpleasant sexual experience?'

## Premorbid personality

The premorbid personality is an indication of the patient's personality and character before the onset of mental illness. Patients may be asked directly about their personality before they became ill, or it may be useful to ask a close family member or friend about a patient's premorbid personality.

For example:

*A young schizophrenic man, with prominent negative symptoms of lack of motivation and interest, and poverty of thought, was described by his mother as being outgoing, intelligent and ambitious before becoming ill.*

## Mental state examination

The mental state examination (MSE) describes an interviewer's impression of many aspects of a patient's mental functioning at a certain period of time. Whereas the psychiatric history remains relatively constant, the MSE may fluctuate from day to day or hour to hour. It is useful to try and gather as much evidence as possible about the MSE while doing the psychiatric history, instead of viewing this as a separate section. In fact, the MSE begins the moment you meet the patient. In addition to noting their appearance, you should observe how patients first behave on meeting you. This includes their body language and the way that they respond to your attempts to establish rapport.

By the time you have finished the psychiatric history, you should have completed many aspects of the MSE, and you should just need to ask certain key questions to finish this process off. The individual aspects of the MSE, which are summarized in Figure 26.1, are now discussed in more detail.

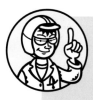 You should not just be recording patients' answers to questions while doing the psychiatric history section of the assessment. You should also be observing the way they speak, their posture, their facial expressiveness, their state of relaxation and their movements as well as displays of emotion such as tearfulness, smiling, anger and anxiety, all of which contribute to the mental state examination.

## Appearance

- Physical state: how old does the patient appear? Do they appear physically unwell? Are they sweating? Are they too thin or obese?
- Clothes and accessories: are clothes clean? Do clothes match? Are clothes appropriate to the weather and circumstances or are they bizarre? Is the patient carrying strange objects?
- Self-care and hygiene: does the patient appear in a state of self-neglect (e.g. unshaven, dirty tangled hair, malodorous, dishevelled)? Is there any evidence of injury or self-harm (e.g. multiple cuts to wrists or forearms)?

## Behaviour and psychomotor function

This section focuses on all motor behaviour, including abnormal movements such as tremors, tics, and twitches as well as displays of suspiciousness, aggression or fear, and catatonic features. Documenting patients' behaviour at the start of, and during, the interview is an integral part of the mental

state examination and should be done in as much detail as possible, e.g.

*Mrs LM introduced herself appropriately, although only made fleeting eye contact. She sat rigidly throughout the first half of the interview, mostly staring at the floor and speaking very softly. She became tearful halfway through the interview when talking about her lack of self-esteem. After this her posture relaxed, her eye contact improved and there were moments when she smiled. There were no abnormal movements.*

The term 'psychomotor' is used to describe a patient's motor activity as a consequence of their concurrent mental processes. Psychomotor abnormalities include *retardation* (slow, monotonous speech; slow or absent body movements) and *agitation* (inability to sit still; fidgeting, pacing or hand-wringing; rubbing or scratching skin or clothes).

 Remember that patients on conventional antipsychotics may display abnormal movements due to extra-pyramidal side-effects (EPSE), that is:

- Parkinson-like symptoms – muscular rigidity, bradykinesia (lack of or slowing of movement) and resting tremor.
- Acute dystonia – involuntary sustained muscular contractions or spasms.
- Akathisia – subjective feeling of inner restlessness and muscular discomfort.
- Tardive dyskinesia – rhythmic, involuntary movements of head, limbs and trunk, especially chewing, grimacing of mouth and protruding, darting movements of tongue.

## Rapport

Note whether you are able to establish a good rapport with patients. What is their attitude towards you? Do they make good eye contact or do they look around the room or at the floor? Patients may be described as cooperative, cordial, uninterested, aggressive, defensive, guarded, suspicious, fearful, perplexed, preoccupied, disinhibited (that is, a lowering of normal social inhibitions, e.g. being over-familiar, or making sexually inappropriate comments), etc.

## Speech

Speech should be described in terms of:

- Rate of production: e.g. pressure of speech in mania; long pauses and poverty of speech in depression.
- Quality and flow of speech: volume, dysarthria (articulation difficulties), dysprosody (unusual speech rhythm, melody, intonation or pitch), stuttering.

Note that disorganized, incoherent or bizarre speech is usually regarded as a thought disorder and is, therefore, described under the thought section.

## Mood and affect

*Mood* refers to a patient's sustained, subjectively experienced emotional state over a period of time. In the context of the mental state examination *affect* means the observed, external expression of emotion – as perceived by another person; affect is sometimes called the 'objective' assessment of mood.

Mood is assessed by asking patients how they are feeling. So, a patient's mood might be depressed,

elated, anxious, guilty, frightened, angry, etc. Figure 26.2 refers to typical questions that may be used to elicit depressed, elated or anxious moods.

Affect is assessed by observing patients' posture, facial expression, emotional reactivity and speech. There are two components to consider when assessing affect:

1. The appropriateness or congruity of the observed affect to the patient's subjectively reported mood, e.g. a schizophrenic woman who reports feeling suicidal with a happy facial expression would be described as having an *incongruous* affect.
2. The range of affect or range of emotional expressivity. In this sense affect may be:
   a. Within the normal range
   b. Blunted: a noticeable reduction in the normal intensity of emotional expression as evidenced by a monotonous voice and minimal facial expression
   c. Flat: very little or no emotional expression.

Note that a *labile* mood refers to a fluctuating mood state that alternates between extremes, e.g. a young man with a mixed affective episode alternates between feeling overjoyed with pressure of speech and miserable with suicidal ideation.

| Typical questions used to elicit specific psychiatric symptoms | |
| --- | --- |
| **Questions used to elicit . . .** | **Chapter/page** |
| Depressive symptoms | Ch. 1; p. 7 |
| Mania/hypomania | Ch. 2; p. 13 |
| Suicidal ideation | Ch. 3; p. 19 |
| Delusions | Ch. 4; p. 31 |
| Hallucinations | Ch. 4; p. 30 |
| Symptoms of anxiety | Ch. 5; p. 36 |
| Obsessions and compulsions | Ch. 7; p. 46 |
| Somatoform disorders | Ch. 8; p. 52 |
| Memory and cognition | Ch. 9; pp. 55, 62 |
| Problem drinking | Ch. 10; p. 72 |
| Symptoms of anorexia and bulimia | Ch. 12; p. 80 |
| Symptoms of insomnia | Ch. 21; p. 130 |

**Fig. 26.2** Typical questions used to elicit specific psychiatric symptoms.

## Anxiety/obsessive-compulsive phenomena

Obsessive-compulsive and anxiety symptoms (free-floating anxiety, panic attacks, phobias, ruminatory thoughts) need not be the presenting complaint to be present to a clinically significant degree. These symptoms are common to many psychiatric disorders and, if not specifically asked about them, patients may fail to mention them. Also record stress reactions, dissociative symptoms, and depersonalization and derealization here (see Ch. 6). Figure 26.2 refers to typical questions that may be used to elicit obsessive-compulsive and anxiety symptoms.

Remember that over 20% of depressed patients can have obsessive-compulsive symptoms, which occur simultaneously at or after the onset of depression. So, make a point of specifically asking about them.

## Perception

At this stage of the assessment, the interviewer will probably have elicited hallucinations following the patient's presenting complaint. However, this is not always the case, so it is important that you specifically enquire about abnormal perceptual experiences. (Perceptual abnormalities are defined and classified on p. 22, Ch. 4.) If patients admit to problems with perception, it is important to ascertain:

- Whether the abnormal perceptions are genuine hallucinations, pseudohallucinations, illusions or just intrusive thoughts.
- From which sense organ the hallucinations appear to arise, that is, are they auditory, visual, olfactory, gustatory or somatic hallucinations – see p. 23.
- Whether auditory hallucinations are elementary or complex. If complex, are they experienced in the first person (audible thoughts, thought echo), second person (critical, persecutory, complimentary or command hallucinations) or third person (voices arguing or discussing the patient, or giving a running commentary)?

It is also important to note whether patients seem to be responding to hallucinations during the interview, as evidenced by them laughing inappropriately as though they are sharing a private joke, or suddenly tilting their head as though listening, or quizzically looking at hallucinatory objects around the room.

Figure 26.2 refers to typical questions that may be used to elicit hallucinations.

## Thinking

In Chapter 4, p. 24, thought disorders were simply classified by dividing them into two broad groups: abnormal beliefs and disorganized thinking.

### *Abnormal beliefs:* **delusions** *and* **overvalued ideas**

It is diagnostically significant to classify delusions as:

- Primary or secondary.
- Mood congruent or mood incongruent.
- Bizarre or non-bizarre.
- And according to the content of the delusion (summarized in Fig. 4.2, p. 25).

See pp. 24–26, Ch. 4, for a detailed discussion.

***Disorganized thinking*** Disorganized thinking includes *circumstantial* and *tangential thinking, loosening of association (derailment/ knight's move thinking), neologisms* and *idiosyncratic word use, flight of ideas, thought blocking, perseveration, echolalia,* and *irrelevant answers* – see p. 26, Ch. 4, for the definitions of these terms. Whenever possible, record patients' disorganized speech word for word, as it can be very difficult to label disorganized thinking with a single technical term and written language may be easier to evaluate than spoken language.

Figure 26.2 refers to typical questions that may be used to elicit delusions.

## Cognition

Cognitive tests were discussed fully in Chapter 9, including tests of memory function and the Mini-Mental State Examination (MMSE), which tests orientation, registration, attention, calculation, language, executive functioning and visuospatial skills. Figures 9.2 and 9.10 refer to these memory function tests and the MMSE.

## Insight

Insight describes patients' understanding of the nature and degree of their mental illness as well as the recognition of the need for treatment. Insight may range from a complete denial of mental illness with the refusal to accept any form of treatment to a genuine understanding, and acceptance, of the course, nature and impact of the illness on oneself and others.

## Risk assessment

Although it is extremely difficult to make an accurate assessment of risk based on a single assessment, clinicians are expected to, as far as is possible, establish some idea of a patient's risk to:

- Self: through self-harm, suicide or self-neglect. Chapter 3 explains the assessment of suicide risk in detail.
- Others: includes violent or sexual crime, stalking and harassment. Chapter 25, p. 160, discusses key principles in assessing dangerousness.
- Children: includes physical, sexual or emotional abuse as well as neglect or deprivation. Child abuse is discussed in more detail in Chapter 23, p. 152.
- Property: includes arson and physical destruction of property.

The risk assessment is an extremely important part of the mental state examination, especially the risk of harm to self, as many patients with depression will have had suicidal thoughts or intent. Make a special point of mentioning your assessment of risk to examiners, admitting that your opinion is only based on one assessment.

## Physical examination

The psychiatric examination includes a general physical examination, with special focus on the neurological and endocrine system. Always remember to look for signs relevant to the psychiatric history, e.g. signs of liver disease in patients who abuse alcohol, signs of self-mutilation in patients with a personality disorder or signs of intravenous drug use (track marks) in patients who use drugs. Also, examine for side-effects of psychiatric medication, e.g. parkinsonism, tardive dyskinesia, dystonia and hypotension. In an exam situation, although only a short, focused physical may be practical, it should always be done. And always make a point of mentioning your positive findings when summarizing the case.

## The formulation: presenting the case

The 'formulation' is the term psychiatrists use to describe the integrated summary and understanding of a particular patient's problems. It usually includes:

- Description of the patient.
- Differential diagnosis.
- Aetiology.
- Management.
- Prognosis.

### Description of the patient

The patient may be described: (1) in detail by recounting all of the information obtained under the various headings in the psychiatric history and mental state examination; or (2) in the form of a case summary. The case summary consists of one or two paragraphs and contains only the salient features of a case, specifically:

- Identifying information.
- Main features of the presenting complaint.
- Relevant background details, e.g. past psychiatric history, positive family history.
- Positive findings in the mental state examination and physical examination.

Figure 26.3 shows a case summary in a case formulation.

When presenting your differential diagnosis, remember that two or more psychiatric disorders can coexist (e.g. depression and alcohol abuse). In this event, it is important to ascertain whether the conditions are independent or related (e.g. alcohol abuse that has developed secondary to the depressive symptoms of emptiness and difficulty sleeping).

### Differential diagnosis

The differential diagnosis is mentioned in order of decreasing probability. Only mention conditions that you have obtained evidence for in your assessment, as you should be able to provide reasons for and against all the alternatives on your list. Figure 26.3 provides an example of a typical differential diagnosis.

## Aetiology

The exact cause of most psychiatric disorders is very often unknown and most cases seem to involve a complex interplay of biological, social and psychological factors. In clinical practice, psychiatrists are especially concerned with the question: 'What factors led to this particular patient presenting with this specific problem at this specific point in time?' That is, what factors predisposed to the problem, what factors precipitated the problem and what factors are perpetuating the problem? Figure 26.3 illustrates an aetiology grid that is very helpful in structuring your answers to these questions in terms of biological, social and psychological factors – the emphasis should be on *considering* all the blocks in the grid, not necessarily on filling them.

## Management
### Special investigations

Special investigations are considered part of the management plan and are performed based on findings from the psychiatric assessment. It is useful to divide them into *physical*, *social* and *psychological* investigations – see pp. 7–8, Chapter 1, for an example. Appropriate special investigations that are relevant to the specific conditions have been given in the chapters in Section I. Familiarize yourself with these, as you should be able to give reasons for any special investigation you propose.

| Differential diagnosis | |
|---|---|
| **Diagnosis** | **Comments** |
| 1. Schizophrenia | For: symptoms present for more than 1 month<br>For: ICD-10 and first-rank symptoms of delusions of control or passivity (thought insertion); delusional perception; and third person, running commentary hallucinations<br>For: clear and marked deterioration in social and work functioning |
| 2. Schizoaffective disorder | For: typical symptoms of schizophrenia<br>Against: no prominent mood symptoms |
| 3. Mood disorder: either manic or depressive episode with psychotic features | Against: on mental state examination, mood was mainly suspicious as opposed to lowered or elevated, and appeared secondary to delusional beliefs<br>Against: no other prominent features of mania or depression<br>Against: mood-incongruent delusions and hallucinations |
| 4. Substance-induced psychotic disorder | Against: long duration of symptoms<br>Against: no evidence of illicit substance or alcohol use |
| 5. Psychotic disorder secondary to a medical condition | Against: no signs of medical illness or abnormalities on physical examination |

| Aetiology | | | |
|---|---|---|---|
| | **Biological** | **Psychological** | **Social** |
| Predisposing (what made the patient prone to this problem?) | Family history of schizophrenia | - | - |
| Precipitating (what made this problem start now?) | The peak age of onset for schizophrenia for men is between 18–25yrs | - | Break up of relationship<br>Recently started college |
| Perpetuating (what is maintaining this problem?) | Poor compliance with medication due to lack of insight | High expressed emotion family | Lack of social support |

**Fig. 26.3** Example of a case formulation (Differential diagnosis, Aetiology, Management) *Continued over*

## Management

1. Special investigations: social, psychological and physical.
2. Management plan below.

| Term | Biological | Psychological | Social |
|---|---|---|---|
| Immediate to short term | Antipsychotic medication, with benzodiazepines if necessary | Establish therapeutic relationship Support for family (carers) | Admission to hospital Allocation of care coordinator (care programme approach) Help with financial, accommodation, social problems |
| Medium to long term | Review progress in out-patient clinic Consider another antipsychotic then clozapine for non-response Consider depot medication for compliance problems | Relapse prevention work Consider cognitive-behavioural and family therapy | Regular review under care programme approach (CPA) Consider day hospital Vocational training |

### Prognosis

Assuming Mr PP has a diagnosis of schizophrenia, it is likely his illness will run a chronic course, showing a relapsing and remitting pattern. Being a young man with a high level of education, Mr PP is particularly at risk for suicide, especially following discharge from hospital. Good prognostic factors include a high level of premorbid functioning and the absence of negative symptoms.

**Fig. 26.3**—Example of a case formulation, cont'd

**Case summary**

Mr PP is a 23-year-old, single man in full-time education, who recently agreed to voluntary hospital admission. He presented with a 6-month history of hearing voices and bizarre beliefs that he was being subjected to government experiments. During this time his college attendance had been uncharacteristically poor, he had terminated his part-time work, and he had become increasingly socially withdrawn. He has no history of past psychiatric illness and denies the use of alcohol or illicit substances; however he did mention that his maternal uncle suffers from schizophrenia. On mental state examination he appeared unkempt and behaved suspiciously. He had delusions of persecution, reference and thought control as well as delusional perception. He also described second person command hallucinations and third person, running commentary hallucinations. He appeared to have no insight into his mental illness as he refused to consider that he might be unwell. There were no abnormalities on physical examination.

## Specific management plan

It may help to structure your management plan by considering biological, social and psychological aspects of treatment – *the biopsychosocial approach* – in terms of immediate to short-term, and medium to long-term management. See Figure 26.3 for an example of this method.

## Prognosis

The prognosis is dependent on two factors:

1. The natural course of the condition, which is based on studies of patient populations; these are

Remember that special investigations do not just include physical investigations (e.g. blood tests), but also include social investigations (e.g. obtaining collateral information from the patient's GP or family, obtaining social worker reports); and psychological investigations (e.g. psychometric testing, mood rating scales).

discussed for each disorder in Part II, Diseases and Disorders.

2. Individual patient factors, e.g. social support, compliance with treatment, co-morbid substance abuse.

See Figure 26.3 for an example.

## Classification in psychiatry

There are two main categorical classification systems in psychiatry:

1. ICD-10: the tenth revision of the International Classification of Diseases, Chapter V (F) – Mental and behavioural disorders (published by the World Health Organization).
2. DSM-IV: the fourth edition of the Diagnostic and Statistical Manual of Mental Disorders (published by the American Psychiatric Association). Note: a revised edition of the DSM-IV text was published in 2000 – DSM-IV-TR (TR, Text Revision).

Both the ICD-10 and DSM-IV make use of a *categorical classification* system, which refers to the process of dividing mental disorders into discrete entities by means of accurate descriptions of specific categories. In contrast, a *dimensional approach* rejects the idea of separate categories, hypothesizing that mental conditions exist on a continuum that merges into normality.

The ICD-10 categorizes mental disorders according to descriptive statements and diagnostic guidelines. The DSM-IV categorizes mental disorders according to *operational definitions*, which means that mental disorders are defined by a series of precise inclusion and exclusion criteria. Note that the research version of the ICD-10 (Diagnostic criteria for research) also makes use of operational definitions.

In general, both the ICD-10 and the DSM-IV propose a *hierarchical* diagnostic system, whereby disorders higher on the hierarchical ladder tend to be given precedence. As a broad rule, organic and substance-related conditions take precedence over conditions such as schizophrenia and mood disorders which take precedence over anxiety disorders. This does not mean that patients may not have more than one diagnosis; they may. It means that clinicians should:

- Always consider a medical, or substance-related, cause of psychological symptoms, before any other.

- Remember that certain conditions have some psychological symptoms in common. For example, schizophrenia commonly presents with features of depression and anxiety, and depression commonly presents with features of anxiety; in both cases, the treatment of the primary condition results in resolution of the symptoms – a separate diagnosis for every symptom is not needed.

The ICD-10 and the DSM-IV share similar diagnostic categories and are, for the most part, technically compatible. Figure 26.4 summarizes the main diagnostic categories in the ICD-10.

The DSM-IV uses a multi-axial diagnostic system with five axes. Axes I and II comprise the entire spectrum of mental disorders. Axis I includes all mental disorders except personality disorders and mental retardation, which fall under Axis II. Axis III includes any concurrent physical disorder or medical condition, whether causative of the mental condition or not. Axis IV includes any social or environmental problems that contribute to the mental condition. Axis V consists of a score from 0 to 100, obtained from a global assessment of functioning (GAF) scale.

The term 'neurosis' is no longer used in the DSM-IV, although retained in the ICD-10 as the group heading title for the anxiety disorders: *F4 – Neurotic, stress related and somatoform disorders*. When first introduced, 'neurosis' was the label given to all 'diseases of the nerves'. However, in modern times, it generally refers to mental disorders:

- That do not have an organic or substance-related aetiology.
- In which contact with reality is maintained (that is, non-psychotic disorders).
- That are characterized by symptoms within the range of normal experience, e.g. anxiety. It is best to avoid using this vague term. Instead, use the specific term that accurately describes the condition, e.g. generalized anxiety disorder or obsessive-compulsive disorder.

## ICD-10 categorical classification

| ICD-10 code* | ICD-10 categories | Examples of included diagnoses |
|---|---|---|
| F0 | Organic, including symptomatic, mental disorders | Dementia<br>Delirium<br>Amnesic syndrome<br>Organic mental and personality disorders |
| F1 | Mental and behavioural disorders due to psychoactive substance use | Intoxication and withdrawal states<br>Harmful use<br>Dependence syndrome<br>Psychotic disorder |
| F2 | Schizophrenia, schizotypal and delusional disorders | Schizophrenia<br>Schizotypal disorder<br>Delusional disorder<br>Acute and transient psychotic disorder<br>Schizoaffective disorder |
| F3 | Mood (affective) disorders | Depressive or manic episode<br>Bipolar affective disorder<br>Recurrent depressive disorder<br>Cyclothymia<br>Dysthymia |
| F4 | Neurotic, stress-related and somatoform disorders | Phobias<br>Panic disorder<br>Generalized anxiety disorder<br>Post-traumatic stress disorder<br>Adjustment disorder<br>Dissociative disorders<br>Somatization and hypochondriacal disorder |
| F5 | Behavioural syndromes associated with physiological disturbance and physical factors | Eating disorders<br>Sleep disorders<br>Sexual dysfunction |
| F6 | Disorders of adult personality and behaviour | Personality disorders<br>Gender identity disorders<br>Disorders of sexual preference (paraphilias) |
| F7 | Mental retardation | Mental retardation (learning disability) |
| F8 | Disorders of psychological development | Specific developmental disorders<br>Pervasive developmental disorders |
| F9 | Behavioural and emotional disorders with onset usually occurring in childhood and adolescence | Hyperkinetic disorder (attention deficit hyperactivity disorder – ADHD)<br>Conduct disorder<br>Emotional disorders<br>Elective mutism<br>Tic disorders<br>Non-organic enuresis and encopresis |

*Note that the 'F' refers to the chapter in the ICD-10 on mental and behavioural disorders, that is, Chapter V (or F).

**Fig. 26.4** ICD-10 categorical classification.

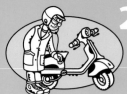
Psychotropic (mind-altering) medication can be divided into the following groups:

- Antidepressants.
- Mood stabilizers.
- Antipsychotics.
- Anxiolytics and hypnotics.
- Other.

Despite its simplicity this arbitrary method of grouping drugs is flawed because many drugs from one class are now used to treat disorders in another class, e.g. antidepressants are first-line therapies for many anxiety disorders.

## Antidepressants

### History

Antidepressants were first used in the late 1950s, with the appearance of the tricyclic antidepressant (TCA) imipramine and the monoamine oxidase inhibitor (MAOI) phenelzine. Research into TCAs throughout the 1960s and 1970s developed many more tricyclic agents and related compounds. A major development in the late 1980s was the arrival of the first selective serotonin reuptake inhibitor (SSRI), fluoxetine (Prozac®). There has since been considerable expansion of the SSRI class, as well as a revival of the MAOIs through the development of the reversible MAOI (RIMA) moclobemide.

### Classification and mechanism of action

At present we classify antidepressants according to their pharmacological actions, as we do not as yet have an adequate explanation as to what exactly makes the antidepressants work. Although there are at least eight different types of antidepressants, the collective action of all antidepressants is to boost the levels of one or more monoamine neurotransmitters in the synaptic cleft. Figure 27.1 illustrates the mechanism of action of antidepressants at the synaptic cleft. Latest research has focused on monoamine neurotransmitter activation of 'second messenger' signal transduction mechanisms. This results in the production of transcription factors that lead to the activation of genes controlling the expression of 'brain-derived neurotrophic factor' (BDNF). BDNF is neuroprotective and could be the 'final common pathway' of antidepressant action. Figure 27.2 summarizes the classification and pharmacodynamics of the important antidepressants.

Certain tricyclic antidepressants, such as clomipramine, have more potency for blocking the serotonin reuptake pump; whereas others are more selective for noradrenaline (norepinephrine) over serotonin, e.g. desipramine, nortriptyline, maprotiline. Most, however, block both noradrenaline (norepinephrine) and serotonin reuptake.

## Indications of antidepressants

Tricyclic antidepressants are used in the treatment of:

- Depression – see pp. 86–87.
- Anxiety disorders – see pp. 98–99.
- Obsessive-compulsive disorder (clomipramine) – see pp. 98–99.
- Other: chronic pain, nocturnal enuresis (see p. 151), narcolepsy (see p. 132), eating disorders.

SSRIs are used in the treatment of:

- Depression – see pp. 86–87.
- Anxiety disorders – see pp. 98–99.
- Obsessive-compulsive disorder – see pp. 98–99.
- Bulimia nervosa (fluoxetine) – see p. 121.

MAOIs are used in the treatment of:

- Depression (especially atypical depression, i.e. hypersomnia, overeating, anxiety) – see pp. 86–87.
- Anxiety disorders – see pp. 98–99.
- Other: eating disorders, chronic pain.

## Side-effects and contraindications

### Tricyclic antidepressants

Figure 27.3 summarizes the common side-effects of the TCAs, most of which are related to the

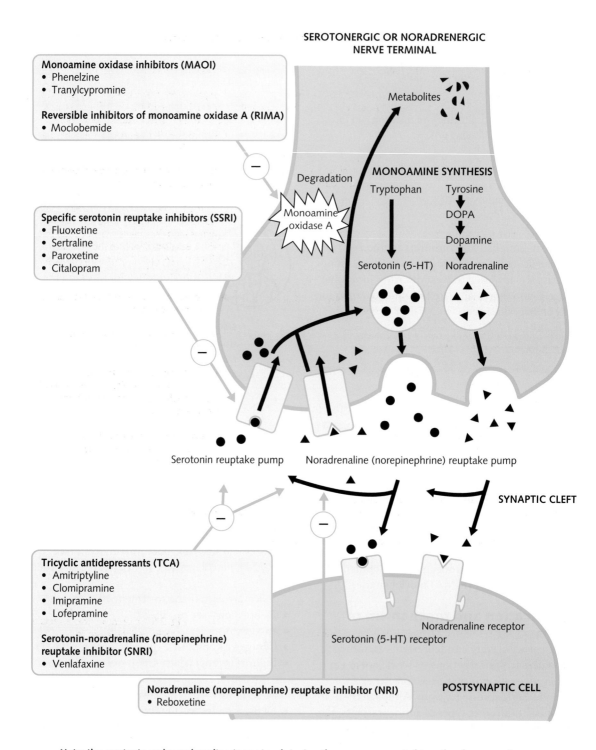

**SEROTONERGIC OR NORADRENERGIC NERVE TERMINAL**

**Monoamine oxidase inhibitors (MAOI)**
• Phenelzine
• Tranylcypromine

**Reversible inhibitors of monoamine oxidase A (RIMA)**
• Moclobemide

Metabolites

Degradation

**MONOAMINE SYNTHESIS**

Tryptophan     Tyrosine

Monoamine oxidase A

DOPA

Dopamine

**Specific serotonin reuptake inhibitors (SSRI)**
• Fluoxetine
• Sertraline
• Paroxetine
• Citalopram

Serotonin (5-HT)     Noradrenaline

Serotonin reuptake pump     Noradrenaline (norepinephrine) reuptake pump

**SYNAPTIC CLEFT**

**Tricyclic antidepressants (TCA)**
• Amitriptyline
• Clomipramine
• Imipramine
• Lofepramine

**Serotonin-noradrenaline (norepinephrine) reuptake inhibitor (SNRI)**
• Venlafaxine

Noradrenaline receptor

Serotonin (5-HT) receptor

**Noradrenaline (norepinephrine) reuptake inhibitor (NRI)**
• Reboxetine

**POSTSYNAPTIC CELL**

Note: the serotonin and noradrenaline (nerepinephrine) pathways are presented together for convenience; they do not occur in the same nerve terminal

**Fig. 27.1** Mechanism of action of antidepressants at the synaptic cleft.

## Classification and pharmacodynamics of the antidepressants

| Class of antidepressant | Examples | Mechanism of action |
| --- | --- | --- |
| Tricyclic antidepressant (TCA) | Amitriptyline, dosulepin (dothiepin), lofepramine, clomipramine, imipramine | Presynaptic blockade of both noradrenaline (norepinephrine) and serotonin reuptake pumps (to a lesser extent – dopamine) Also blockade of muscarinic, histaminergic and α-adrenergic receptors |
| Selective serotonin reuptake inhibitor (SSRI) | Fluoxetine, sertraline, paroxetine, citalopram, fluvoxamine | Selective presynaptic blockade of serotonin reuptake pumps |
| Serotonin-noradrenaline (norepinephrine) reuptake inhibitor (SNRI) | Venlafaxine | Presynaptic blockade of both noradrenaline (norepinephrine) and serotonin reuptake pumps (also dopamine in high doses) but with negligible effects on muscarinic, histaminergic or α–adrenergic receptors (in contrast to TCAs) |
| Monoamine oxidase inhibitor (MAOI) | Phenelzine, tranylcypromine, isocarboxazid | Non-selective and irreversible inhibition of monoamine oxidase A and B |
| Reversible inhibitor of monoamine oxidase A (RIMA) | Moclobemide | Selective and reversible inhibition of monoamine oxidase A |
| Noradrenergic and specific serotonergic antidepressant (NaSSA) | Mirtazapine | Presynaptic alpha 2 receptor blockade (results in increased release of noradrenaline (norepinephrine) and serotonin from presynaptic neurons) |
| Noradrenaline (norepinephrine) reuptake inhibitor (NRI) | Reboxetine | Selective presynaptic blockade of noradrenaline (norepinephrine) reuptake pumps |

Others:
Tetracyclic antidepressants: mianserin, maprotiline
Serotonin 2A antagonist/serotonin reuptake inhibitor (SARI): nefazodone and trazodone

**Fig. 27.2** Classification and pharmacodynamics of the antidepressants.

**Fig. 27.3** Common side-effects of tricyclic antidepressants.

## Common side-effects of tricyclic antidepressants

| Mechanism | Side-effects |
| --- | --- |
| Anticholinergic: muscarinic receptor blockade | Dry mouth Constipation Urinary retention Blurred vision |
| Alpha–adrenergic receptor blockade | Postural hypotension (dizziness, syncope) |
| Histaminergic receptor blockade | Weight gain Sedation |
| Cardiotoxic effects | QT interval prolongation, ST segment elevation, heart block, arrhythmias |

multi-receptor blocking effects of these drugs. Some patients benefit from the sedative properties of TCAs. Those with prominent sedative effects include amitriptyline, clomipramine, dosulepin (dothiepin) and trazodone (tricyclic-related compound). Those with less sedative effects include lofepramine and imipramine. Due to their cardiotoxic effects, some TCAs, especially dosulepin (dothiepin) and amitriptyline, are dangerous in overdose; whereas, lofepramine and trazodone are relatively safer. Lofepramine, a newer TCA, is also associated with fewer antimuscarinic effects.

**Contraindications: recent myocardial infarction, arrhythmias, severe liver disease and mania.**

## SSRIs

SSRIs have fewer anticholinergic effects than the TCAs and are less sedating. Due to the absence of cardiotoxic effects, they are the antidepressant of choice in patients with cardiac disease and in those who are at risk of taking an overdose. However, they do have their own side-effects that may be unacceptable to some patients. These are summarized in Figure 27.4. Concerns have been expressed that fluoxetine might be associated with an increased risk of suicide. There is no convincing evidence to support this claim.

**Contraindications: mania.**

Antidepressants should be used with caution in patients with epilepsy, as they tend to lower the seizure threshold.

## MAOIs/RIMA

Due to the risk of serious interactions with certain foods and other drugs, the MAOIs have become

second-line antidepressants. Their inhibition of monoamine oxidase A results in the accumulation of amine neurotransmitters and impairs the metabolism of some amines found in certain drugs (e.g. decongestants) and foodstuffs (e.g. tyramine). Because MAOIs bind *irreversibly* to monoamine oxidase A, amines may accumulate to dangerously high levels, which may precipitate a life-threatening hypertensive crisis. An example of this occurs when the ingestion of dietary tyramine results in a massive release of noradrenaline (norepinephrine) from endogenous stores. This is termed the 'cheese reaction' because some mature cheeses typically contain high levels of tyramine. Note that an early warning sign is a throbbing headache. Figure 27.5 lists the drugs and foodstuffs that should be avoided in patients taking MAOIs.

The RIMA moclobemide *reversibly* inhibits monoamine oxidase A. Therefore, the drug will be displaced from the enzyme as amines levels start to increase. So, although there is a small risk of developing a hypertensive crisis if high levels of tyramine are ingested, no dietary restrictions are required in general.

When other antidepressants that have a strong serotonergic effect (e.g. SSRIs, clomipramine, imipramine) are administered simultaneously with an MAOI, the risk of developing the potentially lethal 'serotonin syndrome' is increased. It resembles the neuroleptic malignant syndrome (see later) and is

### Common side-effects of the SSRIs

Gastrointestinal disturbance (nausea, vomiting, diarrhoea, pain) – early*
Anxiety and agitation – early*
Loss of appetite and weight loss (sometimes weight gain)
Insomnia
Sweating
Sexual dysfunction (anorgasmia, delayed ejaculation)

*Gastrointestinal and anxiety symptoms occur on initiation of treatment and resolve with time.*

**Fig. 27.4** Common side-effects of the SSRIs.

### Drugs and food that may precipitate a hypertensive crisis in combination with MAOIs

**Tyramine-rich foods**
Cheese—especially mature varieties (e.g. Stilton)
Degraded protein: pickled herring, smoked fish, chicken liver, hung game
Yeast and protein extract: Bovril®, Oxo®, Marmite®
Chianti wine, beer
Broad bean pods
Soya bean extract
Overripe or unfresh food

**Drugs**
Adrenaline (epinephrine), noradrenaline (norepinephrine)
Amfetamines
Cocaine
Ephedrine, pseudoephedrine, phenylpropanolamine (cough mixtures, decongestants)
L-dopa, dopamine
Local anaesthetics containing adrenaline (epinephrine)

*Note: the combination of MAOIs and antidepressants or opiates (especially pethidine) may result in the serotonin syndrome.*

**Fig. 27.5** Drugs and food that may precipitate a hypertensive crisis in combination with MAOIs.

characterized by agitation, fever, rigidity, myoclonus, cardiac arrhythmias and coma. Therefore, other antidepressants should not be started for 2 weeks after an MAOI has been stopped (3 weeks in the case of clomipramine and imipramine). Conversely, an MAOI should not be started for 1–2 weeks after the termination of another antidepressant (3 weeks in the case of clomipramine and imipramine; 5 weeks in the case of fluoxetine). The co-administration of opiates and an MAOI can also result in the serotonin syndrome. This is because opiates (especially pethidine and tramadol) have some intrinsic serotonin reuptake inhibitory activity.

MAOIs may have further side-effects similar to the TCAs, including postural hypotension and anticholinergic effects.

**Contraindications (MAOIs): phaeochromocytoma, cerebrovascular disease, hepatic impairment, mania.**

 The abrupt withdrawal of any antidepressant may result in a discontinuation syndrome with symptoms such as gastrointestinal disturbance, agitation, dizziness, headache, tremor and insomnia. SSRIs with short half-lives (e.g. paroxetine, sertraline) and venlafaxine are particular culprits. Therefore, all antidepressants should be gradually tapered down before being withdrawn completely. Although certain antidepressants may cause a withdrawal syndrome, they do not cause a dependence syndrome or 'addiction'.

## Mood stabilizers

These include lithium and the anticonvulsants valproate and carbamazepine. Other anticonvulsants such as lamotrigine, gabapentin, topiramate and vigabatrin are also being investigated for mood stabilizing properties.

## History

In 1949, an Australian, John Cade, discovered that lithium salts caused lethargy when injected into animals, and later reported lithium's antimanic properties in humans. Trials in the 1950s and 1960s led to the drug entering mainstream practice in 1970.

Valproate was first recognized as an effective anti-epileptic in 1963. Along with carbamazepine, it was later shown to be effective in bipolar affective disorder.

## Mechanism of action

It is not known how any of the mood stabilizers work. Lithium appears to modulate the neurotransmitter-induced activation of second messenger systems. Valproate and carbamazepine may exert their effect via the GABA system; carbamazepine is a GABA agonist and valproate inhibits GABA transaminase.

## Indications

Lithium is used in the treatment of:
- Acute mania – see pp. 88–89.
- Prophylaxis of bipolar of affective disorder (prevention of relapse) – see pp. 88–89.
- Treatment-resistant depression (lithium augmentation) – see p. 87.
- Other: adjunct to antipsychotics in schizoaffective disorder and schizophrenia; and aggression/impulsivity – see p. 93 and p. 117.

Valproate is used in the treatment of:
- Epilepsy.
- Acute mania – see p. pp. 88–89.
- Prophylaxis of bipolar of affective disorder (unlicensed indication) – see pp. 88–89.

Carbamazepine is used in the treatment of:
- Epilepsy.
- Prophylaxis of bipolar affective disorder (unresponsive to lithium) – see pp. 88–89.
- Rapid cycling bipolar disorder – see p. 88.
- Other: treatment-resistant mania, depression or schizophrenia; trigeminal neuralgia; impulse control disorders (see p. 117).

 Valproate is available in formulations as sodium valproate, valproic acid and semisodium valproate (Depakote®), which comprises equimolar amounts of sodium valproate and valproic acid.

## Side-effects and contraindications
### Lithium
Lithium has a narrow therapeutic window between non-therapeutic and toxic blood levels:
- Therapeutic levels: 0.5–1.0 mmol/L
- Toxic levels: >1.5 mmol/L
- Dangerously toxic levels: >2 mmol/L

Lithium is only taken orally and is excreted almost entirely by the kidneys. Renal clearance of lithium is decreased with renal insufficiency (e.g. in the elderly, dehydration) and sodium depletion. Certain drugs such as diuretics (especially thiazides), non-steroidal anti-inflammatory drugs (NSAIDs), and ACE-inhibitors can also increase lithium levels and should be prescribed with utmost caution. Furthermore, antipsychotics may synergistically increase lithium-induced neurotoxicity; this is important as lithium and antipsychotics are often co-administered in acute mania. Figure 27.6 summarizes the side-effects and signs of toxicity of lithium.

It follows that the following investigations are needed prior to initiating therapy:
- Full blood count.
- Renal function and electrolytes.
- Thyroid function.
- Pregnancy test.
- ECG.

Blood levels are monitored weekly after starting treatment until a therapeutic level has been stable for 4 weeks. Lithium blood levels should then be monitored every 3 months; renal function every 6 months; and thyroid function every 12 months.

**Contraindications/cautions: pregnancy, breast-feeding (see p. 125), renal insufficiency,** thyroid disease, cardiac conditions, neurological conditions (e.g. Parkinson's or Huntington's disease).

Lithium, carbamazepine and valproate have potentially serious pharmacokinetic and pharmacodynamic interactions with many other drugs. Therefore, before prescribing new medication for patients on these mood stabilizers, check a drug interactions reference, e.g. Appendix 1 in the British National Formulary (BNF).

### Carbamazepine and sodium valproate
Figure 27.7 summarizes the side-effects of carbamazepine and valproate. It is important to check liver and haematological functions prior to, and soon after, starting these drugs due to the risk of serious blood and hepatic disorders.

## Antipsychotics

### History
Antipsychotics or neuroleptics (originally known as 'major tranquillizers') appeared in the early 1950s with the introduction of the phenothiazine, chlorpromazine. Their ability to treat psychotic symptoms had a profound impact on psychiatry, accelerating the movement of patients out of the old asylums and into the community. The efficacy of chlorpromazine in treating psychotic symptoms seemed to be related to

**Fig. 27.6** Side-effects and signs of toxicity of lithium.

| Side-effects and signs of toxicity of lithium | |
|---|---|
| **Side-effects** | **Signs of toxicity** |
| Thirst, polydipsia, polyuria weight gain, oedema<br>Fine tremor<br>Precipitates or worsens skin problems<br>Concentration and memory problems<br>Hypothyroidism<br>Impaired renal function<br>Cardiac: T-wave flattening or inversion<br>Leucocytosis<br>Teratogenicity | **1.5–2 mmol/L:** nausea and vomiting, apathy, coarse tremor, ataxia, muscle weakness<br>**>2 mmol/L:** nystagmus, dysarthria, impaired consciousness, hyperactive tendon reflexes, oliguria, hypotension, convulsions, coma<br><br>Note: the treatment of lithium toxicity is supportive ensuring adequate hydration, renal function and electrolyte balance. Anticonvulsants may be necessary for convulsions and haemodialysis may be indicated in cases of renal failure |

| Side-effects of carbamazepine and valproate | |
|---|---|
| **Valproate** | **Carbamazepine** |
| Increased appetite and weitht gain | Nausea and vomiting |
| Sedation and dizziness | Skin rashes |
| Ankle swelling | Blurred or double vision (diplopia) |
| Hair loss | Ataxia, drowsiness, fatigue |
| Nausea and vomiting | Hyponatraemia and fluid retention |
| Tremor | Haematological abnormalities |
| Haematological abnormalities (prolongation of bleeding time, thrombocytopaenia, leucopaenia) | (leucopaenia, thrombocytopaenia, eosinophillia) |
| | Raised liver enzymes (hepatic or cholestatic jaundice rare) |
| Raised liver enzymes (liver damage very uncommon) | |
| *Note: Serious blood and liver disorders do occur but are rare* | *Note: serious blood and liver disorders do occur but are rare* |

**Fig. 27.7** Side-effects of carbamazepine and valproate.

its blockade of dopamine $D_2$ receptors in the brain. A number of antipsychotics with a similar pharmacodynamic action soon followed, e.g. the butyrophenone, haloperidol, in the 1960s. However, serious side-effects, e.g. extra-pyramidal side-effects (EPSE), soon became apparent with all these drugs. These side-effects were also related to the blockade of dopamine $D_2$ receptors in other parts of the brain.

Clozapine, which has comparatively little activity at $D_2$ receptors, was the first antipsychotic devoid of extra-pyramidal side-effects, and thus was termed 'atypical'. It led to the introduction of several other atypical antipsychotics, including risperidone, olanzapine and quetiapine, which are currently first-line treatments of schizophrenia. The older

The atypical antipsychotics were initially so called because they failed to induce catalepsy (an extra-pyramidal syndrome) when given to animals, as the typical antipsychotics were known to do. 'Atypicals' thus became antipsychotics that were mostly devoid of extra-pyramidal motor effects, the first of which was clozapine. Today, the term atypical has additional meanings. It can also refer to the action of alleviating both negative and positive symptoms, as well as to the capacity to block serotonin 2A (5-HT2$_A$) receptors – a property of most of the atypical agents introduced to date.

antipsychotics such as haloperidol and chlorpromazine became known as the conventional or typical antipsychotics.

## Indications of antipsychotics
### Psychiatric indications
- Schizophrenia, schizoaffective disorder, delusional disorder – see p. 93.
- Depression or mania with psychotic features – see pp. 86–89.
- Psychotic episodes secondary to a medical condition or psychoactive substance use.
- Delirium – see p. 108 (caution in alcohol withdrawal as lowers seizure threshold).
- Behavioural disturbance in dementia – see p. 106.
- Severe agitation, anxiety and violent or impulsive behaviour – see p. 95.

### Non-psychiatric indications
- Motor tics (Gilles de la Tourette's syndrome) – see p. 151.
- Nausea and vomiting, e.g. prochlorperazine.
- Intractable hiccups and pruritus, e.g. chlorpromazine, haloperidol.

## Classification
Figure 27.8 summarizes the classification of the antipsychotics, which might be useful when trying to understand the side-effects that are particular to certain specific types of antipsychotics – see side-effects.

## Mechanism of action and side-effects
### Conventional (typical) antipsychotics
The efficacy of the conventional antipsychotics in treating psychotic symptoms is thought to be due to

**Fig. 27.8** Classification of the antipsychotics.

| Classification of the antipsychotics | |
|---|---|
| **Chemical class** | **Examples** |
| **Conventional/ Typical Antipsychotics** | |
| Phenothiazines | Aliphatic side chain: chlorpromazine (Largactil®), promazine (Sparine®)<br>Piperidine side chain: thioridazine (Melleril®), pipotiazine (Piportil Depot®)<br>Piperazine side chain: trifluoperazine (Stelazine®), fluphenazine (Modecate®) |
| Butyrophenones | Haloperidol (Serenace®, Haldol®) |
| Thioxanthenes | Flupentixol (Depixol®)<br>Zuclopenthixol (Clopixol®) |
| Substituted benzamides | Sulpiride (Dolmatil®) |
| Diphenylbutylpiperidines | Pimozide (Orap®) |
| **Atypical Antipsychotics** | |
| Dibenzodiazepines | Clozapine (Clozaril®) |
| Thienobenzodiazepines | Olanzapine (Zyprexa®) |
| Benzisoxazoles | Risperidone (Risperdal®) |
| Dibenzothiazepines | Quetiapine (Seroquel®) |
| Substituted benzamides | Amisulpride (Solian®) |

their ability to block dopamine $D_2$ receptors in the mesolimbic dopamine pathway. Unfortunately, these drugs block all the dopamine $D_2$ receptors in the entire brain, resulting in their characteristic side-effects. In addition, these drugs also cause side-effects by blocking muscarinic, histaminergic and α-adrenergic receptors. Figure 27.9 summarizes both the useful and troublesome clinical effects of $D_2$-receptor antagonism as well as the side-effects caused by the blockage of other receptors. Learn this table well; these effects are often asked for in exams. Note that certain types of conventional antipsychotics are associated with specific side-effects:

- The phenothiazines with an aliphatic side chain (e.g. chlorpromazine) have strong sedative effects and moderate anticholinergic effects and moderate EPSE.
- The phenothiazines with a piperidine side chain (e.g. thioridazine) have strong anticholinergic effects and moderate sedative effects, but weak EPSE.
- The phenothiazines with a piperazine side chain (e.g. trifluoperazine, fluphenazine) have strong

EPSE, but weak sedative and anticholinergic effects.

- The conventional antipsychotics in other classes (e.g. butyrophenones, thioxanthenes) and the depot preparations resemble the phenothiazines with a piperazine side chain, i.e. they have strong EPSE and weaker sedative and anticholinergic effects.

The tricyclic antidepressants and the conventional antipsychotics are multi-receptor blockers; therefore, both groups of drugs cause anticholinergic (dry mouth, constipation, blurred vision, urinary retention), anti-adrenergic (postural hypotension) and anti-histaminergic (sedation, weight gain) side-effects.

Figure 27.10 summarizes the antipsychotic-induced extra-pyramidal side-effects and

| Dopamine d$_2$-receptor antagonism | | |
|---|---|---|
| Location of dopamine D$_2$ receptors | Function | Clinical effect of dopamine D$_2$-receptor antagonism |
| Mesolimbic pathway | Involved in delusions/hallucinations/thought disorder, euphoria and drug dependence | Treatment of psychotic symptoms |
| Mesocortical pathway | Mediates cognitive and negative symptoms of schizophrenia | Worsening of negative and cognitive symptoms of schizophrenia |
| Nigrostriatal pathway (basal ganglia/striatum) | Controls motor movement | Extra-pyramidal side-effects (EPSE) – see Fig. 27.10: <br> • Parkinsonian symptoms <br> • Acute dystonia <br> • Akathisia <br> • Tardive dyskinesia <br> • Neuroleptic malignant syndrome |
| Tuberoinfindibular pathway | Controls prolactin secretion – dopamine inhibits prolactin release | Hyperprolactinaemia <br> • Galactorrhoea (breast milk production) <br> • Amenorrhoea and infertility <br> • Sexual dysfunction |
| Chemoreceptor trigger zone | Controls nausea and vomiting | Anti-emetic effect: some phenothiazines, e.g. prochlorperazine (Stemetil®) are very effective in treating nausea and vomiting |
| Other side-effects | | |
| Anticholinergic: muscarinic receptor blockade | Dry mouth, constipation, urinary retention, blurred vision | |
| Alpha-adrenergic receptor blockade | Postural hypotension (dizziness, syncope) | |
| Histaminergic receptor blockade | Sedation, weight gain | |
| Cardiac effects | Prolongation of QT-interval, arrhythmias, myocarditis, sudden death | |
| Dermatological effects | Photosensitivity, skin rashes (especially chlorpromazine: blue-grey discoloration in the sun) | |
| Other | Lowering of seizure threshold, hepatotoxicity, cholestatic jaundice, pancytopenia, agranulocytosis | |

**Fig. 27.9** The clinical and side-effects of conventional antipsychotics.

The extra-pyramidal side-effects (EPSE): parkinson-like motor symptoms and acute dystonia, are due to a relative deficiency of dopamine and an excess of acetylcholine induced by dopamine antagonism in the nigrostriatal pathway. This is why anticholinergic drugs are effective treatments and why piperidine phenothiazines, which inherently have a strong anticholinergic action, do not cause such severe EPSE.

treatment. Note that atypical antipsychotics may also be associated with EPSE, especially in high doses.

Certain antipsychotics are available in a slow-release form, as an intramuscular depot preparation that can be administered every 2–4 weeks, e.g. fluphenazine decanoate (Modecate®), flupentixol decanoate (Depixol®), pipotiazine palmitate (Piportil®). They are used for patients who are poorly compliant with oral therapy.

## Atypical antipsychotics

Although the pharmacodynamic actions of the atypical antipsychotics are diverse most of

**Antipsychotic-induced extra-pyramidal side-effects and treatment**

| Extrapyramidal side-effect | Description | Treatment |
| --- | --- | --- |
| Parkinsonian motor symptoms | Muscular rigidity, bradykinesia (lack of, or slowing, of movement), resting tremor<br>Generally occurs within a month of starting antipsychotic | Anticholinergics, e.g. procyclidine (i.v. for acute onset)<br>Consider reducing dose of antipsychotic or switching to antipsychotic with fewer EPSE (e.g. atypical) |
| Acute dystonia | Involuntary sustained muscular contractions or spasms, e.g. neck (spasmodic torticollis), clenched jaw (trismus), protruding tongue, eyes roll upwards (oculogyric crisis)<br>More common in young men<br>Usually occurs within 72 hours of treatment | |
| Akathisia | Subjective feeling of inner restlessness and muscular discomfort<br>Occurs within 6–60 days | Propranolol or short-term benzodiazepines<br>Consider reducing dose of antipsychotic or switching to antipsychotic with fewer EPSE (e.g. atypical) |
| Tardive dyskinesia (TD) | Rhythmic, involuntary movements of head, limbs and trunk, especially chewing, grimacing of mouth and protruding, darting movements of tongue<br>Develops in up to 20% of patients who receive long-term treatment with conventional antipsychotics | No effective treatment<br>Withdraw antipsychotic if possible<br>Clozapine might be helpful<br>Consider benzodiazepines<br>Do not give anticholinergics (may worsen TD) |
| Neuroleptic malignant syndrome | Life-threatening condition characterized by:<br>*Motor signs:* severe muscular rigidity<br>*Mental signs:* fluctuating consciousness<br>*Autonomic disturbance:* hyperthermia, unstable blood pressure, rapid pulse, sweating<br>*Blood tests:* high creatinine kinase levels<br>Usually occurs within 4–11 days of initiation of treatment or change of dosage | Stop antipsychotic<br>Dantrolene to reduce muscle spasm<br>Bromocriptine to reverse dopamine blockade<br>Cool patient, monitor vital signs, renal function and electrolytes |

**Fig. 27.10** Antipsychotic-induced extra-pyramidal side-effects and treatment.

The atypical antipsychotic clozapine is a very effective antipsychotic but, due to the life-threatening risk of bone marrow suppression with agranulocytosis (1% of patients), is only used in treatment-resistant schizophrenia. Patients should be registered with a clozapine monitoring service and have a full blood count (FBC) with differential prior to starting treatment. This is followed by regular FBCs in an out-patient clinic.

the atypical antipsychotics block both serotonin 2A receptors (5-HT2$_A$) and dopamine D$_2$ receptors. Atypicals also have differing affinities for other receptors including muscarinic, histaminergic and α-adrenergic receptors, which accounts for their varied side-effect profiles. Figure 27.11 summarizes some of the important side-effects associated with the atypical antipsychotics.

## Anxiolytic and hypnotic drugs

A hypnotic drug is one that induces sleep. An anxiolytic or sedative drug is one that reduces anxiety. This differentiation is not particularly helpful as anxiolytic drugs can induce sleep when given in higher doses and hypnotics can have a calming effect when given in lower doses, e.g. the

### Important side-effects of the atypical antipsychotics

| Drug | Side-effect |
|------|-------------|
| Clozapine | Agranulocytosis (regular white blood cell count essential) Risk of seizures in high doses Hypersalivation Weight gain Moderate risk of diabetes |
| Risperidone | Can cause EPSE, especially at higher doses Weight gain Increased prolactin |
| Olanzapine | Weight gain Sedation High risk of diabetes |
| Amisulpiride | Increased prolactin |

**Fig. 27.11** Important side-effects of the atypical antipsychotics.

In the past, the antipsychotics have been referred to as the 'major tranquillizers' and the anxiolytics as the 'minor tranquillizers'. This is misleading because: (1) these drugs are not pharmacologically related; (2) the antipsychotics do far more than just tranquillize; and (3) the effect and use of anxiolytics is in no way minor.

benzodiazepines, which are anxiolytic in low doses and hypnotic in high doses. All of these drugs can result in tolerance, dependence and withdrawal symptoms. Furthermore, their effects, when used in combination or with alcohol, are additive. The benzodiazepines are the most important drugs in this group.

## History

In the 1960s the benzodiazepines replaced the often-abused barbiturates as the drugs of choice for the treatment of anxiety and insomnia. However, this initial enthusiasm was tempered by the observation that they were associated with serious dependence and withdrawal syndromes. Today, benzodiazepines are recognized as highly effective and relatively safe drugs when prescribed judiciously with good patient education.

## Classification

From a clinical perspective, it is important to classify benzodiazepines according to their strength, their length of action and their routes of administration. Figure 27.12 summarizes these qualities in some common benzodiazepines.

## Mechanism of action

Benzodiazepines potentiate the action of GABA (γ-aminobutyric acid), the main inhibitory neurotransmitter in the brain. They bind to specific benzodiazepine receptors on the $GABA_A$ receptor complex, which results in an increased affinity of the complex for GABA. This results in increased activity of chloride ion channels with the flow of chloride

### Classification of the benzodiazepines

| Drug | Dose equivalent to 5 mg diazepam | Length of action | Half-life | Routes of administration |
|------|----------------------------------|------------------|-----------|--------------------------|
| Temazepam | 10 mg | Short acting | 11 h | Oral |
| Oxazepam | 15 mg | Short acting | 8 h | Oral |
| Lorazepam | 0.5 mg | Short acting | 15 h | Oral, i.m.*, i.v. |
| Chlordiazepoxide | 15 mg | Long acting | 100 h | Oral |
| Diazepam | 5 mg | Long acting | 100 h | Oral, per rectum, i.v. Only i.m. if no alternative |

*Lorazepam is the only benzodiazepine that has predictable absorption when given intramuscularly.*

**Fig. 27.12** Classification of the benzodiazepines.

into the neuron, thereby hyperpolarizing the post-synaptic membrane. Benzodiazepines are effective hypnotics, anxiolytics, anticonvulsants and muscle relaxants.

## Indications of benzodiazepines

- Insomnia, especially short-acting benzodiazepines – see p. 131.
- Anxiety disorders – see pp. 98–99.
- Alcohol withdrawal, especially chlordiazepoxide – see pp. 110–111.
- Akathisia – see Figure 27.10.
- Acute mania or psychosis (sedation) – see p. 88 and p. 95.
- Other: epilepsy prophylaxis, seizures, muscle spasm (diazepam), anaesthetic premedication.

## Side-effects of benzodiazepines

- Patients should be warned about the potential dangers of driving or operating machinery due to drowsiness, ataxia and reduced motor coordination.
- Benzodiazepines should be used with caution in patients with chronic respiratory disease (e.g. COPD, sleep apnoea) as they may depress respiration.
- Risk of developing dependence, especially with prolonged use and shorter acting drugs.
- Benzodiazepines are seldom fatal in overdose. Flumazenil, a benzodiazepine receptor antagonist, may be helpful in differentiating benzodiazepine-induced loss of consciousness from other causes.

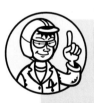 Alcohol, opiates, barbiturates, tricyclic antidepressants, antihistamines and other sedative-hypnotics may all enhance the effects of benzodiazepines; therefore, moderate doses of benzodiazepines in combination with some of these substances can result in respiratory depression.

## Other hypnotic and anxiolytic agents

- The short-acting hypnotics: zopiclone, zolpidem and zaleplon, also act at benzodiazepine receptors, although they are structurally different to the benzodiazepines. Like temazepam, they have a short half-life and do not cause a hangover on the following day.
- Buspirone is a $5-HT_{1A}$ receptor agonist that is used to treat generalized anxiety disorder. It is unrelated to the benzodiazepines, does not have hypnotic, anticonvulsant or muscle relaxant properties, and is not associated with dependence or abuse. Response to treatment may take up to 2 weeks, unlike the benzodiazepines which have an immediate anxiolytic effect. It is, therefore, less useful in patients who, having been treated with benzodiazepines in the past, expect rapid relief of anxiety.
- Sedating antihistamines, e.g. diphenhydramine (Nytol®) are available for insomnia without a prescription. Unfortunately, their long duration of action may lead to drowsiness the following day.
- Clomethiazole, meprobamate and chloral hydrate are no longer first-line sedative-hypnotics due to their adverse effects – see p. 110.

## Other drugs used in psychiatry

*Alcohol dependence:* acamprosate, disulfiram – see p. 111.

*Opiate dependence:* methadone, buprenorphine, lofexidine, naltrexone – see pp. 112–113.

*Dementia:* cholinesterase inhibitors (donepezil, rivastigmine, galantamine), memantine – see p. 106.

*Psychostimulants:* methylphenidate, dexamfetamine – see p. 149.

## Electroconvulsive therapy

### History

The idea that seizures could improve psychiatric symptoms arose from the observation that convulsions led to an improvement of psychotic symptoms in patients with both epilepsy and schizophrenia. This led to seizures being induced pharmacologically with intramuscular camphor in the early 1930s. An electric stimulus was later discovered to be a safe and effective way of inducing seizures, although it proved to be a crude and often dangerous procedure without modern-day anaesthetic induction agents and muscle relaxants. Today, ECT is a safe and often life-saving treatment for patients with serious mental illness.

## Indications

ECT is predominantly used for depression. Although antidepressants are usually the first-line treatment, ECT is considered for the following forms of depression:

- With life-threatening poor fluid intake.
- With strong suicidal intent.
- With psychotic features or stupor.
- When antidepressants are ineffective or not tolerated.

Although ECT may precipitate a manic episode in patients with bipolar affective disorder, it is an effective treatment for established mania. ECT is also an effective treatment for certain types of schizophrenia, specifically catatonic states, positive psychotic symptoms and schizoaffective disorder. ECT is also used for puerperal psychosis (see Ch. 20) with prominent mood symptoms where a rapid improvement is necessary to reunite the mother with her baby.

## Administration and mechanism of action

ECT is administered 2–3 times per week. Most patients need between 4 and 12 treatments. An anaesthetist administers a short-acting induction agent and muscle relaxant that ensure about 5 minutes of general anaesthesia. During this time, a psychiatrist applies two electrodes to the patient's scalp, in a bilateral or unilateral placement, and delivers an electric current of sufficient charge to effect a generalized seizure of at least 15 seconds in duration.

It is still not clear how ECT works. It causes a release of neurotransmitters as well as hypothalamic and pituitary hormones; it also affects neurotransmitter receptors and second-messenger systems, and results in a transient increase in blood–brain barrier permeability.

## Side-effects

The mortality from ECT is the same as that for any minor surgical procedure under general anaesthesia. Loss of memory is a common complaint, particularly for events surrounding the ECT. However, some patients may have impairment of some autobiographical memory. Unfortunately, there are few studies that examine the longterm effects of ECT.

Memory impairment might be reduced by unilateral electrode placement (as opposed to bilateral). Minor complaints such as confusion, headache, nausea and muscle pains are experienced by 80% of patients. Anaesthetic complications (e.g. arrhythmias, aspiration) can be reduced by good preoperative assessment. Prolonged seizures may occur, especially in patients who are on drugs that lower the seizure threshold, e.g. antidepressants and antipsychotics. In contrast, benzodiazepines increase the seizure threshold, making it more difficult to induce a seizure of adequate length.

## Contraindications

There are no absolute contraindications to ECT. Relative contraindications include:

- Heart disease (recent myocardial infarction, heart failure, ischaemic heart disease).
- Raised intracranial pressure.
- Risk of cerebral bleeding (hypertension, recent stroke).
- Poor anaesthetic risk.

# 28. Psychological Therapy

## What is it?

Psychological therapy or psychotherapy describes the interaction between a therapist and a client that leads to beneficial changes in the client's thoughts, feelings and behaviours. Psychological therapy, which is sometimes called 'talking therapy', may be useful in alleviating specific symptoms (e.g. social phobia), or in helping a client improve their overall sense of well-being.

## Who does it?

Members of different professional disciplines, including clinical psychologists, psychiatrists, occupational therapists, mental health nurses, art and drama therapists and counsellors, may all practise psychotherapy, provided they have had adequate training and supervision.

## What approaches are there?

There are many different schools of thought and approaches to psychotherapy. Research has shown efficacy for many different types of psychotherapies for many conditions. This has led to the idea that the success of psychotherapy might be due to certain common therapeutic factors as opposed to specific theories or techniques. A comprehensive review of psychotherapy research showed that common factors, that are operable in any model of therapy, account for 85% of the therapeutic effect, whereas, theoretical orientation only accounts for 15% (Lambert 1992). Common therapeutic factors include client factors (personal strengths, social supports), therapist–client relationship factors (empathy, acceptance, warmth) and the client's expectancy of change.

The single factor most commonly associated with a good therapeutic outcome is the strength of the client–therapist relationship (therapeutic alliance), regardless of the modality of therapy.

## Counselling and supportive psychotherapy

Psychotherapy is sometimes distinguished from counselling, although they exist on a continuum from counselling and supportive psychotherapy, which represent the least complex forms of intervention, to psychodynamic psychotherapy and sophisticated cognitive therapy, which represent the more complex interventions – and which require more specialized training.

Counselling is usually brief in duration and is recommended for clients with minor mental health or interpersonal difficulties or for those experiencing stressful life circumstances, e.g. grief counselling for bereavement. The emphasis is on helping clients utilize their own strengths, with the therapist being reflective and empathic. It also includes providing information and advice and will therefore be undertaken by all healthcare professionals at some time.

In *person-centred counselling* (developed by Carl Rogers), the therapist assumes an empathic and reflective role, allowing clients to discover their own insights, with the basic premise that the client ultimately knows best (non-directive counselling). *Problem-solving counselling* is more directive and focused as clients are actively assisted in finding solutions to their problems.

There is evidence that counselling confers some benefit for anxiety and depression in primary care settings but not for more severe mental disorders.

## Psychodynamic psychotherapy

Sigmund Freud introduced psychoanalytic theory in the late 19th century. Figure 28.1 summarizes some of his ideas. Psychoanalysis has changed somewhat since then with the contributions of many other influential theorists, e.g. Carl Jung, Alfred Adler and Melanie Klein. It is assumed in psychoanalytic theory that it is mainly *unconscious* thoughts, feelings and fantasies that give rise to distressing symptoms. These are said to arise in childhood, if an individual does not progress adequately through the various stages of psychological development.

The essential aim then of psychoanalysis or psychodynamic psychotherapy is to make symptom-causing, unconscious processes conscious. It is the therapist's role to identify and interpret these repressed processes, of which patients are unaware, and then to help them understand these in the context of a safe, caring relationship. The methods used to access these repressed processes include:

- Free association: with prompting, the client reports the first thoughts that come to mind.
- Hypnosis.
- The interpretation of dreams and fantasy material.
- The analysis of defence mechanisms: individuals are said to employ defences when

anxiety-producing aspects of the self that are unconscious, threaten to break through to the conscious mind, potentially giving rise to intolerable feelings, e.g. repression (anxiety-provoking feelings, thoughts or fantasies are pushed into the unconscious), projection (one's own unacknowledged feelings are attributed to someone else).

- The analysis of transference and counter-transference: *transference* occurs when the patient inappropriately transfers feelings or attitudes experienced in an earlier significant relationship onto the therapist, e.g. a male patient becomes angry with his therapist who he sees as cold and uncaring, unconsciously reminding him of his mother. *Counter-transference* occurs when the therapist inappropriately transfers feelings or attitudes experienced in an earlier significant relationship onto the patient.

Although the terms *psychoanalytic* and *psychodynamic* are often used interchangeably, the following therapeutic techniques are distinguished:

- The term *psychoanalysis* is traditionally used to describe the therapy where clients see their analyst five times per week for a non-specified period of time; therapy is conducted with clients on a couch in the recumbent position with the analyst out of view. The analyst hardly says anything except to make an 'interpretation'.
- The term *psychodynamic psychotherapy* usually describes the therapy, which although based on psychoanalytic theory, has client and therapist sitting face-to-face for about one session per week. Therapy tends to be more interactive than psychoanalysis. *Brief insight-oriented psychotherapy* (also called *focal psychotherapy*) is a shorter version of psychodynamic therapy (6–9 months) and tends to only focus on problems affecting current functioning. Psychodynamic psychotherapy may be conducted on an individual basis or in a group setting (see later).

---

### Some of Freud's ideas.

#### The structural model

Freud believed that the psychic apparatus (personality) consisted of three parts:

- Id (the pleasurable): the unconscious part, which is governed by the pleasure principle, and demands immediate satisfaction. It is primitive, instinctive, animalistic and hedonistic.
- Superego (the ideal): the ethical and moral part that sets rigid standards for behaviour. It is usually internalized from the parent's moral code and gives rise to feelings of guilt – as a kind of conscience.
- Ego (the actual): the conscious and cognitive part of the mind that is in touch with reality. It mediates between the demands of the id, the superego and external reality.

#### Psychosexual development

Freud believed that adult personality types were linked to five stages of development: *oral* (birth to 1 year), *anal* (1–3 years), *phallic* (3–6 years), *latency* (6 years to puberty) and *genital* (maturation). Excessive frustration or gratification in any stage could lead to an individual becoming *fixated* in that stage, which would present as specific neuroses, e.g. so-called: oral or anal personality

**Fig. 28.1** Some of Freud's ideas.

Transference and counter-transference often occur in settings outside of a psychodynamic psychotherapy. Patients may inappropriately react to healthcare professionals as if they were some significant figure from the past. An example is when patients express unwarranted anger towards doctors or nurses when they do not receive immediate attention; this may be anger that was initially experienced towards neglectful parents. Similarly, health workers may misplace feelings from their own earlier relationships onto patients.

## Behaviour therapy

Behaviour therapists are concerned with changing maladaptive behaviour patterns that have arisen through inappropriate learning (classical or operant conditioning). They are not concerned with the patient's inner experience or conflicts, and treatment only aims to replace unhelpful behaviour with more adaptive behaviour. Figure 28.2 summarizes some of the techniques used in behaviour therapy. Please see Chapter 22 for the specific techniques used in the psychosexual disorders.

## Cognitive behavioural therapy

Cognitive-behavioural therapy (CBT), which is also referred to as cognitive therapy, was developed by Aaron T. Beck, and is based on the assumption that how individuals think about or interpret things (i.e. their *cognitions*) subsequently determines how they feel and behave. Cognitive techniques include eliciting *automatic thoughts* and *dysfunctional assumptions*, and then testing their validity.

***Automatic thoughts***   Automatic thoughts are the many thoughts that involuntarily enter an individual's mind in response to specific situations, e.g. 'He doesn't like me'; 'I'm such an idiot'; 'I'm so boring'.

***Dysfunctional assumptions***   *Dysfunctional assumptions* are the faulty 'rules' that individuals live by, which, when broken, as they inevitably are, lead to psychological distress, e.g. 'If I don't come first, then I am completely useless'; 'If I hurt someone, then I am evil'.

Using an example, Figure 28.3 summarizes some important aspects of the cognitive model.

CBT also draws on principles from behavioural theory, e.g. dysfunctional assumptions may be

---

**Some techniques used in behaviour therapy**

| Behavioural technique | Clinical uses | Description |
|---|---|---|
| Exposure | Phobias and avoidance, post-traumatic stress disorder | Systematic desensitization: a hierarchy of increasingly threatening situations is created, e.g. spider in another room →spider in the same room →spider near the patient → spider on the patient's hand. Patients imagine, or are exposed to, the least threatening situation while practising relaxation techniques. When anxiety relief has been achieved, patients are then exposed to increasingly threatening situations. There is evidence that real life exposure is more effective, although sometimes impractical.<br>Flooding: patients are instantly exposed to the highest level of their anxiety hierarchy (i.e. flooded) until their anxiety diminishes, e.g. throwing patient with a fear of water in the deep end of a swimming pool (flooding by imagination is termed implosion therapy) |
| Exposure with response prevention | OCD | Patients are encouraged to resist carrying out compulsions until the urge diminishes. They are then exposed to more severe compulsion-evoking situations |
| Relaxation | Anxiety | Progressive relaxation of muscle groups; breathing exercises; visualizing relaxing images and situations (*guided imagery*) |
| Modelling | Phobias and avoidance, OCD | Patients observe the therapist being exposed to the phobic stimulus, then attempt the same |
| Activity scheduling and target setting | Depression | Patients are encouraged to structure their day with certain activities, as depression-induced reduced activity can lead to a further lowering of mood due to reduced stimulation and opportunity for positive experiences |

OCD, obsessive-compulsive disorder

**Fig. 28.2** Some techniques used in behaviour therapy.

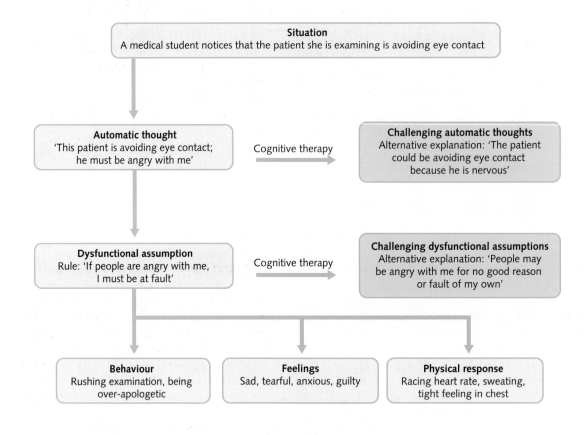

**Fig. 28.3** Illustration of some aspects of the cognitive model.

challenged by behavioural experiments (testing irrational thoughts against reality).

Note that CBT differs from psychodynamic psychotherapy in the following ways:

- CBT tends to be time-limited (12–25 sessions).
- CBT is goal-oriented and predominantly focuses on present problems – it is less concerned with the details of how problems developed or unconscious drives.
- The client and CBT therapist are strongly collaborative, deciding together on the session's agenda and case formulation.
- CBT involves patients doing 'homework assignments'.
- Due to its structured format, CBT is more amenable to efficacy studies.

The other forms of therapy that incorporate elements of CBT are summarized in Figure 28.4.

Beck classically described how depressed patients suffered from a *cognitive triad* of symptoms:
- Negative view of oneself, e.g. 'I am a worthless failure'.
- Negative view of one's environment, e.g. 'The world is harsh and pointless'.
- Negative view of the future, e.g. 'There is nothing for me to live for'.

| Some therapies incorporating elements of cognitive-behavioural therapy (CBT) | | |
|---|---|---|
| **Therapy type** | **Description** | **Developer** |
| Dialectical behaviour therapy (DBT) | An intensive and demanding form of therapy that has shown promising results in the treatment of borderline personality disorder and self-harm | Marsha Linehan |
| Cognitive analytic therapy (CAT) | An brief integrative therapy combining elements of both cognitive behaviour and psychoanalytic theories | Anthony Ryle (specifically in response to the NHS's need for therapies of short duration) |
| Rational emotive behaviour therapy (REBT) | Consists of encouraging patients to challenge and dispel 'irrational thoughts' | Albert Ellis |

NHS, National Health Service (UK)

**Fig. 28.4** Some therapies incorporating elements of cognitive-behavioural therapy (CBT).

## Interpersonal therapy

Interpersonal therapy (IPT) is based on the assumption that problems with interpersonal relationships and social functioning are significant contributors to the development of mental illness, as well as being a consequence of mental illness, particularly depression. IPT attempts to enable patients to evaluate their social interactions and improve their interpersonal skills in all social roles, from close family and friendships to community and work-related roles. Main areas of focus include: (1) role disputes; (2) role transitions; (3) interpersonal deficits; and (4) loss or grief. IPT is similar to CBT in that it tends to focus on current problems and is brief in duration (12–16 sessions). It was developed by Weissman and Klerman, and was largely influenced by Harry Stack Sullivan's *Interpersonal Psychiatry*.

## Group therapy

Group therapy may be practised according to different theoretical orientations, from supportive to cognitive-behavioural to psychodynamic approaches. Most groups meet once weekly for an hour and consist of one or two therapists and a selection of about 8–10 patients. Therapy can run from months (CBT orientation) to years (psychodynamic orientation). Group therapy allows patients (and therapists) the opportunity to observe and analyse their psychological and behavioural responses to other individuals in the group in a 'safe' social setting. It is thought that group therapy owes its effectiveness to a number of 'curative factors', e.g. *universality*, which describes the process of patients realizing that they are not alone in having particular problems.

## Family therapy

Instead of focusing on the individual patient, this form of therapy treats the family as a whole. It may include just parents and siblings or extended family. It is hoped that improved family communication and conflict resolution will result in an improvement of the 'symptomatic patient'. Similarly to group therapy, there are many different orientations, most notably the psychodynamic, structural and systems approach.

## Milieu therapy (therapeutic community)

Therapeutic communities are cohesive residential communities that consist of a group of about 30 patients who are resident for between 9 and 18 months. During this time residents are encouraged to take responsibility for themselves and others, e.g. by allowing them to be involved in running the unit. They may be useful for patients with personality disorders (especially antisocial and borderline types) and behavioural problems. An example is the Henderson Hospital in London.

The term *eclectic therapy* refers to the practice of using a mixture of psychotherapeutic theories and techniques (e.g. psychodynamic, interpersonal and cognitive-behavioural therapy) in understanding and treating the same patient. Many therapists use it to create a therapy package uniquely tailored to the individual.

## What is it used for?

The psychological treatment options for specific conditions have been discussed in each of the relevant chapters in these conditions. The main treatment options with the strongest evidence base, along with relevant cross-references, have been summarized in Figure 28.5. Note, however, that the lack of evidence for certain psychological treatments does not mean that they are not effective.

| Main indications of psychological treatments | | |
|---|---|---|
| **Psychiatric condition** | **Main psychological treatment used** | **Cross-reference** |
| Stressful life events, illnesses, bereavements | Counselling | See p. 99 |
| Depression | Cognitive-behaviour therapy, interpersonal therapy<br>Other: psychodynamic therapy, group therapy | See p. 87 |
| Anxiety disorders (including OCD) | Cognitive-behavioural therapy | See pp. 98–99 |
| Post-traumatic stress disorder | Systematic desensitization<br>Eye movement desensitization<br>Other: psychodynamic therapy, hypnotherapy | See p. 99 |
| Schizophrenia | Cognitive-behavioural therapy<br>Family therapy | See p. 94 |
| Eating disorders | Cognitive-behavioural therapy<br>Interpersonal therapy<br>Family therapy | See p. 121 |
| Borderline personality disorder | Dialectical behaviour therapy<br>Psychodynamic therapy<br>Cognitive analytic therapy<br>Therapeutic communities | See pp. 116–117 |
| Alcohol dependence | Cognitive-behavioural therapy<br>Group therapy | See p.111 |

OCD, obsessive-compulsive disorder

**Fig. 28.5** Main indications of psychological treatments.

# 29. Mental Health Legislation

Severe mental illness can place patients at risk of deliberate self-harm, self-neglect or exploitation from others. It can also make them a danger to others. When they lose insight into their condition and refuse hospitalization or psychiatric treatment, mental health and law enforcement officers may need to enact mental health legislation in order to protect patients' interests, as well as those of the public. The following legislation is applicable in the UK:

- England and Wales: Mental Health Act 1983.
- Scotland: Mental Health (Scotland) Act 1984.
- Northern Ireland: Mental Health (Northern Ireland) Order 1986.

## England and Wales Mental Health Act 1983

In England and Wales, the Mental Health Act of 1983 (MHA) provides a legal framework for the detention and care of mentally disordered patients in hospital. The MHA is divided into ten parts, each of which is divided into groups of paragraphs or 'Sections'. The principal parts are as follows:

- Part I: sets out the application and extent of the act and defines 'mental disorder'.
- Part II: compulsory admission to hospital and guardianship.
- Part III: patients concerned with criminal proceedings.
- Part IV: consent to treatment.

Note: the government are in the process of reforming the MHA and have put forward proposals in the new Mental Health Bill, published in July 2002. You should be aware there is widespread opposition to the proposals, and the Royal College of Psychiatrists have 'extreme anxieties about its ethical basis, practicality and effectiveness' (see the discussion on DSPD in Ch. 25, and http://www.rcpsych.ac.uk/college/parliament/MHBill.htm).

### Part I: definitions
Part I of the MHA specifies four types of mental disorder under which individuals may be detained:
1. Mental illness: this is not defined by the MHA and is left as a *'matter for clinical judgement'*.

This 'mental illness' should be of such a nature or degree as to warrant the detention of patients:
- In the interests of their health, or
- In the interests of their safety, or
- For the protection of other people.

2. Mental impairment: *'means a state of arrested or incomplete development of the mind which includes significant impairment of intelligence and social functioning and is associated with abnormally aggressive or seriously irresponsible conduct'*.
3. Severe mental impairment: as for mental impairment, but with *'severe impairment of intelligence and social functioning'*.
4. Psychopathic disorder: *'means a persistent disorder or disability of mind (whether or not including significant impairment of intelligence) which results in abnormally aggressive or seriously irresponsible conduct'*.

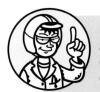

Note that the Mental Health Act 1983 does not regard dependence on alcohol or drugs, promiscuity, sexual deviancy or 'immoral conduct' alone as evidence of a mental disorder.

Certain officials and bodies are designated to carry out specific duties related to implementation of the MHA. Some of these are summarized in Figure 29.1.

### Part II: civil sections
Part II of the MHA incorporates Sections 2–34 and relates to compulsory admission to hospital. Figure 29.2 summarizes the most important sections in this part. The usual sequence of events for detention under Section 2 or 3 of the MHA is as follows:
- The approved social worker (ASW), or nearest relative, having personally seen the patient within 14 days, will make an *application* for assessment.
- The application must be supported following an assessment and *recommendation* of two doctors, one of whom should be Section 12 approved (this is usually a psychiatrist). It is recommended that one of the doctors have had previous acquaintance

**Mental Health Act (MHA) officials**

| Official or body | Definition | Main duties |
|---|---|---|
| Approved social worker (ASW) | A social worker approved by the local social services authority as being competent to carry out MHA duties | To assess patients and then to make application for MHA Section if appropriate |
| Section 12 approved doctor | A doctor approved under Section 12 of the MHA as having the appropriate expertise in the diagnosis and treatment of mental disorder, usually MRCPsych-qualified psychiatrists, or doctors with more than 3 years' experience in psychiatry | To assess patients and then to provide a recommendation for MHA Section if appropriate |
| Mental Health Act Commission (MHAC) | An independent body that protects the interests of patients detained under the MHA | Monitors and regulates MHA practice and procedures |
| Mental health review tribunal | A panel which includes a lawyer, a doctor and a layperson | Can discharge patients from hospital, following the hearing of their appeals in a formal tribunal |
| Mental Health Act managers ('hospital managers') | The body responsible for the of runningthe hospital – usually the board of the NHS Trust | Receives appeals from patients, and requests for discharge by the nearest relative. May discharge patients at any time |

*NHS, UK National Health Service.*

**Fig. 29.1** Mental Health Act (MHA) officials.

**Civil Sections enabling compulsory admission**

| Section | Aim | Duration | Application | Recommendation |
|---|---|---|---|---|
| *Section 2* Admission for assessment | Compulsory detention for assessment. Used when diagnosis and response to treatment are unknown. May be converted to a Section 3 if longer admission needed. Medication may be given as part of the assessment process | 28 days | Approved social worker (ASW) or nearest relative | Two doctors (at least one must be Section 12 approved) |
| *Section 3* Admission for treatment | Compulsory detention for treatment. Used when diagnosis and treatment response is established. May be extended | 6 months | ASW or nearest relative | Two doctors (at least one must be Section 12 approved) |
| *Section 4* Emergency admission for assessment | Emergency admission to hospital for assessment when there is no time to wait for Section 2 procedures in the community | 72 hours | ASW or nearest relative | One doctor |
| *Section 5(2)* Doctor's holding power | Detention of a hospital in-patient receiving any form of treatment in order to give time to complete a Section 2 or 3 | 72 hours | - | Doctor responsible for patient's care or other nominated doctor |
| *Section 5(4)* Nurse's holding power | Urgent detention of an in-patient receiving treatment for a mental disorder when doctor unable to attend | 6 hours | - | Registered nurse trained in mental health |

**Fig. 29.2** Civil Sections enabling compulsory admission.

with the patient (this is usually the patient's general practitioner).

- Patients are then informed of the Section and their rights, and may apply to have their case reviewed by a mental health review tribunal or the hospital managers.
- Patients may be discharged from their Section by the:
  a. Responsible medical officer (usually the consultant psychiatrist),
  b. Hospital managers (Mental Health Act managers)
  c. Mental health review tribunal
  d. Nearest relative, who must give the hospital managers 72 hours' written notice. Note that the consultant psychiatrist may issue a 'barring certificate' to stop a nearest relative discharging a patient who is a danger to himself or others.
- Patients may be granted leave from hospital for a specified period of time with certain conditions (e.g. 4 hours, escorted by a responsible adult) under Section 17 by their responsible medical officer (RMO).

Note the term 'informal' applies to hospital patients who not are detained on a Section, that is, patients who have agreed to voluntary admission. About 90% of psychiatric admissions are on an informal basis.

Section 5(2) – doctor's holding power – may be enacted by *any* hospital doctor provided they are either the responsible medical officer (RMO), e.g. the consultant, or another doctor nominated by the RMO, e.g. a specialist registrar or senior house officer. This means that a psychiatrist need not see suspected mentally ill patients on a medical or surgical ward before they can be detained under this Section.

## Part III: forensic sections

Part III of the MHA incorporates Sections 35–55 and relates to mentally ill patients involved in criminal proceedings or under sentence. Figure 29.3 summarizes the most important sections in this part.

## Part IV: consent to treatment

This part of the MHA clarifies the extent to which treatments can be imposed on detained patients. Patients on a Section 3 or 37 (long-term treatment orders) can be treated with standard psychiatric medication for 3 months with or without their

| Forensic Sections | | | |
| --- | --- | --- | --- |
| Section | Aim | Duration | Application |
| Section 35 Remand to hospital for report on mental condition | To prepare a report on the mental condition of an individual who is charged with an offence that could lead to imprisonment | 28 days, with option to extend to 12 weeks | Crown or Magistrates' Court, on evidence of one medical doctor* |
| Section 36 Remand to hospital for treatment | To treat an individual who is charged with an offence that could lead to imprisonment | 28 days, with option to extend to 12 weeks | Crown Court, on the evidence of two medical doctors* |
| Section 37 Hospital order | Detention and treatment of an individual convicted of an imprisonable offence (similar to Section 3) | Initially 6 months, with option to extend | Crown or Magistrates' Court, on evidence of two medical doctors* |
| Section 41 Restriction order | Leave and discharge of Section 37 patients may only be granted with approval of the Home Office (recorded as 37/41) – applied to serious persistent offenders | As for Section 37 | Crown Court only, on evidence of one medical doctor* |

*One doctor must be Section 12 approved

**Fig. 29.3** Forensic Sections.

consent. However, after 3 months and in other special cases (see below), an extra Section is required for treatment. These include:

- Section 57 – treatment that requires the patient's consent *and* a second opinion: psychosurgery, and surgical implants of hormones to reduce male sex drive.
- Section 58 – treatment that requires the patient's consent *or* a second opinion: administration of medication after 3 months have elapsed on a Section 3 (or 37), and electroconvulsive therapy (ECT).

In circumstances where *urgent* treatment is required to save the patient's life or to prevent serious suffering or deterioration, the second opinion requirements of Sections 57 and 58 can be waived under Section 62, e.g. emergency ECT for a patient who is not eating or drinking. Section 62 is only used until a second opinion can be obtained.

See also 'Consent to treatment', later.

## Mentally disordered persons in the community

Under Section 135, an approved social worker may apply to a magistrate for a warrant, which will allow the police to enter *private premises* in order to remove someone with a mental disorder and take them to a 'place of safety' (usually a police station or hospital) for further assessment.

Under Section 136, a police constable who finds a person in a *public place* appearing to suffer from a mental disorder may remove him or her to a 'place of safety'. Persons are detained for a period not exceeding 72 hours so that a doctor and social worker can assess them. This may lead to an admission under the Mental Health Act (usually a Section 2 or 3).

## Common law

*Common law* refers to law that is based on court decisions (case law) or customs, rather than laws made in parliament, that is, *statute law*. The Mental Health Act is an example of statutory law; whereas, instituting life-saving treatment on an unconscious patient, who is unable to consent, is justified under common law. Nearly all clinicians will, at some stage, have to act under common law because statutory law does not make provision for many of the difficult clinical scenarios that might require that patients be admitted, treated, or restrained without their consent.

Unfortunately, many doctors and nurses who are not familiar with mental health legislation are often so concerned about infringing patients' rights that they tend to not act at all. So, the regrettable situation arises where the semi-conscious man with a life-threatening alcohol-withdrawal delirium is allowed to leave the ward with no one attempting to stop him. The principle of duty to care is sacrificed for the fear of being accused of assault.

When considering an action under common law, always ask yourself whether your actions would be defensible in court. Your actions should be consistent with what most individuals with your level of training would do in the same situation. And remember that choosing not to act when you should is indefensible, and would be construed as negligent.

 It is permissible under *common law* to restrain and medicate patients who are mentally disordered and who present an imminent danger to themselves or others. However, it is bad practice to repeatedly impose psychiatric medication on informal patients. They should be assessed under the Mental Health Act and treated under the appropriate Section.

## Consent to treatment

Clinicians should provide patients with a clear explanation of the nature and likely benefits of a treatment as well as its potential risks and side-effects. Adults have the right to refuse treatment, even if this refusal results in death or serious disability. When patients refuse essential treatment, clinicians should ascertain whether they have the capacity to consent to treatment and have made a free decision without coercion.

There is no statutory definition of capacity to consent but the expert committee on reform of the Mental Health Act (MHA) 1983 have adopted the *Law Commission's definition of incapacity* which was proposed in 1995. This is summarized in Figure 29.4.

There is no statute law that governs the decision to treat when an adult patient is deemed to not have capacity; therefore, in these cases, the decision to treat should be made according to the patient's best interests, as determined by the responsible medical

---

A person is without capacity if at the time the decision needs to be made he is:

1. Unable by reason of mental disability to make a decision because he is unable to:

   - Understand and believe the relevant information
   - Retain this information
   - Make a decision based on information given.

2. Unable to communicate a choice on that matter because he or she is unconscious or for any other reason.

**Fig. 29.4** The Law Commission's definition of incapacity.

officer, under *common law*. Note that 'best interests' does not just mean medical interests but also includes psychological, social and spiritual interests. It is good practice to consult those close to the patient, although they cannot give or withhold consent.

It is becoming increasingly common for patients to set up an *advanced directive* (also called 'living will'). This set of instructions, issued in advance to medical practitioners, makes patients' preferences known for situations when they are unable to direct their own treatment.

Never hesitate to discuss the issues concerning consent to treatment with knowledgeable colleagues or your medical defence organization if you are uncertain. And remember to keep detailed notes of all the reasons motivating your decisions.

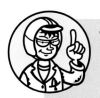

- Note that a having a serious mental illness does not preclude a patient from having the capacity to consent to physical treatment, as long as this illness does not interfere with the understanding of relevant information and the decision-making process.
- The Mental Health Act 1983 makes provision for the compulsory treatment of mental disorders only, not for the compulsory treatment of physical disorders. Therefore, you can never 'section' a patient to treat a physical disorder

and patients are within their rights to refuse physical treatment as long as they are deemed to have capacity. In other words, patients who require urgent physical treatment, but who do not have capacity, are treated without consent under *common law*, not under the Mental Health Act.

## Testamentary capacity

Testamentary capacity is an individual's competence to make a valid will. Psychiatrists may be asked to assess testamentary capacity because it can be impaired by a mental disorder (e.g. dementia). It should be determined whether the testator (person who makes a will) is of 'sound disposing mind' when (1) drawing up the will and (2) executing the will, which means: signing it in the presence of witnesses. Four criteria are used to assess a 'sound disposing mind':

1. The testator understands that he is giving his property after his death to one or more objects of regard, that is, he understands what a will is.
2. He understands the nature of, and is able to recollect the extent of, his property.
3. He is aware of those who might have a reasonable claim to his estate.
4. He is able to weigh up the relative claims and make rational judgements about allocation, that is, an abnormal state of mind should not directly distort the decision-making process.

Note that a psychotic or dementing patient may still have testamentary capacity provided they meet the above criteria.

### Fitness to drive

Both mental illness and psychiatric medication can impair fitness to drive. Clinicians should be aware of the following legal provisions:

- It is the responsibility of the Driver and Vehicle Licensing Authority (DVLA) to make the decision whether an individual is fit to continue driving.
- It is the driver's responsibility to inform the DVLA of any condition that may impair his/her driving ability.
- It is the doctor's responsibility to advise patients to inform the DVLA of any condition that may

interfere with their driving (e.g. psychotic episode, manic episode, dementia). Doctors may subsequently be contacted by the DVLA for further information.

- Doctors may, and indeed have a duty to, breach confidentiality considerations and contact the DVLA medical advisor themselves if patients fail to take this advice and the potential impairment is serious. The same applies to patients who, due to their illness (e.g. dementia, psychosis), are unable, or unlikely, to contact the DVLA.

For further information see:
http://www.dvla.gov.uk/drivers/dmed1.htm.

## Scotland: Mental Health (Scotland) Act 1984

The compulsory admission and treatment orders are similar to those for England and Wales. For most community-based patients, admissions take place under either Section 24 or Section 18 of the Act.

### Section 24: emergency admission to hospital

Section 24 is used in cases of urgent necessity where application for Section 18 would involve undesirable delay. It requires a recommendation by *one* doctor (usually a GP) with the consent of the patient's nearest relative or a mental health officer (MHO), which is similar to an approved social worker. It lasts 72 hours, and there is no appeal process. Patients may not be treated under this Section, but emergency treatment is, of course, possible under common law. It is not renewable; so, at the end of 72 hours, patients either become informal, or are detained on a different Section, usually a Section 26.

### Section 26: short-term detention

This Section follows on from a Section 24 (or Section 25 – detention of patients already in hospital), and thus cannot be used independently to admit a patient to hospital. It lasts for up to 28 days and requires a second recommendation from a senior psychiatrist, with the consent of a relative or mental health officer. Patients may appeal to the sheriff and the Mental Welfare Commission.

### Section 18: long-term detention

Section 18 may follow a Section 26, or may bring someone who has a chronic mental illness directly into hospital from the community. It requires an application from the nearest relative or a mental health officer, and *two* medical recommendations, usually the GP and an approved psychiatrist. Additionally, the Section should be approved by the sheriff. It lasts for up to 6 months but can be renewed further. Patients may be treated without their consent for the first 3 months of this Section. Following this, a certificate of second opinion must be sought from the Mental Welfare Commission. Patients may appeal against the Section at the time of application to the sheriff, or on renewal of the Section.

## Northern Ireland: Mental Health (Northern Ireland) Order 1986

The Mental Health (Northern Ireland) Order 1986 is similar to the Mental Health Acts of England and Wales, although there are some noteworthy differences:

- For the first time in UK legislation, the order defines 'mental illness': ' "Mental illness" means a state of mind which affects a person's thinking, perceiving, emotion or judgement to the extent that he requires care or medical treatment in his own interests or the interest of other persons.'
- The various paragraphs are referred to as Articles, not Sections.
- The order does not allow for the detention of individuals with psychopathic disorder, although individuals may be detained when a personality disorder coexists with mental illness or severe mental impairment.
- There is only one procedure for admission to hospital: All patients compulsorily admitted to hospital will be held for a period of assessment lasting up to 14 days. Following this, they may be detained under Article 12, which allows detention for treatment for up to 6 months beginning with the date of admission. The application for assessment is made by the nearest relative or an approved social worker, and is followed by a medical recommendation, usually by the patient's GP. The order stipulates that a patient admitted for assessment should be examined by a consultant psychiatrist within 48 hours after admission, and, if detained under Article 12, examined by a consultant psychiatrist during both the first and second 7 days of the assessment period.

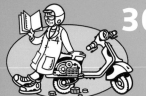

# 30. Mental Health Service Provision

## History

Until the 18th century, the mentally ill in England received no formal psychiatric care, and those who were not looked after by their families were kept in workhouses amd private institutions. In 1845, the Lunatics Act led to the building of an asylum in every county so that those patients with severe mental illness could be cared for in large remote asylum communities. Since the introduction in 1952 of chlorpromazine, the first effective medication for schizophrenia, there has been a significant decline in the numbers of patients in psychiatric hospitals. The attempts to reduce the cost of in-patient care, and the criticism levelled at asylums regarding the 'institutionalization' of patients and the loss of patient autonomy, led to the closure of the large asylums and the rise of community care. Today, most mentally ill patients are assessed and managed in the community, and hospital admission, when indicated, is usually only brief in duration.

## Primary care

Up to 95% of mental illness is seen and managed exclusively in primary care by general practitioners, with mild to moderate mood and anxiety disorders and alcohol abuse being the most common conditions. Depression, which is the most common mental illness treated, is frequently associated with symptoms of anxiety as well as physical complaints.

It is important to note that up to half of all mentally ill patients go undetected in primary care. This is because many of these patients present with physical, rather than psychological, symptoms. Also, some patients are reluctant to discuss emotional issues with their doctor, due to feelings of embarrassment or uncertainty about how they will be received.

Some GPs have the option of referring patients with mild symptoms or those going through a life crisis (e.g. bereavement) to a practice counsellor (see p. 193). Practice and district nurses may be helpful in screening for, and educating patients about, mental illness.

Certain patients require secondary mental health care. GPs usually refer these cases to their local psychiatrist or community mental health team (CHMT). Figure 30.1 lists the common reasons for referral from primary to secondary mental health care.

## Secondary care

### Community mental health teams (CMHTs)

In the UK, specialist psychiatric care in the community is mostly coordinated by regional CMHTs, which consist of a multidisciplinary team of psychiatrists, community mental health nurses (CPNs), social workers, psychologists, occupational therapists and support workers. Team members usually operate from a base which is easily accessible to the community they serve, although local GP surgeries are also used to see patients. Patients who are unable to come to the CMHT member's location are often seen at home.

### Care programme approach (CPA)

The approach taken by the secondary psychiatric services is called the care programme approach (CPA), which was introduced by the Department of Health in 1991. This approach applies to all patients under specialist psychiatric care and includes community-, hospital- and prison-based patients. The key components of the CPA are:

- The systematic assessment of patients' health and social care needs.
- The formation of an agreed care plan which addresses these identified needs.
- The allocation of a *care coordinator* (previously called 'keyworker') to keep in touch with the patient to monitor and coordinate the care of these needs. This is usually a CPN, social worker or psychiatrist.
- Regular review meetings, which include all relevant professionals, patients and their carers, to adjust the care plan, if necessary.

Patients may be placed on a *standard* or *enhanced* CPA according to the severity of their needs.

**Reasons for referral to secondary mental health services**

- Moderate to severe mental illness, e.g. schizophrenia, bipolar affective disorder, severe depressive or anxiety disorders, personality disorder
- Patients who pose a serious risk of harm to self, others or property
- Uncertainty regarding diagnosis
- Poor response to standard treatment, despite adequate dose and compliance
- Specialist treatment required, e.g. psychological therapy, specialist medication regimens

**Fig. 30.1** Reasons for referral to secondary mental health services.

Psychiatric care is unique inasmuch as the diverse and multiple needs of patients with mental health problems make a multidisciplinary approach indispensable. A multidisciplinary team consists of members with medical, psychological, social and occupational therapy expertise.

## Out-patient clinics

Psychiatric out-patient clinics are coordinated by, and take place in, CMHT centres. GP surgeries and, rarely, hospital buildings are also sometimes used for clinic settings. Types of clinics include psychiatrist's clinics for new referrals and follow-up patients, and special purpose clinics, e.g. depot injections clinics, clozapine-monitoring clinics.

## Day hospitals

Day hospitals are non-residential units that patients attend during the day. They are an alternative to in-patient care for patients who, although distressed, are able to go home in the evening and on weekends.

Having a supportive family is helpful in this regard. They may also be used for patients who have just been discharged from hospital, but who still need a high level of support, as a form of 'partial hospitalization'.

## In-patient units

Occasionally, community care is not possible and hospital admission is necessary. Reasons for admission include:

- To provide a safe environment when there is (1) risk of harm to self or others, or (2) grossly disturbed behaviour.
- A period of in-patient assessment is needed, e.g. of response to treatment or when the diagnosis is uncertain.
- It is necessary to institute treatment in hospital, e.g. electroconvulsive therapy, clozapine therapy.

There are various types of in-patient units. These range from a general adult acute ward for uncomplicated admissions, to psychiatric intensive care units (PICUs) for severely disturbed patients who cannot be adequately contained on an open ward. High security units (also called 'special hospitals', e.g. Broadmoor, Rampton) are for mentally ill offenders who pose a grave risk to others.

## Rehabilitation units

These units aim to reintegrate patients, whose social and living skills have been severely handicapped by the effects of severe mental illness and institutionalization, into the community.

## Accommodation

Certain patients, who are unable to live independently due to severe and enduring mental illness, may need *supported accommodation*. Types of supported accommodation range from warden-controlled property to homes with trained staff on hand 24 hours a day.

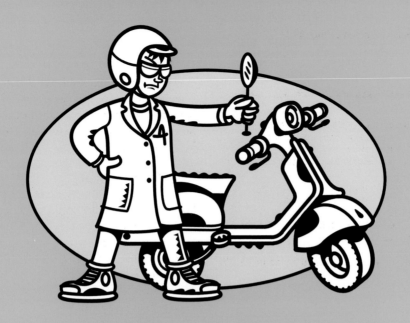

# SELF-ASSESSMENT

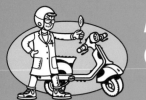

# Multiple-choice Questions

**Indicate whether each answer is true or false.**

## Mood (affective) disorders – Chapters 1, 2, 3, 13

**1. Biological or somatic symptoms of depression include:**

(a) Suicidal thoughts.
(b) Psychomotor retardation.
(c) Hopelessness.
(d) Mood worse in the evening.
(e) Loss of libido.

**2. Regarding anhedonia:**

(a) It means the inability to derive pleasure from activities that were formerly enjoyed.
(b) It occurs in bipolar affective disorder.
(c) It is a core feature of depression.
(d) It is regarded as a psychotic feature of depression.
(e) It occurs in dysthymia.

**3. Regarding the differential diagnosis of depression:**

(a) Dysthymia means depressive episodes that last less than 1 week.
(b) Cyclothymia is characterized by alternating periods of mild elation and mild depression.
(c) A schizoaffective episode is difficult to distinguish from a depressive episode with psychotic features.
(d) Hypothyroidism is an important medical cause of depression.
(e) Antihypertensive medication is a recognized cause of depression.

**4. The following are typical manic symptoms:**

(a) Grandiose delusions.
(b) Psychomotor retardation.
(c) Pressured speech.
(d) Tangential speech.
(e) Delusions of thought insertion.

**5. Manic episodes:**

(a) Always feature psychotic symptoms.
(b) Commonly feature rapidly alternating manic and depressive symptoms.
(c) Are known to feature an extremely irritable mood.
(d) Usually only result in a partial disruption to work or social activities.
(e) Commonly feature a decreased need for sleep as an early symptom.

**6. Strong suicide intent is suggested by the following:**

(a) A woman overdosed on the tricyclic antidepressants that she had stored up over a month.
(b) A man dependent on alcohol took an impulsive overdose while drunk.
(c) The patient phoned an ambulance after taking an overdose.
(d) An elderly man attempted to gas himself in his car.
(e) A woman was found unconscious in her car on an abandoned country road.

**7. Patients who have survived a suicide attempt:**

(a) Must always be admitted to a psychiatric hospital for further assessment.
(b) Should not be asked about ongoing suicidal ideas for fear of provoking a further attempt.
(c) Are more often female than male.
(d) Are at increased risk of suicide if they are dependent on alcohol or suffer from anorexia nervosa.
(e) Have a lower risk of subsequent completed suicide if they are divorced men over the age of 45.

**8. Regarding the aetiology of depression:**

(a) The monoamine theory suggests a shortage of acetylcholine and GABA.
(b) Only the efficacy of monoamine oxidase inhibitors (MAOIs) may be explained by the monoamine theory.
(c) Twin and family studies have shown that there is no genetic component to depression.
(d) Low expressed emotion (EE) by family members contributes to the risk of relapse.
(e) Having three or more children at home under the age of 14 is a risk factor.

**9. Regarding the treatment of depression:**

(a) The SSRIs are the most effective antidepressants.
(b) SSRIs should be prescribed with caution to suicidal patients, as they are cardiotoxic in overdose.
(c) Antidepressants should be continued for at least 6 months to reduce relapse.
(d) Lithium is used to augment antidepressants.
(e) Cognitive-behavioural therapy (CBT) is as effective as antidepressants in moderate depression.

**10. The following increase the risk of developing depression:**

(a) Borderline personality disorder.
(b) Loss of one's mother before the age of 11.
(c) A family history of depression.
(d) Divorce.
(e) Taking an antidepressant and L-tryptophan together.

**11. Regarding bipolar affective disorder (BAD):**

(a) It affects twice as many women as men.
(b) There is a stronger genetic component in the aetiology of BAD than in unipolar depression.
(c) Antidepressants are contraindicated.
(d) Lithium is usually stopped when the manic episode has resolved.
(e) The clinical features of bipolar depression are indistinguishable from those in unipolar depression.

# Psychotic disorders – Chapters 4, 14

**12. Delusions:**

(a) Are symptoms of psychosis.
(b) Are characteristic of personality disorder.
(c) Never correspond to reality.
(d) Are easily understood within a person's cultural background.
(e) Are always bizarre in content.

**13. Hallucinations:**

(a) May occur in a normal bereavement reaction.
(b) On waking from sleep are termed hypnagogic.
(c) Are frequently misinterpretations of external stimuli.
(d) Are always pathological.
(e) Are typical of paranoid schizophrenia.

**14. The following are forms of thought disorder:**

(a) Word salad.
(b) Neologisms.
(c) Thought-echo.
(d) Flight of ideas.
(e) Waxy flexibility.

**15. Motor symptoms of schizophrenia include:**

(a) Mannerisms.
(b) Formication.
(c) Stupor.
(d) Waxy flexibility.
(e) Stereotypies.

**16. Schizophrenia:**

(a) Was coined by Bleuler and means 'splitting of the mind'.
(b) Is much more common in men.
(c) Has been related to limbic dopamine depletion.
(d) Is entirely a genetic disease.
(e) Is characterized by first-rank symptoms described by Schneider.

**17. The following are characteristic of schizophrenia:**

(a) Flight of ideas.
(b) Second person auditory hallucinations.
(c) Grandiose delusions.
(d) Delusional perception.
(e) Running commentary auditory hallucinations.

**18. The following are subtypes of schizophrenia:**

(a) Hebephrenic.
(b) Paranoid.
(c) Schizotypal.
(d) Borderline.
(e) Residual.

**19. The following conditions may cause psychotic symptoms:**

(a) Epilepsy.
(b) Human immunodeficiency virus (HIV) infection.
(c) Acute intermittent porphyria.
(d) Hyperglycaemia.
(e) Vitamin deficiency.

**20. Regarding the epidemiology of schizophrenia:**

(a) The lifetime risk of developing schizophrenia is 1%.
(b) Women tend to have a later age of onset than men.
(c) There is an increased incidence in rural compared to urban areas.
(d) In the UK, the incidence rate is higher for African-Caribbeans than for Caucasians.
(e) There is a higher prevalence in higher socioeconomic classes.

**21. Regarding the aetiology of schizophrenia:**

(a) The risk of developing schizophrenia is increased if more family members are affected.
(b) The concordance rate for monozygotic twins is 100%.
(c) Families that are over-critical or over-involved contribute to relapse.
(d) Schizophrenia is associated with ventricular enlargement and reduced brain size.
(e) Schizophrenia is not associated with complications during pregnancy.

**22. Regarding the treatment of schizophrenia:**

(a) Atypical antipsychotics are less effective than typicals in treating negative symptoms.
(b) Clozapine is indicated for treatment-resistant schizophrenia.
(c) Benzodiazepines are of limited value in the acute phase.
(d) Compliance is usually increased by switching to intramuscular depot antipsychotics.
(e) A delay in starting treatment results in a worse prognosis.

**23. Regarding the prognosis of schizophrenia:**

(a) There is a high risk of suicide.
(b) Men tend to do better than women.
(c) Most patients will have repeated psychotic episodes.
(d) An early age of onset is associated with a worse outcome.
(e) Negative symptoms are associated with a good response to treatment.

# Anxiety disorders – Chapters 5, 6, 7, 8, 15

### 24. Free-floating anxiety:

(a) Occurs only in predictable situations such as in aeroplanes or at sea.
(b) Characteristically features avoidance.
(c) Has an acute onset and is experienced in discrete episodes lasting 5–10 minutes.
(d) Is an essential feature of panic disorder.
(e) Is strongly associated with agoraphobia.

### 25. Panic attacks:

(a) Always occur as a response to a phobic stimulus.
(b) Are integral to the diagnosis of generalized anxiety disorder (GAD).
(c) Are invariably accompanied by strong autonomic symptoms.
(d) Are associated with hallucinatory voices saying, 'You are dying'.
(e) Are associated with the use of amfetamines.

### 26. Regarding bereavement:

(a) A normal bereavement reaction may feature typical symptoms of depression.
(b) Most bereavement reactions should be treated with antidepressants.
(c) Marked psychomotor retardation is a feature of normal bereavement.
(d) A normal bereavement reaction seldom extends beyond 6 months.
(e) Hallucinations, other than transiently seeing or hearing the deceased, suggest abnormal bereavement.

### 27. Regarding post-traumatic stress disorder (PTSD):

(a) Avoidance of stimuli associated with the stressor is a characteristic feature.
(b) Symptoms usually develop immediately after, or within a few minutes of, a traumatic stressor.
(c) Increased arousal is prominent with an exaggerated startle response and hypervigilance.
(d) Hallucinations may occur.
(e) Co-morbid substance abuse is a common problem.

### 28. Regarding patients with numerous physical complaints:

(a) In somatization disorder, patients believe they have a serious physical illness.
(b) In hypochondriacal disorder, symptoms are produced intentionally or feigned.
(c) In body dysmorphic disorder or dysmorphophobia, patients have a delusional belief that there is a defect in their appearance.
(d) Malingering is differentiated from factitious disorder by the intensity of the feigned symptoms.
(e) Individuals with depressed mood often present with numerous somatic complaints.

### 29. Obsessions:

(a) Are recognized by patients as a product of their own mind.
(b) May occur in one in five patients with depression.
(c) Are usually rational and ego-syntonic.
(d) May lead to compulsive acts which heighten anxiety.
(e) Are recognized features of obsessive-compulsive personality disorder.

### 30. Regarding panic disorder with agoraphobia:

(a) Benzodiazepines are indicated for acute panic attacks.
(b) Cognitive-behavioural therapy commonly features exposure therapy.
(c) Patients tend to feel better when large crowds surround them.
(d) Avoidance may lead to sufferers becoming housebound.
(e) Fluoxetine is contraindicated.

### 31. Regarding social phobia:

(a) It is more common in women.
(b) It may feature panic attacks.
(c) It is often associated with avoidance.
(d) Psychoanalysis is considered first-line psychological treatment.
(e) Benzodiazepines are considered first-line for chronic pharmacological treatment.

### 32. Regarding obsessive-compulsive disorder (OCD):

(a) Men and women are equally affected.
(b) Nortriptyline is the treatment of choice.
(c) Inhibition of serotonin uptake seems to be the essential component of effective drug therapy.
(d) It has a peak age of onset in adolescence to early adulthood.
(e) It may be diagnosed if symptoms do not cause distress or impair functioning.

### 33. Regarding the treatment of anxiety disorders:

(a) Venlafaxine is effective in generalized anxiety disorder (GAD).
(b) Cognitive behavioural therapy (CBT) is an effective treatment for most anxiety disorders.
(c) SSRIs are first-line treatment for specific phobias.
(d) Tricyclic antidepressants (TCAs) are as effective as SSRIs in panic disorder.
(e) Antidepressants can cause increased anxiety in the first few days of treatment.

# Alcohol and substance-related disorders – Chapters 10, 17

### 34. The following are features of the alcohol dependence syndrome:

(a) Increased tolerance to alcohol.
(b) Preferring spirits to beer or cider.

(c) Withdrawal symptoms.
(d) Drinking is given priority over family and career.
(e) Rapid reinstatement after abstinence.

### 35. Symptoms of the alcohol withdrawal syndrome include:

(a) Nausea and vomiting.
(b) Shaking.
(c) Cold dry skin.
(d) Impaired consciousness.
(e) Low mood.

### 36. Complications of excessive alcohol use include:

(a) Decreased carbohydrate deficient transferrin (CDT).
(b) Amnesic syndrome.
(c) Psychotic symptoms.
(d) Red blood cell microcytosis.
(e) Increased risk of committing violent offences.

### 37. Regarding the treatment of alcohol dependence:

(a) Out-patient alcohol detoxification includes vitamin $B_1$ supplementation.
(b) Increasing the cost of alcohol is generally ineffective at decreasing overall consumption.
(c) Clomethiazole is unsafe in patients who continue to drink.
(d) Chlorpromazine ameliorates withdrawal symptoms and reduces the risk of developing seizures.
(e) Disulfiram enhances GABA transmission.

### 38. Regarding alcohol-related disorders:

(a) All individuals who drink heavily on a regular basis have alcohol dependence.
(b) Chronic, heavy alcohol use is associated with the development of dementia.
(c) Korsakoff's syndrome is usually reversible with high doses of thiamine.
(d) Alcohol-induced psychotic disorder may resemble schizophrenia.
(e) The risk of suicide is higher in problem drinkers.

### 39. In the treatment of substance dependence:

(a) Clean needles and injecting equipment should be offered.
(b) Lofexidine is a centrally acting α-adrenoceptor agonist used in amfetamine dependence.
(c) Methadone is preferable to heroin because of its increased safety in overdose.
(d) Buprenorphine is a partial opiate agonist.
(e) Benzodiazepines are withdrawn gradually by a small amount every few weeks.

### 40. Regarding the use of illicit substances:

(a) Ecstasy, amfetamines and cannabis can all cause psychosis.
(b) The benzodiazepine withdrawal syndrome seldom causes serious physical consequences.

(c) Cocaine withdrawal often causes serious physical consequences.
(d) Naltrexone may induce withdrawal in patients who are dependent on methadone.
(e) Heroin is the most commonly used illicit drug in England.

### 41. Delirium tremens:

(a) Can be managed in the community.
(b) Is associated with lilliputian hallucinations.
(c) Usually occurs within 5 days of cessation of drinking.
(d) Is associated with tachycardia and pupil dilatation.
(e) Is primarily treated with antipsychotic medication.

## Cognitive disorders and old age psychiatry – Chapters 9, 16, 24

### 42. The following are characteristic of delirium:

(a) Impairment of consciousness.
(b) Normal sleep–wake cycle.
(c) Prominent perceptual abnormalities, especially visual hallucinations.
(d) Gradual onset with progressive deterioration over months to years.
(e) A medical cause is seldom found.

### 43. The following are characteristic of dementia:

(a) Memory impairment in the absence of other cognitive deficits.
(b) Global impairment of cognitive function and personality without an impairment of consciousness.
(c) Absence of a recognized medical cause.
(d) Stupor.
(e) Early loss of memory for personal information.

### 44. The following symptoms and causes of dementia are correctly paired:

(a) Multi-infarct dementia – uneven or stepwise deterioration in cognitive function.
(b) Frontotemporal dementia – motor signs of parkinsonism.
(c) Dementia with Lewy bodies (DLB) – recurrent visual hallucinations.
(d) Alzheimer's disease – early disinhibition and emotional blunting.
(e) Huntington's disease – jerky movements of the face and body.

### 45. In the cognitive assessment:

(a) Asking the patient to name the prime minister tests procedural or implicit memory.
(b) The *digit span test* tests short-term (primary) memory.
(c) A score of 20 on the Mini-Mental State Examination (MMSE) is diagnostic of Alzheimer's disease.
(d) Asking the patient what they had for breakfast tests long-term memory.
(e) Marked difficulty naming objects suggests a subcortical dementia.

**46. Regarding dementia:**

(a) New variant Creutzfeldt–Jakob disease (nvCJD) typically presents in young adults and causes death over a period of 18 months.
(b) Dementia with Lewy bodies (DLB) has a better prognosis than Alzheimer's disease.
(c) Parkinson's disease and HIV encephalopathy can both cause a subcortical form of dementia.
(d) Huntington's disease has autosomal recessive inheritance and is caused by an excessive number of trinucleotide (CAG) repeat sequences.
(e) Pick's disease features 'knife-blade atrophy' of the frontal and temporal lobes.

**47. Regarding Alzheimer's disease (AD):**

(a) Postmenopausal hormone replacement therapy (HRT) is a risk factor.
(b) The cholinergic hypothesis explains the efficacy of anticholinergic drugs.
(c) Computed tomography (CT) invariably makes the diagnosis.
(d) Seldom develops in individuals with trisomy 21 (Down's syndrome).
(e) Most cases result from transmission of an autosomal dominant gene.

**48. The following neuropathological signs are associated with Alzheimer's disease (AD):**

(a) Generalized brain atrophy, especially in the frontal and temporal regions.
(b) Many small infarctions in the white matter.
(c) Extracellular β-amyloid plaques.
(d) Intracellular neurofibrillary tangles.
(e) Small ventricles and narrow sulci.

**49. The following are associated with an increased risk of developing dementia:**

(a) Two copies of the ApoE 4 allele.
(b) Possession of the amyloid precursor protein gene (APP).
(c) Diabetes.
(d) Infection with the human immunodeficiency virus (HIV).
(e) Development of tremor, rigidity and bradykinesia.

**50. The following are associated with increasing age:**

(a) Increased risk of parasuicide, but decreased risk of completed suicide.
(b) Increased incidence of bipolar affective disorder.
(c) Increase in lean body mass and decrease in total body fat.
(d) Depressive pseudodementia.
(e) Increased risk of postural hypotension with tricyclic antidepressants.

**51. Regarding mental disorders in the elderly:**

(a) Numerous physical complaints are often a sign of depression.
(b) Late-onset schizophrenia (paraphrenia) is characterized predominantly by hallucinations.

(c) Electroconvulsive therapy (ECT) is generally ineffective for severe depression.
(d) Late-onset schizophrenia is far more common in men.
(e) Mania frequently presents after a stroke.

# Personality disorders – Chapters 11, 18

**52. The following are associated with antisocial (dissocial) personality disorder:**

(a) Increased risk of violent crime.
(b) Conduct disorder in childhood.
(c) Exaggerated capacity to experience guilt.
(d) Decreased risk of suicide.
(e) Substance abuse.

**53. Regarding borderline personality disorder (BPD):**

(a) It is associated with deliberate self-harm.
(b) It is associated with childhood sexual abuse.
(c) It is associated with unstable relationships and single marital status.
(d) It is more prevalent in young men.
(e) It is grouped in Cluster B in the DSM-IV (dramatic, emotional or erratic).

**54. The following personality disorders (PDs) and characteristics are correctly paired:**

(a) Obsessive-compulsive (anankastic) PD – preoccupation with orderliness, perfectionism and control.
(b) Histrionic PD – dramatic, exaggerated expressions of emotion.
(c) Paranoid PD – odd beliefs or magical thinking.
(d) Schizoid PD – neither enjoys nor desires close or sexual relationships.
(e) Narcissistic PD – frantic efforts to avoid abandonment.

**55. The following are correctly paired:**

(a) Trichotillomania – pathological fire setting.
(b) Kleptomania – pathological stealing.
(c) Organic personality disorder – frontal lobe tumour.
(d) ICD-10 – dimensional approach.
(e) Schizotypal personality disorder – odd beliefs or magical thinking.

**56. The following statements are true:**

(a) The prevalence of personality disorder in prisons is no greater than in community samples.
(b) Schizotypal disorder is more common in the relatives of patients with schizophrenia.
(c) Patients with personality disorder never show clinically significant improvement.
(d) Patients with personality disorder are at increased risk for developing depression.
(e) Psychopathic disorder is an ICD-10 term.

**57. Regarding the treatment of personality disorder:**

(a) Hospital admission is contraindicated.
(b) Dialectical behaviour therapy (DBT) is effective in borderline personality disorder.
(c) Lithium or antipsychotics may be helpful in treating aggression and impulsivity.
(d) Motivated patients may benefit from a therapeutic community.
(e) Cognitive analytic therapy (CAT) is a recognized treatment for borderline personality disorder.

# Eating, sleep, psychosexual and puerperal disorders – Chapters 12, 19, 20, 21, 22

**58. The following are characteristic of anorexia nervosa (AN):**

(a) A body mass index of 17.5 kg/m$^2$ or less.
(b) An overvalued idea of dread of fatness.
(c) Absence of binge eating behaviour.
(d) Widespread endocrine abnormalities (e.g. amenorrhoea).
(e) Amenorrhoea if using oral contraception.

**59. Patients with bulimia nervosa (BN):**

(a) Must have a body mass index of 17.5 kg/m$^2$ or less.
(b) Must have an overvalued idea of dread of fatness.
(c) May have Russell's sign.
(d) May be overweight.
(e) May have hyperkalaemic, hypochloraemic alkalosis as a consequence of repeated vomiting.

**60. Poor caloric intake may lead to the development of:**

(a) Osteoporosis.
(b) Lanugo.
(c) Hypercholesterolaemia.
(d) Erosion of dental enamel.
(e) Infertility.

**61. Regarding the difference between anorexia (AN) and bulimia nervosa (BN):**

(a) Bulimia has an earlier age of onset.
(b) Anorexia is more prevalent in the general population.
(c) Bulimia has an increased prevalence in higher socioeconomic classes.
(d) The prognosis for bulimia tends to be better.
(e) The aetiology of anorexia is known.

**62. Regarding the treatment of eating disorders:**

(a) Fluoxetine may reduce bingeing and purging behaviour.
(b) Family therapy may be effective for adolescents living with their parents.
(c) A late age of onset indicates a good prognosis in anorexia nervosa.
(d) Under no circumstances may patients be force-fed.
(e) Psychotherapy forms the mainstay of treatment.

**63. The following sleep disorders and symptoms are correctly paired:**

(a) Circadian rhythm sleep disorder – being tired when one should be awake and being awake when one should be sleeping.
(b) Obstructive sleep apnoea (OSA) – awaking from sleep in a state of extreme panic or terror.
(c) Somnambulism – obstruction of the upper airways during sleep.
(d) Sleep (night) terrors – remembering a nightmare in vivid detail.
(e) Parasomnias – abnormal episodes that occur during sleep.

**64. Regarding hypersomnia:**

(a) Primary hypersomnia is diagnosed when there is a known medical or psychiatric cause.
(b) Narcolepsy features attacks of refreshing sleep and catatonia.
(c) It improves when mirtazapine or trazodone are prescribed.
(d) It is invariably a feature of depression.
(e) It may be caused by all the parasomnias.

**65. Regarding postnatal blues:**

(a) It occurs in 50% of postpartum women.
(b) It meets the ICD-10 criteria for a depressive episode.
(c) It usually requires treatment with antidepressants.
(d) It might be due to a fall in progesterone post-delivery.
(e) Symptoms peak between the third and fifth day post-delivery.

**66. Regarding puerperal psychosis (PP):**

(a) It is closely related to bipolar affective disorder (BAD).
(b) Psychosocial factors are very important in its aetiology.
(c) There is a 30% chance of experiencing a recurrence after future childbirths.
(d) It is more likely to develop in women with a history of depression or mania.
(e) It develops in about one in eight childbirths.

**67. Regarding postnatal depression (PND):**

(a) It occurs in about 10% of postpartum women.
(b) It may be treated with lithium in breast-feeding mothers.
(c) Stressful life events, lack of close relationships and a young maternal age are important risk factors.
(d) Electroconvulsive therapy (ECT) is contraindicated.
(e) A previous history of non-pregnancy related depression is a risk factor.

**68. Regarding sexual dysfunction:**

(a) It may be described according to abnormalities of the normal sexual response cycle.
(b) It may be improved or worsened by antidepressants.
(c) The 'squeeze technique' may be helpful in men with hypoactive sexual desire.
(d) Lack of sexual interest and anorgasmia are two of the

most common problems in women.

(e) 'Sensate focus', as part of sex therapy, places a high priority on achieving orgasm.

### 69. The following psychosexual disorders and descriptions are correctly paired:

(a) Fetishism – sexual arousal through inanimate objects.
(b) Transsexualism – sexual arousal by cross-dressing.
(c) Vaginismus – involuntary spasm of the muscles surrounding the outer third of the vagina.
(d) Gender identity disorder – a desire to have sex with a member of the same sex.
(e) Sexual sadism – sexual arousal by the infliction of suffering on oneself.

## Child and adolescent psychiatry – Chapter 23

### 70. Regarding autism in children:

(a) There is a serious impairment in social interaction.
(b) There is frequently an inflexible adherence to routines and rituals.
(c) Evidence indicates that the MMR vaccine (mumps, measles, rubella) is a causal factor.
(d) Many have significant mental retardation (learning disability).
(e) Girls are more often affected.

### 71. Regarding children with attention-deficit/hyperactivity disorder (ADHD):

(a) Symptoms may only be present at school.
(b) It is more common in boys.
(c) Symptoms never persist into adulthood.
(d) Symptoms usually present early, before the age of 6.
(e) Methylphenidate improves school performance in most cases.

### 72. Regarding conduct disorder:

(a) It involves behaviour that violates the law or the basic rights of others.
(b) There is an equal sex ratio.
(c) It is associated with the later development of schizoid personality disorder.
(d) There is often associated illicit substance misuse in later life.
(e) It is a milder variant of oppositional defiant disorder (ODD).

### 73. Regarding the emotional problems in childhood:

(a) Separation anxiety can be normal for 1-year-old children.
(b) Separation anxiety disorder (SAD) often results in truancy.
(c) School refusal is the refusal to go to school because of anxiety in spite of parental pressure.
(d) School refusal is associated with conduct disorder.
(e) Emotional disorders frequently feature hallucinations.

### 74. Regarding patients with mental retardation (learning disability):

(a) Impaired adaptive functioning is essential to the diagnosis.
(b) They have a higher prevalence of schizophrenia.
(c) The prevalence is higher in males.
(d) Less than half of all cases are mild.
(e) Mild cases are likely to have a specific cause.

### 75. Regarding the treatment of acquired disorders of childhood:

(a) Gilles de la Tourette's syndrome can be treated with haloperidol.
(b) Antipsychotics are first-line treatments for attention-deficit/hyperactivity disorder (ADHD).
(c) In non-organic enuresis, parental education and behaviour therapy (star charts, pad and buzzer) are first-line treatments.
(d) Methylphenidate can cause suppression of growth.
(e) Children with Gilles de la Tourette's syndrome may need treatment for obsessive-compulsive disorder (OCD).

### 76. The following are risk factors for child abuse:

(a) A child with low birth weight.
(b) A child who is hyperactive.
(c) High socioeconomic class.
(d) Parents with mental illness.
(e) Parents who have children late in life.

### 77. Regarding the pervasive developmental disorders:

(a) They are characterized by severe impairments in social interactions and restricted, stereotyped interests.
(b) They usually manifest after age 5.
(c) Asperger's syndrome is similar to autism but without marked language or cognitive impairment.
(d) Rett's syndrome has an equal sex incidence.
(e) Childhood disintegrative disorder (Heller's syndrome) occurs after 2 years of normal development.

## Forensic psychiatry – Chapter 25

### 78. The following are associated with violent crime:

(a) Alcohol and substance use.
(b) Obsessive-compulsive disorder (OCD).
(c) Antisocial personality disorder.
(d) History of violent offences.
(e) Schizophrenia.

### 79. A male on trial will not be found guilty of murder under the following circumstances:

(a) He is under the age of 10.
(b) He is deemed 'insane' under the M'Naghten Rules.
(c) A defence of 'diminished responsibility' is successful.
(d) His actions are deemed to be due to an epileptic phenomenon.
(e) He has an ICD-10 diagnosis of schizophrenia.

# Pharmacological and psychological therapy, ECT – Chapters 27, 28

### 80. Regarding antidepressants:

(a) SSRIs are more effective in treating depressive symptoms than tricyclic antidepressants (TCAs).
(b) TCAs and SSRIs are effective in treating obsessive-compulsive disorder (OCD)
(c) SSRIs have fewer anticholinergic effects than the TCAs and are less sedating.
(d) SSRIs are known to cause anorgasmia.
(e) They lower the seizure threshold.

### 81. Regarding lithium:

(a) Lithium undergoes extensive liver metabolism.
(b) Lithium is relatively safe in pregnancy and breast-feeding.
(c) Lithium therapy commonly leads to low TSH levels.
(d) Lithium decreases the efficacy of antidepressants.
(e) Lithium is a powerful anticonvulsant.

### 82. Regarding anxiolytic and hypnotic drugs:

(a) Benzodiazepines exert their action by binding to a dopamine receptor.
(b) Zopiclone, zolpidem and zaleplon are long-acting compounds.
(c) Buspirone is associated with dependence.
(d) Benzodiazepines are often fatal in overdose.
(e) Oxazepam has predictable absorption when given intramuscularly.

### 83. Regarding MAOIs:

(a) Eating mature cheese and yeast extracts frequently results in a hypertensive crisis in patients prescribed moclobemide.
(b) Tricyclic antidepressants (TCAs) are routinely combined with phenelzine to treat severe depressive episodes.
(c) Phenelzine reversibly inhibits monoamine oxidase B.
(d) In combination, tranylcypromine and lorazepam results in the potentially lethal 'serotonin syndrome'.
(e) They are relatively safe in combination with pethidine.

### 84. Clozapine:

(a) Requires regular white blood cell counts to detect agranulocytosis.
(b) Is a potent $D_2$ receptor antagonist.
(c) Is less likely to cause extra-pyramidal side-effects (EPSE) than haloperidol.
(d) May cause seizures in high doses.
(e) Is more likely to be effective against negative symptoms of schizophrenia than typical antipsychotics.

### 85. The following antipsychotics and chemical classes are correctly paired:

(a) Haloperidol – butyrophenone.
(b) Chlorpromazine – thioxanthene.
(c) Flupentixol – phenothiazine.
(d) Trifluoperazine – phenothiazine.
(e) Sulpiride – dopamine reuptake inhibitor.

### 86. Regarding mood stabilizers:

(a) Carbamazepine has proven efficacy in rapid cycling bipolar affective disorder.
(b) Valproate is licensed for the treatment of acute mania.
(c) They are safe in pregnancy.
(d) They control mania, but make depressive episodes more frequent.
(e) They are known to have many potentially serious drug interactions.

### 87. The following are typical side-effects of conventional antipsychotics:

(a) Galactorrhoea.
(b) Vomiting.
(c) Akathisia.
(d) Hypertension.
(e) Shortening of the QT interval on electrocardiogram (ECG).

### 88. Regarding antipsychotic-induced extra-pyramidal side-effects:

(a) Acute dystonia should be treated promptly with intramuscular propranolol.
(b) An oculogyric crisis indicates tardive dyskinesia.
(c) Anticholinergics are used to treat parkinsonian motor symptoms.
(d) Neuroleptic malignant syndrome (NMS) is characterized by hyperthermia, unstable blood pressure and flaccid paralysis.
(e) Tardive dyskinesia (TD) responds promptly to anticholinergics.

### 89. The following statements about diazepam are true:

(a) Naloxone is an antagonist.
(b) It has a half-life of about 15 hours.
(c) Its effects are enhanced by alcohol, opiates and tricyclic antidepressants.
(d) It is often used in suppository form for acute seizures.
(e) It has an immediate anxiolytic effect.

### 90. Regarding electroconvulsive therapy (ECT):

(a) Schizophrenia is an absolute contraindication.
(b) It is a recognized precipitant of mania in patients with bipolar affective disorder.
(c) It should only be used when antidepressants have failed.
(d) Loss of memory is a common complaint.
(e) It causes permanent brain damage.

### 91. Regarding psychological treatments:

(a) Psychodynamic therapy makes use of transference in the therapeutic process.
(b) Dialectical behaviour therapy (DBT) is used in the treatment of borderline personality disorder.
(c) Cognitive-behavioural therapy (CBT) aims to interpret unconscious desires.
(d) Systematic desensitization is used in the treatment of phobias and avoidance.

(e) Psychoanalysis is the psychological treatment of choice for obsessive-compulsive disorder.

**92. The following are correctly paired:**

(a) Freud and superego.
(b) Carl Jung and psychodynamic psychotherapy.
(c) Aaron Beck and cognitive therapy.
(d) Automatic thoughts and behaviour therapy.
(e) Psychoanalysis and dream interpretation.

# Psychiatric assessment and diagnosis – Chapter 26

**93. In the psychiatric interview:**

(a) 'Are you having suicidal thoughts?' is a closed question.
(b) The CAGE questionnaire is a tool used to screen for hypochondriacal disorder.
(c) Affect and mood mean the same thing.
(d) The Mini-Mental State Examination (MMSE) should not be used to screen for cognitive impairment.
(e) All patients should be asked whether they have had suicidal thoughts.

**94. Regarding classification in psychiatry:**

(a) The ICD-10 and DSM-IV are two commonly used categorical classification systems.
(b) Organic and substance-related conditions are given diagnostic precedence over mood and anxiety disorders.
(c) The ICD-10 and DSM-IV do not share similar diagnostic categories.
(d) The DSM-IV uses a multi-axial diagnostic system with five axes.
(e) The term 'neurosis' should be used instead of 'generalized anxiety disorder'.

**95. The following terms are paired correctly with the examples:**

(a) Second person auditory hallucination – a voice saying, 'Look how ugly he is!'
(b) Bizarre delusion – a belief that one's husband is having an affair.
(c) Nihilistic delusion – a belief that oneself is non-existent.
(d) Mannerism – patient salutes whenever someone walks past.
(e) Overvalued idea – a man with hypochondriacal disorder is convinced he has a severe neurological disease.

# Mental Health legislation – Chapter 29

**96. Regarding the capacity to consent to treatment:**

(a) Adults have the right to refuse treatment, even if this refusal results in death.
(b) When patients refuse essential treatment for physical illness, clinicians must assess their capacity to consent to treatment.

(c) Patients who are unable to grasp the implications of their illness are deemed to be without capacity.
(d) A close relative of an unconscious patient has the choice to stop life-saving treatment.
(e) Psychiatrists should consent for all patients with severe schizophrenia.

**97. Regarding detention under the 1983 Mental Health Act (England and Wales):**

(a) Section 2 is an admission for assessment and lasts for up to 28 days.
(b) Section 3 is an admission for treatment and lasts for 1 year unless it is renewed.
(c) The responsible doctor may detain a hospital patient for up to 72 hours under Section 5(2).
(d) One doctor and one social worker are needed to detain a patient under Section 3.
(e) The police may detain a seemingly mentally ill patient for assessment under Section 136.

**98. The following statements about the 1983 Mental Health Act (MHA) are true:**

(a) Mental illness is not defined.
(b) Severe alcohol dependence alone may be treated under Section 3.
(c) Patients may be given treatment against their will under Section 3.
(d) Psychiatrists may discharge their patients from Section before it expires.
(e) The Mental Health Act (1983) allows for compulsory treatment of mental and physical disorders.

# Mental health service provision – Chapter 30

**99. Regarding the care programme approach (CPA):**

(a) The allocation of a care coordinator is a key component.
(b) GPs should offer it to all their patients in primary care.
(c) It involves a systematic assessment of patients' needs with the formation of a care plan that addresses these.
(d) It involves regular review meetings.
(e) It is not needed for patients who are in hospital.

**100. Regarding mental health service provision:**

(a) Psychiatrists treat most of their patients in hospital.
(b) GPs should refer most of their mentally ill patients to a community mental heath team (CMHT).
(c) Rates of institutionalization have increased over the last 30 years.
(d) Day hospitals may be helpful for patients who have just been discharged from hospital.
(e) A CMHT consists of psychiatrists and mental health nurses only.

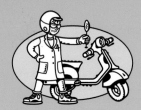
For each scenario described below, choose the single most likely diagnosis from the list of options. Each option may be used once, more than once, or not at all.

**1. Mood symptoms**

A. Grandiose delusions.
B. Diurnal variation of mood.
C. Blunted affect.
D. Psychomotor agitation.
E. Circumstantial speech.
F. Manic stupor.
G. Pressure of speech.
H. Anhedonia.
I. Mixed affective episode.
J. Tangential speech.

1. A 35-year-old mother of three says that she does not enjoy anything anymore, even horse riding, which had always been a great source of pleasure.

2. A depressed man, who has stopped eating, shows little facial expression or emotion, and speaks slowly with a monotonous tone.

3. A woman with long-standing bipolar affective disorder alternates, over the course of 2 days, between tearfulness with psychomotor retardation and elated mood with pressure of speech.

4. A young man with an amfetamine-induced manic episode is unable to stay focused in his initial train of thought, and jumps from one topic to the next, without ever returning to the original point.

5. A man who has severe depression with psychotic features is unable to sit still for longer than a few minutes without standing up and pacing around the room, all the time hand wringing and fidgeting with his clothes.

**2. Psychotic symptoms**

A. Reflex hallucinations.
B. Echolalia.
C. Lilliputian hallucinations.
D. Formication.
E. Hypnagogic hallucinations.
F. Word salad.
G. Mood-incongruent delusion.
H. Nihilistic delusion.
I. Hypnopompic hallucinations.
J. Running commentary, third person auditory hallucinations.

1. A 22-year-old man describes two female voices that incessantly remark on everything he does, e.g. 'He is now getting up. He has just turned on the light. He is getting angry. He wants to punch the wall'.

2. A heavy drinker presents to his general practitioner in a confused and drowsy state saying that he can see tiny people jumping up and down.

3. An otherwise asymptomatic 33-year-old woman is concerned because she regularly hears someone calling out her name when lying in bed at night.

4. A man with schizoaffective disorder, depressive type, is convinced that he does not exist.

5. A patient with a relapse of schizophrenia presents with speech that is completely incomprehensible as it is a mixture of strange, idiosyncratic words and phrases.

## 3. Anxiety

A. Dissociation.
B. Specific phobia.
C. Social phobia.
D. Agoraphobia.
E. Post-traumatic stress disorder.
F. Adjustment disorder.
G. Generalized (free-floating) anxiety.
H. Hypochondriacal disorder.
I. Obsessions.
J. Somatization disorder.

1. A 32-year-old woman is referred by her GP with a problem of chronic anxiety. She says that she cannot help worrying about 'anything and everything'. She is worried about her job security, finances, marriage and children. Her anxiety fluctuates from mild to moderate severity and is present for most of the day.

2. A psychiatrist visits a middle-aged man who is housebound due to anxiety. The man says that he is terrified of leaving home, and will only do so on rare occasions when accompanied by his wife. His problems started 5 years previously when he had a spontaneous panic attack while standing in a crowded train station. Since then, he has become increasingly afraid of venturing out in case he has another panic attack.

3. A 41-year-old women is a frequent visitor to her GP. She has had numerous special investigations for a multitude of physical symptoms, including abdominal pain, dysmenorrhoea, dysuria and difficulty swallowing. She refuses to accept her GP's explanation that there is no physical cause for her symptoms. She is now requesting a referral to a neurologist because she has a persistent tingling sensation in her legs.

4. A 28-year-old woman, who has recently given birth, is referred to a psychiatrist because she is having distressing thoughts. She says that many times during the day a thought will enter her head that she should smother her baby. She finds the thought of this reprehensible and can hardly bring herself to admit it. She tries to resist these thoughts, but this makes her even more anxious.

5. A young man seeks help because he is terrified of heights, and cannot bear to be more than one flight of stairs above the ground.

## 4. Dementia

A. Alzheimer's disease.
B. Frontotemporal dementia.
C. Dementia with Lewy bodies (DLB).
D. Parkinson's disease.
E. Huntington's disease.
F. Vascular dementia.
G. Creutzfeldt–Jakob disease.
H. Depressive pseudodementia.
I. HIV-related dementia.
J. Normal pressure hydrocephalus.

1. A 66-year-old man with diabetes mellitus and long-standing hypertension is referred to a psychiatrist with memory problems and subtle personality changes. His GP noted a stepwise deterioration in his cognitive functioning. On Mini-Mental State Examination (MMSE), he has a score of 19. On physical examination, he has an upper motor neuron facial nerve palsy on the right and is a little dysarthric.

2. A GP is called to a nursing home to assess an elderly woman who has been diagnosed with dementia. She has recently had a number of falls associated with syncope, and, at times, has appeared to be suffering from visual hallucinations. Physical examination reveals increased muscle tone and a resting tremor. Despite pressure from nursing staff, the GP is reluctant to prescribe an antipsychotic.

3. Six years ago, a 78-year-old man was referred to a psychiatrist after experiencing increasing difficulty remembering things. At that time, his MMSE score was 22. A dementia work-up, which included a thorough physical examination and comprehensive special investigations, revealed no abnormalities. Since then, his cognitive functioning and personality have gradually deteriorated. He is now unable to care for himself.

4. A psychiatrist refers a 63-year-old retired solicitor for a SPECT scan, following a rapid deterioration of her personality, characterized by coarse social conduct and tactlessness. Her husband had commented that she seemed 'emotionally distant' and 'much quieter than usual'. On examination, she had an MMSE score of 24 and noticeable perseveration. An earlier CT-scan revealed 'knife-blade atrophy'.

5. A 65-year-old man with recurrent depressive disorder is admitted to a psychiatric ward with psychomotor retardation, social withdrawal, difficulty thinking and poor concentration. His wife is concerned because his memory has deteriorated suddenly. His MMSE score is 18.

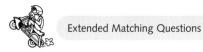 

### 5. Substance misuse

A. Naltrexone.
B. Lysergic acid diethylamine (LSD).
C. Disulfiram.
D. Thiamine.
E. Methadone.
F. Acamprosate.
G. Ketamine.
H. Buprenorphine.
I. Flumazenil.
J. Chlordiazepoxide.

*For each of the descriptions below, select TWO drugs from the above list. Each answer may only be selected once.*

1. Two drugs used in the acute treatment of alcohol withdrawal (detoxification).

2. Two drugs strongly associated with hallucinations.

3. Two drugs used to help prevent relapse in the treatment of alcohol dependence.

4. Two drugs used as 'substitute drugs' in the maintenance treatment of opiate dependence.

5. Two receptor antagonists that can precipitate severe withdrawal in patients with substance dependence.

### 6. Psychiatric diagnoses

A. Cyclothymia.
B. Recurrent depressive disorder.
C. Depressive episode with psychotic symptoms.
D. Dysthymia.
E. Mania with psychotic symptoms.
F. Mania without psychotic symptoms.
G. Bipolar affective disorder.
H. Paranoid schizophrenia.
I. Delusional disorder.
J. Schizoaffective disorder.

1. A 48-year-old man has a chronic psychiatric history, which has included five admissions to a psychiatric hospital. During the first admission, a diagnosis of hypomania was made. The last four admissions were characterized by severe depression associated with strong suicidal ideation.

2. A young drama student presents to the mental health services for the first time with greatly elevated mood, insomnia and increased energy. She believes that she is a famous actress with legions of adoring fans. She has none of Schneider's first-rank symptoms.

3. A man with numerous previous psychotic episodes is admitted to hospital with a relapse. He describes low mood, anhedonia and fatiguability. He is observed to have psychomotor retardation. On mental state examination, he describes thought withdrawal as well as running commentary third person auditory hallucinations.

4. A 30-year-old woman is prescribed clozapine for a treatment-resistant psychotic illness. She believes that aliens have poisoned her water supply and have her on 24-hour surveillance. She has second person auditory hallucinations telling her that people are watching her. She does not have disorganized speech or negative symptoms. Her mood seems euthymic, despite the distressing nature of her delusions.

5. A 45-year-old woman has attended a psychiatric out-patient clinic, at infrequent intervals, since early adulthood, but has never been admitted to hospital. Her condition is stabilized on sodium valproate and 50 mg of sertraline daily. When unwell, she feels either mildly elated with increased energy or mildly depressed with low self-esteem. She has never met ICD-10 criteria for either a depressive episode or hypomania.

**7. Epidemiology of mental illness**

A. 0.5%.
B. 1%.
C. 5%.
D. 10–25%.
E. 35%.
F. 50%.
G. 75%.
H. 100%.

*For each of the population groups below, select the most appropriate prevalence/lifetime risk from the above list. The same answer may be selected more than once.*

1. The lifetime risk of recurrent depressive disorder in women.

2. The lifetime risk of bipolar affective disorder in men.

3. The lifetime risk of schizophrenia in men.

4. The lifetime risk of schizophrenia in a monozygotic twin if the other twin is affected.

5. The prevalence of dementia in people over the age of 65.

6. The prevalence of postnatal blues (baby blues) in postpartum women.

**8. Psychiatric medication in context**

A. Chlordiazepoxide.
B. Amitriptyline.
C. Lorazepam.
D. Lithium.
E. Haloperidol.
F. Olanzapine.
G. Clozapine.
H. Diazepam.
I. Procyclidine.
J. Fluoxetine.

1. A 57-year-old man, while recovering from a serious myocardial infarction, is diagnosed with a moderate depressive episode.

2. A woman with an alcohol withdrawal delirium becomes acutely agitated and aggressive. After considering important medical causes of agitation, the treating doctor prescribes intramuscular tranquillizing medication because the woman refuses oral medication.

3. A young man with recently diagnosed schizophrenia has not responded to 2 months of treatment with risperidone, followed by 2 months of treatment with quetiapine, both at maximum dose.

4. A 34-year-old man has treatment-resistant depression with numerous biological symptoms. He has tried numerous different antidepressants in high doses and in combination, but with little improvement. His psychiatrist suggests antidepressant augmentation.

5. A 29 year-old man, on a flupentixol depot injection, who is poorly compliant with oral antipsychotics, requests help for 'stiff legs, difficulty moving and trembling hands'.

**9. Side-effects of psychiatric medication**

A. Tardive dyskinesia.
B. Hypothyroidism.
C. Akathisia.
D. Neuroleptic malignant syndrome.
E. Acute dystonia.
F. Agranulocytosis.
G. Serotonin syndrome.
H. Hypertensive crisis.
I. Prolongation of QT-interval.
J. Parkinsonian symptoms.

1. A 22-year-old man with treatment-resistant schizophrenia has recently started clozapine. On day 14 of treatment, he develops a high fever with chills, as well as myalgia, headache, abdominal pain and a sore throat. On examination, his muscular tone is normal.

2. A woman with atypical depression has responded well to phenelzine. Three months after starting treatment, she takes a standard over-the-counter decongestant in response to a blocked nose and flu-like symptoms. A few hours later, she develops a throbbing headache and palpitations.

3. A young man, recently diagnosed with hebephrenic schizophrenia, is given 5 mg haloperidol intramuscularly because he refuses to take any oral medication. A few hours later, a nurse notices that he appears in extreme discomfort. His eyes are deviated upwards and to the side, his face seems contorted in a painful grimace, and his neck is twisted at an awkward angle to his body.

4. A middle-aged woman with schizoaffective disorder suddenly loses consciousness and is rushed to hospital with a suspected cardiac arrhythmia. The casualty doctor notes that she takes very high doses of numerous psychiatric medications including amitriptyline, thioridazine and haloperidol, as well as a fluphenazine depot injection 3-weekly.

5. A 67-year-old woman with paranoid schizophrenia has been on a monthly pipotiazine depot injection for most of her adult life. At a routine clinic appointment, her psychiatrist notices that she has developed rhythmic, involuntary chewing movements, and protruding, darting movements of her tongue.

**10. Mental state examination**

A. Flight of ideas.
B. Second person auditory hallucinations.
C. Third person auditory hallucinations.
D. Persecutory delusions.
E. Panic attack.
F. Delusions of control.
G. Thought insertion.
H. Delusions of reference.
I. Grandiose delusions.
J. Hypochondriacal disorder.
K. Generalized anxiety.
L. Anhedonia.

1. Have you ever been so frightened that your heart was pounding and you thought you might die?

2. Do your voices ever talk directly to you or give you commands?

3. Are you afraid that someone is trying to harm or poison you?

4. Does it seem as though you are being controlled or influenced by some external force?

5. Have you noticed that people are doing or saying things that have a special meaning for you?

6. Have you noticed your thoughts racing in your head?

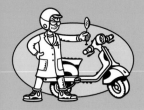
1.  (a) Anhedonia is an important biological symptom of depression. What does it mean?
    (b) Name five other biological symptoms of depression.

2.  (a) Explain the difference between deliberate self-harm, suicide and parasuicide.
    (b) Name four factors that suggest strong suicide intent.

3.  (a) Delusions of control are one of Schneider's first rank symptoms. What are they?
    (b) Explain the importance of recognizing first-rank symptoms.

4.  (a) How does generalized anxiety differ from the anxiety experienced in panic attacks?
    (b) Name three anxiety disorders associated with panic attacks.

5.  (a) What are obsessions and compulsions?
    (b) What questions would you use to elicit obsessions and compulsions on mental state examination?

6.  (a) Explain how you would distinguish between the somatoform disorders, and factitious disorder and malingering.
    (b) What is the difference between somatization disorder and hypochondriacal disorder?

7.  (a) Explain the essential differences between delirium, dementia and the amnesic syndrome.
    (b) How do you manage an alcohol-withdrawal delirium?

8.  What does the 'alcohol dependence syndrome' mean and what are its main characteristics?

9.  (a) What do you understand by the term 'personality disorder'?
    (b) Borderline personality disorder is in Cluster B in the DSM-IV. What does this mean?

10. (a) Name the four essential requirements for a diagnosis of anorexia nervosa.
    (b) In addition to reduced caloric intake, patients with anorexia may induce vomiting. What electrolyte abnormalities occur in patients who repeatedly induce vomiting?

11. (a) What is 'cyclothymia'?
    (b) An elderly man with cyclothymia is treated with amitriptyline. Name five common side-effects associated with this tricyclic antidepressant.

12. (a) What is meant by 'psychomotor agitation'?
    (b) Psychomotor agitation or aggressive behaviour frequently occurs in mentally and physically ill patients. Name five conditions that often present in this way.

13. (a) What are the differences between typical and atypical antipsychotics?
    (b) Name five antipsychotic-induced extra-pyramidal side-effects.
    (c) How would you manage these conditions?

14. (a) What three conditions should you consider when a woman presents with psychiatric symptoms in the puerperium?
    (b) What is the prevalence of each condition?
    (c) What is the clinical presentation of a puerperal psychosis?

15. (a) How are psychiatric disorders in children classified?
    (b) What are the three main characteristics of autism?
    (c) What are the causes of school refusal and how does it differ from truancy?

16. (a) On mental state examination, what is the difference between *mood* and *affect*?
    (b) Affect is assessed by observing patients' posture, facial expression, emotional reactivity and speech. What components should you consider when describing affect?
    (c) What does labile mood mean?

17. (a) Under what circumstances should electroconvulsive therapy (ECT) be considered in the treatment of depression?
    (b) A young woman with severe depression is concerned about side-effects from ECT. How would you respond to her?
    (c) What is the danger in giving a patient with bipolar affective disorder ECT?

18. (a) Name three conditions in which lithium is used.
    (b) What are the common side-effects of lithium?
    (c) Lithium has a narrow therapeutic index and is excreted almost exclusively by the kidneys. What investigations are needed prior to initiating therapy?
    (d) How often should lithium levels be checked?

19. (a) What is primary insomnia?
    (b) How would you manage a patient with primary insomnia?

20. (a) What are the differences and similarities between Section 2 and Section 3 of the Mental Health Act (1983) in England and Wales with reference to:
    • Aims of the Section
    • Duration
    • Application and recommendations.
    (b) What is a Section 5(2)?

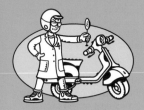

1. A 56-year-old man tells his general practitioner that he has been feeling depressed and anxious for most of the time over the last 3 years. He says that he is unable to sleep unless he has drunk at least a bottle of wine. He describes an unhappy marriage, in part, due to his loss of interest in sex.

   - Based on the presenting complaint, what conditions would be in your differential diagnosis?
   - Describe how you would further assess this man to narrow your differential diagnosis.

2. A 32-year-old man with bipolar affective disorder complains of difficulty sleeping over the past 3 weeks. He is on several psychiatric drugs, including an SSRI, which he started recently. He uses cannabis occasionally. He is unemployed and has little structure to his day. He is overweight and suffers from arthritis and gastro-oesophageal reflux disease.

   - Discuss the possible causes of this man's sleep disturbance.
   - Describe non-pharmacological measures that might be helpful in this case.

3. A 28-year-old man, who is well known to the local psychiatric services, arrives at casualty at 1 a.m. and asks to see a psychiatrist, insisting that he has taken an aspirin overdose. He says that if he is not admitted to hospital he will go home and kill himself. On examination, the casualty doctor can smell alcohol on his breath and notes that he has numerous self-harm scars on both his forearms.

   - Discuss the factors you should consider when assessing this man's risk of suicide with reference to:
     a. Lethality of suicidal attempt
     b. Mental state examination
     c. Risk factors for suicide
     d. Social and psychiatric support in the community.

4. A 19 year-old-man is brought to see his general practitioner by his parents who have become concerned about his behaviour. He has been asking his parents repeatedly whether there is something wrong with him, and then refusing to believe them, saying strange things like, 'There are imbalances and improbabilities underfoot'. At times, it appears as though he is talking to himself. Over the previous week, his parents have heard him shifting furniture in his room throughout the night.

   - What questions would you ask in order to elicit delusions and hallucinations?
   - How would you rule out organic and substance-related causes of psychosis?
   - You suspect that this man may need to be assessed and treated under mental health legislation. Describe the process, as you would explain it to him and his parents.

5. A 37-year-old man with a history of several depressive episodes is brought into casualty by his girlfriend. She is concerned because he has been acting 'completely out of character' for the last few days. He has been sleeping very little, spending large amounts of money, and embarking on numerous risky business ventures. The patient is adamant that there is nothing wrong with him saying that he has never felt better or more invigorated. He says that he is 'insulted to be dragged along here and interrogated by the junior ranks'. He takes citalopram, which has recently been increased to 40 mg daily.

   - What is the most likely diagnosis?
   - Discuss the factors you would take into account when considering whether this man should be admitted to hospital.
   - What change would you make to his current medication?

6. A 22-year-old woman tells her general practitioner that she is becoming increasingly reluctant to socialize due to anxiety. She is not significantly depressed and has no psychotic symptoms. She is not taking any medication and does not abuse alcohol or any illicit substances.

   - What anxiety disorders would you include in a wide differential diagnosis?
   - What questions would you ask in order to narrow the differential diagnosis?
   - Discuss the treatment options for social phobia and agoraphobia.

7. A 41-year-old woman with a 10-year history of alcohol dependence is scheduled for an elective out-patient detoxification.

   • What are the contraindications to out-patient detoxification?
   • What are the dangers of inadequately managed alcohol detoxification?
   • How do you treat a Wernicke's encephalopathy?

8. As a casualty doctor, you are asked to assess a man who, according to his wife, has taken an overdose of 48 paracetamol tablets with a bottle of whisky. He appears inebriated and confused and is unable to give a coherent account of himself. He will not allow you to do a paracetamol blood level and refuses any form of treatment. His psychiatric notes reveal a history of severe depression. You decide that he is at risk of serious liver damage if he is not treated promptly.

   • The duty psychiatrist tells you that you cannot treat this man's suspected paracetamol poisoning under mental health legislation. What are the principles that govern your further actions?
   • What factors are important in determining his capacity to consent to treatment?

9. As a general practitioner, you are asked to see an 18-year-old woman who was brought into the surgery by her mother. The mother says that she is very concerned because her daughter is eating 'next to nothing' and is exercising excessively. The young woman is clearly upset but says nothing. In an attempt to get her to talk more freely, you ask to speak to her alone. The young woman looks very thin.

   • What questions should you ask in order to clarify the extent of this woman's eating problems?
   • You discover that the woman regularly vomits after episodes of binge eating. You measure her body mass index to be 16 kg/m². What medical complications, related to starvation and vomiting, should you be concerned about?

10. As a casualty doctor, you are asked to see a young man, who is described as 'threatening and menacing' by the nursing staff. He was brought to the department by the police and is known to suffer from paranoid schizophrenia. You can hear him shouting 'Leave me alone! Go away!' down the corridor.

    • Describe how you would manage this agitated patient with reference to:
      a. Environmental interventions
      b. Behavioural interventions
      c. Medical interventions
    • With help from the duty psychiatrist, you diagnose an acute psychotic episode and administer 5 mg of haloperidol and 2 mg of lorazepam intramuscularly under common law. What side-effects should you monitor the man for?

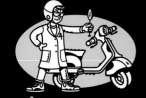

# MCQ Answers

## Mood (affective) disorders – Chapters 1, 2, 3, 13

**1.** (a) False – thoughts of suicide or self-harm are not regarded as biological symptoms.
  (b) True – psychomotor agitation or retardation are somatic symptoms.
  (c) False – hopelessness is a *cognitive* symptom of depression.
  (d) False – depression *worse in the morning* is an important biological symptom.
  (e) True – see p. 5.

**2.** (a) True – see p. 4.
  (b) True – anhedonia may be evident in a depressive or mixed episode.
  (c) True – low mood, loss of interest or pleasure and fatiguability are the three core symptoms of depression.
  (d) False – it is a biological symptom of depression.
  (e) True – dysthymia features typical symptoms of depression, although these are seldom severe enough to meet the criteria for a depressive episode.

**3.** (a) False – dysthymia is a chronically depressed mood that is seldom severe enough to satisfy the formal criteria for a depressive episode and does not present with discrete episodes as in genuine recurrent depressive disorder.
  (b) True – see p. 12.
  (c) True – see p. 6.
  (d) True – see p. 7.
  (e) True – especially methyldopa and beta-blockers.

**4.** (a) True – see p. 11.
  (b) False – this is typical of depression.
  (c) True – see p. 10.
  (d) True – see p. 10.
  (e) False – this is typical of schizophrenia.

**5.** (a) False – the ICD-10 specifies two types of manic episode: *mania without psychotic symptoms* and *mania with psychotic symptoms*.
  (b) False – rapidly alternating manic and depressive symptoms are termed *mixed affective episodes*, and are not common.
  (c) True – manic patients may have an elevated or irritable mood.
  (d) False – the ICD-10 specifies that manic episodes disrupt work and social activities *completely*.
  (e) True – this is a very important early warning sign of mania or hypomania.

**6.** (a) True – suicide intent is suggested by forward planning, as well as dangerous method – tricyclics are known to be lethal in overdose.
  (b) False – impulsive self-harm in the context of alcohol intoxication probably indicates lower suicide intent, although might indicate increased risk of future suicide. Remember that the risk of completed suicide in the alcohol-dependent patient is much higher than in the general population.
  (c) False – suicide intent is suggested by *not* seeking help after the attempt.
  (d) True – this is a dangerous method.
  (e) True – precautions taken to avoid discovery or rescue suggests suicide intent.

**7.** (a) False – parasuicidal patients should always receive a thorough clinical assessment, but may be sent home if their risk is manageable in the community.
  (b) False – asking about ongoing suicidal ideation is an important part of the mental state examination.
  (c) True – women engage in more parasuicidal acts, although men are more likely to complete suicide.
  (d) True – both alcohol dependence and anorexia nervosa are risk factors for suicide.
  (e) False – male sex, age over 45 and divorced marital status are risk factors for completed suicide.

**8.** (a) False – it suggests a shortage of serotonin, noradrenaline (norepinephrine) and dopamine.
  (b) False – the efficacy of almost all antidepressants may be explained by the monoamine theory.
  (c) False – they have shown that there is a genetic component to depression.
  (d) False – high EE contributes to the risk of relapse.
  (e) True – see p. 85.

**9.** (a) False – antidepressants have a similar efficacy, but varying side-effect profiles.
  (b) False – SSRIs are relatively safe in overdose; tricyclic antidepressants are cardiotoxic in overdose.
  (c) True – patients with recurrent episodes need treatment for even longer
  (d) True – see p. 87.
  (e) True – see p. 87.

**10.** (a) True – see p. 85.
  (b) True – see p. 85.
  (c) True – a history of depression in first-degree relatives is a significant risk factor.
  (d) True – adverse life events have been shown to increase the risk of developing depression.
  (e) False – L-tryptophan is used to augment antidepressants in treatment-resistant depression.

11. (a) False – the sex ratio of BAD is equal.
    (b) True.
    (c) False – may be used with utmost caution for depressive episodes.
    (d) False – lithium is used for both initial and maintenance treatment and is usually long term.
    (e) True.

12. (a) True – the narrowest clinical definition of psychosis is: delusions and hallucinations.
    (b) False – overvalued ideas, not delusions, may be present in personality disorder.
    (c) False – although a delusion may actually be true (e.g. partner having an affair), the reasons given for believing it are faulty.
    (d) False – delusions are out of keeping with the person's social and cultural background.
    (e) False – the content of delusions may be bizarre or non-bizarre.

13. (a) True – these are transient and always involve images of the deceased, and are strictly speaking pseudohallucinations.
    (b) False – hypnagogic hallucinations occur as a person goes to sleep.
    (c) False – *illusions* are misperceptions of real external stimuli.
    (d) False – hallucinations may occur in normal people, e.g. hypnagogic and hypnopompic hallucinations.
    (e) True – paranoid schizophrenia is characterized by the presence of delusions and/or hallucinations, i.e. positive symptoms.

14. (a) True – *word salad* describes speech that becomes a mixture of incoherent words and phrases.
    (b) True – *neologisms* are new words created by the patient.
    (c) False – *thought echo* is a form of first person auditory hallucination.
    (d) True – *flight of ideas* occurs when thinking is markedly accelerated resulting in a stream of connected concepts.
    (e) False – *waxy flexibility* is a catatonic phenomenon.

15. (a) True – *mannerisms* are apparently goal-directed movements, e.g. waving, saluting, that are performed repeatedly or at socially inappropriate times.
    (b) False – *formication* is the sensation of insects crawling on or just below the skin; it is a tactile hallucination.
    (c) True – *catatonic stupor* is a presentation of akinesis (lack of voluntary movement), mutism and extreme unresponsiveness in an otherwise alert patient.
    (d) True – in *waxy flexibility*, patients can be 'moulded' like wax.
    (e) True – *stereotypies* are complex movements that do not appear to be goal-directed, e.g. rocking back and forth, gyrating.

16. (a) True – see p. 91.
    (b) False – men have only a slightly higher incidence than women.
    (c) False – the dopamine hypothesis suggests that schizophrenia is secondary to *overactivity* of the mesolimbic dopamine pathway.
    (d) False – although there is a significant genetic factor involved, evidence indicates that the environment also plays an important role.
    (e) True – Schneider defined the first-rank symptoms of schizophrenia.

17. (a) False – although flight of ideas may occur in schizophrenia, they are more indicative of mania.
    (b) False – second person auditory hallucinations are not characteristic of schizophrenia as they often occur in *mood disorders with psychotic symptoms*.
    (c) False – grandiose delusions also typically occur in *mania with psychotic symptoms* and, therefore, are not characteristic of schizophrenia.
    (d) True – delusional perception is a first-rank symptom of schizophrenia and part of the ICD-10 criteria.
    (e) True – hallucinatory voices giving a running commentary or discussing the patient among themselves are both first-rank symptoms of schizophrenia and part of the ICD-10 criteria.

18. (a) True – the subtypes of schizophrenia are paranoid, hebephrenic (disorganized), catatonic and residual.
    (b) True – see (a).
    (c) False – although *schizotypal disorder* is characterized by eccentric behaviour and peculiarities of thinking and appearance, it is not schizophrenia.
    (d) False – this is a personality disorder subtype.
    (e) True – see (a).

19. (a) True – especially temporal lobe epilepsy.
    (b) True – see p. 30.
    (c) True – see p. 30.
    (d) True – hyperglycaemia may cause a delirium, which may feature psychotic symptoms.
    (e) True – especially vitamin $B_{12}$, niacin (pellagra) and thiamine deficiencies (Wernicke's encephalopathy).

20. (a) True – see p. 91.
    (b) True – see p. 91.
    (c) False – the incidence is increased in urban areas.
    (d) True – see p. 91.
    (e) False – there is an increased prevalence in lower socioeconomic classes – classes IV and V.

21. (a) True – see p. 92.
    (b) False – the concordance rate for monozygotic twins is 50%.
    (c) True – this is termed high expressed emotion.
    (d) True – see p. 92.
    (e) False – there is strong evidence that schizophrenia is associated with complications during pregnancy and birth.

**22.** (a) False – they are probably more effective.
(b) True – see p. 93.
(c) False – they are helpful for the short-term relief of behaviour disturbance, insomnia, aggression and agitation.
(d) True – see p. 93.
(e) True – see p. 95.

**23.** (a) True – 10% of patients will commit suicide.
(b) False – women have a better prognosis.
(c) True – only about 20% of patients have a single episode.
(d) True – see p. 95.
(e) False – positive symptoms respond well to treatment; negative symptoms indicate a worse prognosis.

**24.** (a) False – free-floating anxiety is not associated with a specific external threat or situation but is rather excessive worry about many normal life events.
(b) False – avoidance describes the change in behaviour in response to a real or imagined threat, and is characteristic of phobic disorders.
(c) False – free-floating anxiety has a gradual onset, does not occur in discrete episodes and tends to last for hours, days or longer.
(d) False – the key element of panic disorder is panic attacks, although patients may have anticipatory anxiety.
(e) False – panic disorder is strongly associated with agoraphobia.

**25.** (a) False – panic attacks can occur spontaneously (unprovoked) or as a response to a phobic stimulus.
(b) False – the key element of GAD is long-standing, free-floating anxiety.
(c) True – see p. 34.
(d) False – although, strong autonomic symptoms during an attack may lead patients to believe they are dying.
(e) True – see p. 37.

**26.** (a) True – see p. 42.
(b) False – most bereavement reactions are normal and do not require treatment.
(c) False – this probably indicates the development of a depressive episode.
(d) True – see p. 42.
(e) True – hallucinatory experiences *other than* patients thinking that they transiently see or hear the deceased are not considered part of the normal bereavement reaction.

**27.** (a) True – see p. 41.
(b) False – this describes the onset of an *acute stress reaction*. The symptoms of PTSD usually develop within 6 months of a traumatic stressor.
(c) True – see p. 41.
(d) True – hallucinations are one of the ways in which patients repetitively re-experience the traumatic event.

(e) True – this is important because alcohol and substance intoxication or withdrawal may present with similar symptoms to PTSD.

**28.** (a) False – the essential feature of somatization disorder is multiple, recurrent, frequently changing physical symptoms. Patients with hypochondriacal disorder believe they have a serious physical disease.
(b) False – physical or psychological symptoms are produced intentionally or feigned in both *factitious disorder* and *malingering*.
(c) False – the psychopathology of body dysmorphic disorder (and hypochondriacal disorder) takes the form of an *overvalued idea*, not a delusion.
(d) False – factitious disorder and malingering are differentiated by the patient's *motivation* for simulating symptoms. In factitious disorder, patients are focused on the *primary internal gain* of assuming the sick role. In malingering, patients are focused on a *secondary external gain*.
(e) True – these tend to be episodic and resolve with the treatment of the depression.

**29.** (a) True – obsessions are recognized as being the product of their own mind even though they are involuntary and often repugnant.
(b) True – over 20% of depressed patients can have obsessive-compulsive symptoms, which occur simultaneously at or after the onset of depression.
(c) False – obsessions are experienced as *ego-dystonic* and insight is generally retained into the fact that they are *irrational*.
(d) False – compulsions are often performed in response to obsessions in an attempt to reduce anxiety.
(e) False – most patients with obsessive-compulsive personality disorder do not have obsessions or compulsions.

**30.** (a) True – see Fig. 15.2, p. 99.
(b) True – see Fig. 15.2, p. 99.
(c) False – agoraphobia is a fear of entering crowded spaces where an immediate escape is difficult or in which help might not be available in the event of having a panic attack.
(d) True – see p. 35.
(e) False – SSRIs are first-line treatments.

**31.** (a) False – anxiety disorders tend to be more common in women apart from social phobia and obsessive-compulsive disorder where the prevalence is about equal.
(b) True – the situationally induced anxiety of all the phobic disorders may be so severe as to take the form of a *panic attack*.
(c) True – all phobic disorders are associated with a prominent avoidance of the feared situation.
(d) False – cognitive-behavioural therapy (CBT) is first-line psychological treatment.
(e) False – SSRIs are first-line treatment. Benzodiazepines are considered in treatment-resistant cases.

**32.** (a) True – see p. 98.
   (b) False – nortriptyline is predominantly a noradrenergic agent. In OCD serotonergic drugs such as the SSRIs and clomipramine are most effective
   (c) True – see p. 98.
   (d) True – see p. 98.
   (e) False – the ICD-10 criteria state that obsessions or compulsions should be a source of distress or interfere with the patient's functioning.

**33.** (a) True – both venlafaxine and the SSRIs have proven efficacy in GAD.
   (b) True – CBT has proven efficacy in most anxiety disorders and often has a synergistic effect with medication.
   (c) False – pharmacotherapy is not standard treatment for specific phobias.
   (d) True – TCAs are as effective as SSRIs but less well tolerated.
   (e) True – restlessness, jitteriness and an initial increase in anxiety symptoms may occur in the first few days of treatment with either the SSRIs or the TCAs.

**34.** (a) True – see Fig. 10.4, p. 69.
   (b) False – see (a).
   (c) True – see (a).
   (d) True – this indicates increased salience of drinking; see (a).
   (e) True – see (a).

**35.** (a) True – see Fig. 10.5, p. 70.
   (b) True – see (a).
   (c) False – sweating is a key feature of alcohol withdrawal; see (a).
   (d) False – this would indicate an *alcohol withdrawal delirium* (delirium tremens); see (a).
   (e) True – mood disturbance is a key feature of alcohol withdrawal; see (a).

**36.** (a) False – an *increase* in carbohydrate deficient transferrin (CDT) is considered the best single screening test for excessive alcohol use.
   (b) True – alcohol-induced amnesic syndrome, or *Korsakoff's syndrome*, occurs as a result of a thiamine (vitamin $B_1$) deficiency.
   (c) True – both hallucinations and delusions can occur in the context of heavy alcohol consumption.
   (d) False – excessive alcohol use causes red blood cell *macrocytosis*.
   (e) True – alcohol use is strongly associated with violent crime.

**37.** (a) True – thiamine (vitamin $B_1$) is given in order to avert a Wernicke's encephalopathy.
   (b) False – increasing the cost of alcohol through taxation is the most effective strategy in reducing overall consumption.
   (c) True – see p. 110.
   (d) False – chlordiazepoxide does this. Antipsychotics such as chlorpromazine actually lower the seizure threshold.
   (e) False – disulfiram blocks alcohol oxidation, leading to an accumulation of acetaldehyde. Acamprosate enhances GABA transmission.

**38.** (a) False – not all patients who drink heavily meet the criteria for the alcohol dependence syndrome.
   (b) True – see p. 69.
   (c) False – only about 20% of patients with Korsakoff's syndrome recover.
   (d) True – see p. 70
   (e) True – the lifetime risk of suicide in problem drinkers is 3–4%, which is 60–120 times greater than the normal population.

**39.** (a) True – see p. 113.
   (b) False – lofexidine is a centrally acting α-adrenoceptor agonist used in opiate dependence.
   (c) False – methadone can be lethal in overdose; it is a longer acting oral opiate that helps to stabilize the user's life and prevent the complications of injecting.
   (d) True – see p. 113.
   (e) True – see p. 113.

**40.** (a) True – see p. 71.
   (b) False – benzodiazepine withdrawal is potentially fatal, and may include hallucinations, convulsions and delirium.
   (c) False – both cocaine and amfetamines can be stopped abruptly.
   (d) True – naltrexone is an opiate antagonist and therefore blocks opiate receptors.
   (e) False – cannabis is the most commonly consumed drug in England; heroin is the most frequently reported drug of misuse.

**41.** (a) False – delirium tremens is a life-threatening condition that requires emergency hospital admission.
   (b) True – *lilliputian hallucinations* are visual hallucinations of miniature humans or animals.
   (c) True – delirium tremens develops 24 hours to 1 week after drinking cessation, peaking at 72–96 hours.
   (d) True – delirium tremens is associated with autonomic arousal.
   (e) False – delirium tremens is primarily treated with benzodiazepines.

**42.** (a) True – the essential feature of a delirium is an impairment of consciousness with a reduced ability to focus or maintain attention.
(b) False – sleep abnormalities in delirium can range from daytime drowsiness and night-time hyperactivity to a complete reversal of the normal cycle.
(c) True – both illusions and hallucinations may occur in delirium.
(d) False – delirium has an acute onset and has a duration of hours to weeks; dementia has a gradual onset with progressive deterioration over months to years.
(e) False – there is invariably an identifiable medical or drug-related cause of delirium.

**43.** (a) False – this describes the amnesic syndrome.
(b) True – see p. 56.
(c) False – there are many recognized medical causes of dementia (see Fig. 9.3, p. 57).
(d) False – dementia is just one of many causes of stupor.
(e) False – memory for personal information is usually retained until late in dementia.

**44.** (a) True – see Fig. 9.4, p. 58.
(b) False – this symptom is typical of DLB (see Fig. 9.4, p. 58).
(c) True – (Fig. 9.4).
(d) False – this symptom is typical of frontotemporal dementia (Fig. 9.4).
(e) True – see p. 59.

**45.** (a) False – this tests explicit or declarative memory. Procedural or implicit memory includes all material which is stored without an individual's awareness, e.g. ability to speak a language or ride a bicycle.
(b) True – see p. 55.
(c) False – the MMSE is used as a screening test for cognitive impairment, of which there are many causes. A score below 25/30 is consistent with dementia but does not indicate the type of dementia.
(d) True – long-term memory features a duration of storage from minutes to decades. It may be divided into recent (e.g. remembering breakfast) and remote (e.g. remembering childhood) memory.
(e) False – difficulty naming objects may be due to agnosia or aphasia, both of which are early features of cortical dementia and preserved until late in subcortical dementia.

**46.** (a) True – this is as opposed to typical CJD, which tends to affect people in their fifties, and has a time course of 6–8 months.
(b) False – the duration of survival is 1–2 years for DLB and 7–9 years for Alzheimer's disease.
(c) True – Parkinson's disease and HIV-related dementia (as well as DLB) have a subcortical presentation.
(d) False – Huntington's disease has autosomal *dominant* inheritance.
(e) True – Pick's disease is a frontotemporal dementia and features paper-thin (knife-blade) atrophy.

**47.** (a) False – HRT appears to be a protective factor.
(b) False – the cholinergic hypothesis explains the efficacy of the cholinesterase inhibitors.
(c) False – there are no specific tests that are diagnostic for AD. CT may be supportive in diagnosing AD and is used to exclude other causes of cognitive impairment.
(d) False – adults with trisomy 21 almost always develop pathological changes similar to AD.
(e) False – most cases are sporadic. In rare cases, AD may be transmitted through an autosomal dominant gene.

**48.** (a) True – see p. 104.
(b) False – this indicates vascular dementia, specifically Binswanger's disease.
(c) True – see p. 104.
(d) True – see p. 104.
(e) False – AD is associated with enlarged ventricles and widened sulci.

**49.** (a) True – increased risk of Alzheimer's disease.
(b) True – increased risk of early-onset AD.
(c) True – increased risk of vascular dementia.
(d) True – increased risk of HIV encephalopathy or opportunistic infections.
(e) True – 30% of patients with Parkinson's disease develop dementia.

**50.** (a) False – the prevalence of parasuicide in the elderly is lower than in adults, but they are at a high risk for completed suicide (p. 155).
(b) False – unlike depression, the incidence of bipolar affective disorder does not increase with age.
(c) False – the elderly have a decreased lean body mass and total body water, and increased body fat.
(d) True – depression in the elderly may present with apparent cognitive impairment; this is termed *depressive pseudodementia*.
(e) True – the elderly have an increased sensitivity to central nervous system drugs.

**51.** (a) True – see p. 155.
(b) False – it is characterized by delusions, although hallucinations may occur.
(c) False – ECT can be very effective.
(d) False – it is far more common in women.
(e) True – see p. 156.

**52.** (a) True – see p. 160.
(b) True – a substantial proportion of adolescents with conduct disorder go on to develop antisocial personality disorder.
(c) False – these individuals commonly have an incapacity to experience guilt for the consequences of their behaviours.
(d) False – antisocial personality disorder is associated with an increased risk of suicide.
(e) True – there is strong evidence linking alcohol and substance abuse with antisocial personality traits.

233

**53.** (a) True – BPD is associated with repetitive self-harm or suicidal behaviour.
  (b) True – there is an association between BPD and childhood sexual abuse.
  (c) True – see p. 116.
  (d) False – BPD is more prevalent in younger age groups and females.
  (e) True – see p. 77.

**54.** (a) True – see p. 77.
  (b) True – see p. 77.
  (c) False – this is a feature of schizotypal PD; individuals with paranoid PD suspect others are exploiting, harming or deceiving them.
  (d) True – see p. 77.
  (e) False – this is a feature of borderline (emotionally unstable) PD; individuals with narcissistic PD have a grandiose sense of self-importance and need for admiration.

**55.** (a) False – pyromania is pathological fire setting. Trichotillomania is repetitive pulling out of one's hair.
  (b) True – see p. 76.
  (c) True – see p. 76.
  (d) False – the ICD-10 classifies personality disorders using a *categorical* approach.
  (e) True – see p. 77.

**56.** (a) False – there is a much higher prevalence in prisons.
  (b) True – see p. 116.
  (c) False – certain disorders respond significantly to treatment and improve over time.
  (d) True – they have a greater incidence of all mental illness.
  (e) False – it is not found in the ICD-10. It is a legal term described in the Mental Health Act 1983.

**57.** (a) False – hospital admission may be necessary during times of crisis.
  (b) True – see p. 116.
  (c) True – see p. 117.
  (d) True – see p. 117.
  (e) True – see p. 116.

**58.** (a) True – this is essential to the diagnosis; see Fig. 12.2, p. 80.
  (b) True – this is essential to the diagnosis; see Fig. 12.2, p. 80.
  (c) False – binge eating may occur in, and does not preclude the diagnosis of, AN.
  (d) True – this is essential to the diagnosis; see Fig. 12.2, p. 80.
  (e) False – women with AN often continue to menstruate if they use oral contraception.

**59.** (a) False – unlike in anorexia nervosa (AN), low body weight is not required to diagnose BN and patients may have a normal or even increased body weight.
  (b) True – the overvalued idea of dread of fatness is essential to the diagnosis of both AN and BN.
  (c) True – Russell's sign describes calluses on the back of hands as a result of repeated teeth trauma from self-induced vomiting.

  (d) True – see (a).
  (e) False – repeated vomiting leads to *hypokalaemic*, hypochloraemic alkalosis.

**60.** (a) True – low body weight leads to reduced FSH and LH; this leads to reduced oestrogen production, which can lead to osteoporosis over time.
  (b) True – starvation is associated with the development of fine, downy hair on the trunk – lanugo.
  (c) True – see p. 81.
  (d) False – this occurs subsequent to repeated vomiting, not poor caloric intake.
  (e) True – see (a).

**61.** (a) False – bulimia has a later age of onset.
  (b) False – bulimia is more prevalent in the general population, affecting 1–3 % of young women. Anorexia has a high prevalence in certain subgroups, e.g. models, ballet dancers.
  (c) False – bulimia has an equal socioeconomic class distribution; there is conflicting evidence as to whether AN is more prevalent in higher socioeconomic classes.
  (d) True – see p. 121.
  (e) False – the aetiology of neither anorexia nor bulimia is known.

**62.** (a) True – see p. 121.
  (b) True – see p. 121.
  (c) False – a late age of onset is a poor prognostic factor.
  (d) False – for patients who have lost all insight it may be necessary to enforce life-saving feeding under mental health legislation.
  (e) True – the use of medication is limited.

**63.** (a) True – it is a lack of synchrony between patients' endogenous circadian rhythm for sleep and that demanded by their environment.
  (b) False – OSA is due to obstruction of the upper airways during sleep in spite of adequate respiratory effort.
  (c) False – somnambulism, or sleepwalking, is complex motor behaviour that occurs during sleep.
  (d) False – in night terrors, children wake in a state of extreme terror and panic, after which there is amnesia for the episode and no recall of any dream or nightmare.
  (e) True – e.g. nightmares, night terrors and sleepwalking.

**64.** (a) False – primary sleep disorders are, by definition, not caused by another medical condition, mental illness or use of a substance.
  (b) False – narcolepsy is characterized by a tetrad of attacks of sleep, *cataplexy*, hypnagogic or hypnopompic hallucinations and sleep paralysis.
  (c) False – these are antidepressants with sedative properties.
  (d) False – only about a fifth of depressed patients experience hypersomnia, which is referred to as an *atypical depressive feature*.

(e) True – parasomnias, which are abnormal episodes that occur during sleep or sleep–wake transitions (e.g. night terrors, sleepwalking), may cause both insomnia and hypersomnia.

65. (a) True – see p. 124.
(b) False – it features only mild depression, anxiety or irritability and episodes of weepiness.
(c) False – it is a self-limiting condition that resolves spontaneously and usually only requires reassurance.
(d) True – the lack of association with life events, demographic factors or obstetric events suggests a biological cause, e.g. a fall in progesterone.
(e) True – see p. 124.

66. (a) True – the clinical presentation, past psychiatric history and family history of patients with PP suggest that it is related to BAD.
(b) False – unlike in postnatal depression, psychosocial factors seem less important in the development of PP.
(c) True – see p. 127
(d) True – patients with PP are more likely to have a past psychiatric history of mood disorder.
(e) False – PP develops in about one in 500 childbirths.

67. (a) True – see p. 125.
(b) False – there is a risk of neonatal lithium toxicity as breast milk contains 40% of the maternal lithium concentration.
(c) True – psychosocial factors seem strongly linked to the development of PND, more so than postnatal blues and puerperal psychosis.
(d) False – ECT is a highly effective treatment and results in a rapid improvement, which is important when mother and baby are separated.
(e) True – a previous history of non-pregnancy related depression, PND as well as postnatal blues are risk factors.

68. (a) True – see p. 136.
(b) True – if depression is causing sexual dysfunction, antidepressants may lead to improvement. However, antidepressants may commonly feature sexual dysfunction as a side-effect.
(c) False – the 'squeeze technique' is used in premature ejaculation.
(d) True – see p. 137.
(e) False – this technique focuses on stages of increasing sexual intimacy and pleasurable physical contact as opposed to the goal of achieving orgasm.

69. (a) True – see p. 139.
(b) False – in *transsexualism*, individuals cross-dress in an attempt to live and be accepted as a member of the opposite sex; whereas, in *transvestic fetishism*, individuals are sexually aroused by cross-dressing.
(c) True – see p. 136.
(d) False – this is a description of homosexuality, which is not a disorder. Gender identity disorder (transsexualism) describes a desire to live and be accepted as a member of the opposite sex.

(e) False – this is a description of *sexual masochism*. Sexual sadism describes arousal from the infliction of suffering on others.

70. (a) True – see p. 147.
(b) True – see p. 147.
(c) False – there is no good evidence that indicates that the MMR vaccine results in autism.
(d) True – 75% have significant mental retardation.
(e) False – the male-to-female ratio is approximately 3–5:1, but girls are more seriously affected.

71. (a) False – symptoms should be evident in more than one situation, e.g. at school and at home.
(b) True – the male-to-female ratio is approximately 3–9:1
(c) False – 15% of patients have symptoms persisting into adulthood.
(d) True – see p. 148.
(e) True – effective in up to 75% of cases.

72. (a) True – see p. 149.
(b) False – more boys are affected with a male-to-female ratio of approximately 3–12:1.
(c) False – it is associated with the development of antisocial (dissocial) personality disorder.
(d) True – see p. 149.
(e) False – ODD describes negativistic, defiant and disruptive behaviour *in the absence* of behaviour that violates the law or the basic rights of others.

73. (a) True – normal separation anxiety occurs in well-adjusted children from 6 months to 2 years.
(b) False – SAD may result in school refusal.
(c) True – see p. 150.
(d) False – truancy is associated with conduct disorder.
(e) False – emotional disorders are characterized by depression or anxiety.

74. (a) True – mental retardation is characterized by subaverage intellectual functioning *and* an impaired ability to adapt to the normal demands of daily living.
(b) True – the prevalence of other psychiatric disorders is three to four times higher in patients with mental retardation than in the general population.
(c) True – the male-to-female ratio is approximately 1.5:1.
(d) False – 85% of cases are mild.
(e) False – in 30–40% of cases, no clear aetiology can be determined; specific causes are more likely to be found in patients with severe or profound mental retardation.

75. (a) True – dopamine antagonists such as haloperidol, pimozide and sulpiride are used to treat tics.
(b) False – central nervous system stimulants such as methylphenidate (Ritalin®) are first-line; antidepressants, clonidine and some antipsychotics are considered second-line options.
(c) False – see p. 151.
(d) True – see p. 149.
(e) True – OCD and ADHD are associated with Tourette's syndrome.

**76.** (a) True – see Fig. 23.4, p.152, for all the risk factors.
(b) True – see (a).
(c) False – poor socioeconomic status and overcrowding are risk factors (see (a)).
(d) True – see (a).
(e) False – young, immature parents are a risk factor (see (a)).

**77.** (a) True – see p. 146.
(b) False – they usually manifest within the first few years of life.
(c) True – see p. 148.
(d) False – Rett's syndrome is almost only seen in girls.
(e) True – see p. 148.

**78.** (a) True – the psychiatric conditions associated with violent crime are alcohol and substance misuse, personality disorders (antisocial and borderline), and schizophrenia.
(b) False – there is no association between OCD and violent crime; patients with OCD tend to find violent thoughts or impulses repugnant and rarely act on these.
(c) True – see (a).
(d) True – a past history of violent behaviour is the best predictor of future violent behaviour.
(e) True – see (a).

**79.** (a) True – in England and Wales, children are only deemed legally responsible for their actions after the age of 14 years.
(b) True – in English law, legal insanity is defined in terms of the M'Naghten Rules.
(c) True – in this case, he would be found guilty of manslaughter.
(d) True – this would indicate an automatism – a very rare defence.
(e) False – individuals with schizophrenia are legally responsible for their actions unless proven otherwise; it is not a defence in itself.

**80.** (a) False – the antidepressants are equally effective if prescribed at the correct dose and taken for an adequate length of time.
(b) True – both clomipramine and the SSRIs are effective in OCD.
(c) True – see p. 182
(d) True – see Fig. 27.4 for side-effects of SSRIs.
(e) True – most antidepressants lower the seizure threshold.

**81.** (a) False – lithium is excreted unchanged, almost entirely, by the kidneys.
(b) False – lithium may cause major congenital malformations and is excreted in significant concentration in breast milk.
(c) False – lithium is associated with hypothyroidism and, therefore, high TSH levels.
(d) False – in treatment-resistant depression, lithium may be used to augment antidepressants.
(e) False – unlike the mood stabilizers, valproate and carbamazepine, lithium has no anticonvulsant properties. Lithium toxicity may cause seizures.

**82.** (a) False – benzodiazepines bind to specific benzodiazepine receptors on the $GABA_A$ receptor complex, which results in an increased affinity of the complex for GABA.
(b) False – these are short-acting hypnotics that are indicated for the treatment of insomnia.
(c) False – unlike the benzodiazepines, buspirone is not associated with abuse or dependence.
(d) False – benzodiazepines are seldom fatal in overdose.
(e) False – lorazepam is the only benzodiazepine that has predictable absorption when given intramuscularly.

**83.** (a) False – moclobemide is a *reversible* inhibitor of monoamine oxidase A (RIMA). Therefore, significantly accumulated amines will be metabolized, as they are able to displace the drug from the enzyme.
(b) False – the combination of an MAOI and another antidepressant increases the risk of developing the potentially lethal 'serotonin syndrome'.
(c) False – phenelzine reversibly inhibits monoamine oxidase A.
(d) False – benzodiazepines and MAOIs are usually safe in combination. MAOIs in combination with other antidepressants may result in the serotonin syndrome.
(e) False – pethidine especially is associated with a rapid, severe, potentially fatal interaction.

**84.** (a) True – see p. 188.
(b) False – clozapine has comparatively little activity at $D_2$ receptors.
(c) True – clozapine is virtually devoid of EPSE.
(d) True – for this reason, the anticonvulsant, sodium valproate, is prescribed when clozapine is used in high doses.
(e) True – typical antipsychotics may worsen negative symptoms; whereas, atypical antipsychotics tend to improve them.

**85.** (a) True – see Fig. 27.8, p. 186.
(b) False – chlorpromazine is a phenothiazine with an aliphatic side chain (see (a)).
(c) False – both flupenthixol and zuclopenthixol are thioxanthenes (see (a)).
(d) True – trifluoperazine is a phenothiazine with a piperazine side chain (see (a)).
(e) False – both sulpiride and amisulpride are substituted benzamides (see (a)).

**86.** (a) True – carbamazepine is particularly effective in patients with rapid cycling bipolar affective disorder.
(b) True – both lithium and semisodium valproate (Depakote®) are licensed in the UK for acute mania.
(c) False – lithium, valproate and carbamazepine are all teratogenic.
(d) False – mood stabilizers, especially lithium, tend to reduce the incidence of depressive episodes.
(e) True – lithium, carbamazepine and valproate have serious pharmacokinetic and pharmacodynamic interactions with many other drugs.

**87.** (a) True – breast milk production is due to hyperprolactinaemia.
(b) False – some phenothiazines, e.g. prochlorperazine, are powerful anti-emetics.
(c) True – akathisia is an extra-pyramidal side-effect and describes a subjective feeling of inner restlessness.
(d) False – due to α-adrenergic receptor blockade, conventional antipsychotics tend to cause postural hypotension.
(e) False – certain antipsychotics, e.g. thioridazine, are known to prolong the QT interval on ECG.

**88.** (a) False – acute dystonia should be treated promptly with anticholinergics – i.v./i.m. if necessary.
(b) False – an oculogyric crisis indicates acute dystonia.
(c) True – see p. 188.
(d) False – NMS is characterized by hyperthermia, unstable pulse and blood pressure, fluctuating consciousness and severe muscular rigidity.
(e) False – TD is resistant to treatment and may be worsened by anticholinergics.

**89.** (a) False – naloxone is an opiate receptor antagonist; flumazenil is a benzodiazepine receptor antagonist.
(b) False – it is a long-acting benzodiazepine with a half-life of about 100 hours.
(c) True – see p. 190.
(d) True – this is helpful when intravenous access is difficult; remember that intramuscular absorption of all benzodiazepines, except lorazepam, is unpredictable.
(e) True – the anxiolytic effect of benzodiazepines is immediate.

**90.** (a) False – ECT is an effective treatment for certain types of schizophrenia: catatonic states, positive psychotic symptoms and schizoaffective disorder.
(b) True – see p. 190
(c) False – it may be used first line when depression is life-threatening, e.g. poor fluid intake, strong suicidal ideation, or when a rapid response is necessary, e.g. puerperal psychosis, psychotic features.
(d) True – especially for events surrounding the ECT, that is, newly laid memories.
(e) False – there is very little evidence to support this claim.

**91.** (a) True – the analysis of transference and counter-transference is one of the methods used to make unconscious processes conscious.
(b) True – DBT has shown promising results in the treatment of borderline personality disorder and self-harm.
(c) False – CBT predominantly focuses on present problems; it does not seek to analyse unconscious desires.
(d) True – see p. 195.
(e) False – CBT, which includes exposure therapy and response prevention, is the treatment of choice for OCD.

**92.** (a) True – Freud suggested that the personality consisted of the id, superego and ego.
(b) True – Carl Jung was an important influence on psychodynamic theory.
(c) True – Aaron Beck was the founder of cognitive therapy.
(d) False – automatic thoughts and dysfunctional assumptions are examined in *cognitive therapy*.
(e) True – according to psychoanalytical theory, the analysis of dreams is important to understanding the unconscious mind.

**93.** (a) True – closed questions force patients to choose between one or two word answers.
(b) False – it used to screen for alcohol dependence.
(c) False – *mood* refers to a patient's sustained, subjectively experienced emotional state over a period of time; *affect* means the observed, external expression of emotion.
(d) False – the MMSE is a good tool to screen for cognitive impairment.
(e) True – this is an important part of the risk assessment.

**94.** (a) True – see pp. 176–177.
(b) True – this is a *hierarchical* diagnostic system.
(c) False – they are for the most part compatible.
(d) True – see pp. 176–177.
(e) False – 'neurosis' is a vague term that is rarely used. It is best to use the specific term that accurately describes the condition, e.g. generalized anxiety disorder.

**95.** (a) False – this is a third person auditory hallucination.
(b) False – this delusion is possible in reality, therefore not bizarre.
(c) True – see p. 25.
(d) True – a mannerism is an apparently goal-directed movement (e.g. waving, saluting) that is performed inappropriately.
(e) True – an overvalued idea is a plausible belief that a patient becomes preoccupied to an unreasonable extent.

**96.** (a) True – see p. 202.
(b) True – see p. 202.
(c) True – see p. 203.
(d) False – relatives of patients who are unable to consent cannot give or withhold consent; the responsible medical officer acts in the patient's 'best interests', which may be determined with help from relatives.
(e) False – a serious mental illness does not preclude a patient from having the capacity to consent to physical treatment, as long as this illness does not interfere with the understanding of relevant information and the decision-making process.

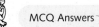 

**97.** (a) True – see p. 200.
    (b) False – Section 3 lasts for 6 months unless it is renewed.
    (c) True – see p. 200.
    (d) False – two doctors, one of whom must be Section 12 approved, and an approved social worker are required.
    (e) True – see p. 202.

**98.** (a) True – it is left as a 'matter for clinical judgement'.
    (b) False – the MHA does not regard dependence on alcohol or drugs, promiscuity, sexual deviancy or 'immoral conduct' alone as evidence of a mental disorder.
    (c) True – see pp. 201–202.
    (d) True – discharge from Section is at the discretion of the responsible medical officer.
    (e) False – the MHA only allows for compulsory treatment of mental, not physical, disorders.

**99.** (a) True – see p. 205.
    (b) False – the CPA applies to all patients under secondary psychiatric care.
    (c) True – see p. 205.
    (d) True – see p. 205.
    (e) False – it applies to community-, hospital- and prison-based patients.

**100.** (a) False – most mentally ill patients are managed in the community (see p. 205.)
    (b) False – 95% of all mental illness is managed in primary care.
    (c) False – with the advent of community psychiatry and closure of the old asylums, institutionalization has declined.
    (d) True – see p. 206.
    (e) False – a CMHT is a multidisciplinary team that includes psychiatrists, nurses, social workers, psychologists, occupational therapists and support workers.

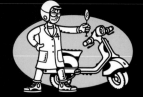
1. **Mood symptoms**

1. **H – Anhedonia**. Anhedonia describes the loss of ability to derive pleasure from activities that were formerly enjoyed. It is one of the core symptoms of depression and is one of the eight symptoms of the somatic syndrome.

2. **C – Blunted affect**. Affect is the *observed, external expression of emotion* – as perceived by another person. There are two components to consider when assessing affect:
   - The appropriateness or congruity of the observed affect to the patient's subjectively reported mood.
   - The range of affect or range of emotional expressivity. In this sense affect may be:
     a. Within the normal range
     b. *Blunted*: a noticeable reduction in the normal intensity of emotional expression as evidenced by a monotonous voice and minimal facial expression
     c. *Flat*: very little or no emotional expression.

3. **I – Mixed affective episode**. *Mixed affective episodes* occur when a patient presents with rapidly alternating manic (elated mood, pressure of speech) and depressive symptoms (tearfulness, psychomotor retardation).

4. **J – Tangential speech**. Tangential speech is characterized by the speaker diverting from the initial train of thought but never returning to the original point, jumping tangentially from one topic to the next. Circumstantial (over-inclusive) speech, on the other hand, means speech that is delayed in reaching its final goal because of the over-inclusion of details and unnecessary asides and diversions; however, the speaker, if allowed to finish, does eventually connect the original starting point to the desired destination.

5. **D – Psychomotor agitation**. The term 'psychomotor' is used to describe a patient's motor activity as a consequence of their concurrent mental processes. Psychomotor changes in depression include *retardation* (slow, monotonous speech; long pauses before answering questions or muteness; leaden body movements and limited facial expression, i.e. blunted affect) and *agitation* (inability to sit still; fidgeting, pacing or hand-wringing; rubbing or scratching skin or clothes).

2. **Psychotic symptoms**

1. **J – Running commentary, third person auditory hallucinations**. *Third person auditory hallucinations* occur when patients hear a voice or voices speaking about them, referring to them in the third person. This may take the form of two or more voices arguing or discussing the patient among themselves; or one or more voices giving a *running commentary* on the patient's thoughts or actions.

2. **C – Lilliputian hallucinations**. This man is confused and drowsy and is experiencing visual hallucinations, which probably indicates a delirium, most likely due to alcohol withdrawal. *Lilliputian hallucinations* are visual hallucinations of miniature people or animals, typically seen in alcohol withdrawal delirium.

3. **E – Hypnagogic hallucinations**. This woman, when trying to fall asleep, is probably having auditory hallucinations. *Hypnagogic* hallucinations are false perceptions in any modality (usually auditory or visual) that occur as a person goes to sleep; whereas, *hypnopompic* hallucinations occur as a person awakens. These occur in normal people and are not indicative of psychopathology.

4. **H – Nihilistic delusion**. A nihilistic delusion is a false belief that oneself, others or the world is non-existent or about to end. In severe cases, negation is carried to the extreme with patients claiming that nothing, including themselves, exists. Nihilistic delusions commonly occur in severe depressive conditions, where it is regarded as a mood-congruent delusion.

5. **F – Word salad**. Loosening of association (derailment/knight's move thinking) occurs when the patient's train of thought shifts suddenly from one very loosely or unrelated idea to the next. In its worst form, speech becomes a mixture of incoherent words and phrases and is termed *word salad*. Loosening of association is characteristic of schizophrenia. Some psychiatrists use the term *formal thought disorder* synonymously with loosening of association.

3. **Anxiety**

1. **G – Generalized (free-floating) anxiety**. Generalized (free-floating) anxiety does not occur in discrete episodes and tends to last for hours, days or even longer and is of mild to moderate severity. It is not associated with a specific external threat or situation (i.e. free-floating) but is rather excessive worry or apprehension about many normal life events (e.g. job security, relationships and responsibilities). It is the key element of generalized anxiety disorder.

2. **D – Agoraphobia**. Agoraphobia is a fear of entering crowded spaces (shops, trains, buses, elevators) where an immediate escape is difficult, or in which help might not be available in the event of having a panic attack. At the worst extreme, patients may become housebound or refuse to leave the house unless accompanied by a close friend or relative. Studies have shown that up to 95% of patients presenting with agoraphobia have a current or past diagnosis of panic disorder.

3. **J – Somatization disorder**. The essential feature of somatization disorder is multiple, recurrent, frequently changing physical symptoms. They should be present for at least 2 years with no adequate physical explanation found. Patients with this disorder

persistently refuse to accept reassurance from doctors that there is no physical cause for their symptoms. Somatization disorder should be distinguished from *hypochondriacal disorder*, where patients believe that they have a serious and progressive physical disease.

4. **I – Obsessions**. Obsessions are involuntary *thoughts, images or impulses*, which have the following characteristics:
  * They are recurrent and intrusive and are experienced by patients as unpleasant or distressing.
  * They enter the mind against conscious resistance. Patients try to resist but are unable to do so.
  * Patients recognize obsessions as being the product of their own mind even though they are involuntary and often repugnant.

  Obsessions are not merely excessive concerns about normal life problems and patients generally retain insight into the fact that their thoughts are irrational. In fact, patients often see their obsessions as foreign to, or against, their 'essence' (*ego-dystonic* or *ego-alien*) – as in this case.

5. **B – Specific phobia**. A *phobia* is an intense, irrational fear of an object, activity or situation (e.g. flying, heights, animals, blood, public speaking). Although they may recognize that their fear is irrational, patients characteristically avoid the phobic stimulus or endure it with extreme distress. It is the degree of fear that is irrational in that the feared objects or situations are not inevitably dangerous and do not cause such severe anxiety in most other people. Specific (simple) phobias are restricted to clearly specific and discernible objects or situations.

## 4. Dementia

1. **F – Vascular dementia**. This man has two serious risk factors for cerebrovascular disease (diabetes mellitus, hypertension), and, on clinical examination, appears to have had a stroke (facial nerve palsy, dysarthria). Furthermore, an uneven or stepwise deterioration in cognitive function is characteristic of vascular dementia. Note that vascular dementia and Alzheimer's disease often occur together.

2. **C – Dementia with Lewy bodies (DLB)**. DLB is characterized by:
  * Day to day (or shorter) fluctuations in cognitive performance.
  * Recurrent visual hallucinations.
  * Spontaneous motor signs of parkinsonism (rigidity, bradykinesia, tremor).
  * Recurrent falls and syncope.
  * Transient disturbances of consciousness.

  Additionally, 50% of patients with dementia with Lewy bodies (DLB) will have a catastrophic reaction to antipsychotics (even atypicals) precipitating irreversible parkinsonism, impaired consciousness, severe autonomic symptoms and a two- to threefold increase in mortality. Benzodiazepines and cholinesterase inhibitors are safer in this group of patients.

3. **A – Alzheimer's disease**. Alzheimer's disease accounts for up to 60% of all cases of dementia. It has a gradual onset and features a progressive cognitive decline with aphasia, agnosia and apraxia. Speech and motor function is usually preserved until late. It is usually diagnosed by exclusion of other causes of dementia. The duration of survival from the time of diagnosis is about 7–9 years.

4. **B – Frontotemporal dementia**. The frontotemporal dementias account for up to 20% of presenile (<65 years) dementia cases. They are characterized by:
  * Early decline in social and personal conduct (disinhibition, tactlessness).
  * Early emotional blunting.
  * Attenuated speech output, echolalia, perseveration, mutism.
  * Early loss of insight.
  * Relative sparing of other cognitive functions.

  They are associated with bilateral atrophy of the frontal and anterior temporal lobes (atrophied paper-thin gyri known as 'knife-blade atrophy'). There are three main histological types (60% – microvacuolar; 25% – Pick's type; 15% – microvacuolar/Pick's type combined with histological signs of motor neuron disease). Pick's bodies are intraneuronal masses of cytoskeletal elements.

5. **H – Depressive pseudodementia**. *Depressive pseudodementia* is the term used when patients present with clinical features resembling a dementia that results from an underlying depression (also called *depression-related cognitive dysfunction*). Depressive pseudodementia is differentiated from dementia by the abrupt onset of cognitive impairment with relatively normal premorbid functioning in association with depressive symptoms. The situation usually responds to antidepressant treatment.

## 5. Substance misuse

1. **D, J – Thiamine, chlordiazepoxide**. In order to ameliorate severe symptoms and reduce the risk of developing seizures or a delirium, a drug with cross-tolerance to alcohol is prescribed, usually in the form of the benzodiazepine, chlordiazepoxide (diazepam and lorazepam are also effective). Initially, high doses are given (up to 40 – 60 mg four times daily), but this is tapered down over 5 to 7 days. In order to avert a Wernicke's encephalopathy, thiamine (vitamin B$_1$) supplements are also administered.

2. **B, G – Lysergic acid diethylamine (LSD), ketamine**. Lysergic acid diethylamine (LSD, acid) is classified as a hallucinogen and is associated with marked perceptual disturbances (also chronic flashbacks), paranoid ideas, and suicidal and homicidal ideas. Ketamine is an anaesthetic agent and is associated with hallucinations, paranoid ideas, thought disorganization and aggression.

3. **C, F – Disulfiram, acamprosate**. Disulfiram leads to an unpleasant systemic reaction after the ingestion of alcohol. It blocks alcohol oxidation, which leads to an accumulation of acetaldehyde. This causes anxiety, flushing, palpitations, headache, and a choking sensation within 20 minutes of alcohol consumption. Acamprosate enhances GABA transmission and appears to reduce the likelihood of relapse after detoxification by reducing craving. Note: although naltrexone is not licensed in the UK for this purpose, it is also used in the treatment of alcohol dependence as it has been shown to reduce craving and relapse rates.

4. **E, H – Methadone, buprenorphine**. Patients with opiate dependence may be offered substitution therapy by converting to the longer-acting oral opiate methadone. It helps stabilize the user's life and prevents the complications of injecting. Methadone may be prescribed indefinitely, but the aim should be gradual reduction with long-term abstinence. Sublingual buprenorphine (Subutex®), a partial opiate agonist, is also used as substitution therapy for patients with moderate dependence. The dose is then gradually reduced to avoid a precipitous withdrawal syndrome.

5. **A, I – Naltrexone, flumazenil**. Naltrexone is an opiate antagonist that is sometimes used to block the euphoriant effects of any continued opiate use in patients who have been detoxified. It induces withdrawal if the patient is still dependent. Flumazenil is a benzodiazepine antagonist, which may be helpful in differentiating benzodiazepine-induced loss of consciousness from other causes. It may precipitate severe withdrawal symptoms in patients dependent on benzodiazepines.

6. **Psychiatric diagnoses**

1. **G – Bipolar affective disorder**. This man has had four depressive episodes and one episode of hypomania. A patient presenting with a second episode of a major mood disturbance (depression or mania) should be diagnosed as having *recurrent depressive disorder* or *bipolar affective disorder*. If a patient has had at least one hypomanic, manic or mixed affective episode in association with any kind of past mood episode (hypomanic, manic, depressive, mixed), then bipolar affective disorder is the correct diagnosis.

2. **E – Mania with psychotic symptoms**. This young woman presents with typical symptoms of mania (elevated mood, insomnia, increased energy). She also has psychotic symptoms in the form of mood-congruent grandiose delusions. The absence of typical symptoms (first-rank symptoms) of schizophrenia precludes a diagnosis of schizoaffective disorder.

3. **J – Schizoaffective disorder**. A diagnosis of schizoaffective disorder is made when patients present with both mood (depression or mania) symptoms and typical schizophrenic symptoms within the same episode of illness. The mood symptoms should meet the criteria for either a depressive or manic episode. Patients should also have at least one, preferably two, of the typical schizophrenic symptoms – symptoms (a) to (d) – as specified in the ICD-10 schizophrenia diagnostic guidelines (see Fig. 4.5). These symptoms should occur simultaneously or at least within a few days of each other.

4. **H – Paranoid schizophrenia**. The presence of bizarre delusions and auditory hallucinations in the absence of prominent mood symptoms indicates a diagnosis of schizophrenia. Prominent positive symptoms (persecutory delusions and hallucinations) in the relative absence of thought disorganization, or negative or catatonic symptoms indicate the paranoid subtype.

5. **A – Cyclothymia**. Cyclothymia usually begins in early adulthood and follows a chronic course with intermittent periods of wellness in between. It is characterized by an instability of mood resulting in alternating periods of mild elation and mild depression, none of which are sufficiently severe or long enough to meet the criteria for either a hypomanic or a depressive episode.

7. **Epidemiology of mental illness**

1. **D – 10–25%**. The lifetime risk of recurrent depressive disorder is 10–25% in women, and 5–12% in men.

2. **B – 1%**. The lifetime risk of bipolar affective disorder in *both* men and women is about 1%.

3. **B – 1%**. The lifetime risk of schizophrenia in *both* men and women is about 1%.

4. **F – 50%**. The concordance rate of schizophrenia for monozygotic twins is 50%. This suggests that although there is a significant genetic factor involved, there must be an environmental factor contributing to the development of schizophrenia as well.

5. **C – 5%**. The prevalence of dementia in persons aged 65 or over is approximately 5% and in those over 80 about 20%. The overall prevalence of dementia in the UK population is approximately 0.3%.

6. **F – 50%**. Postnatal blues (baby blues) occurs in about 50% of postpartum women. The prevalence of postnatal blues, postnatal depression and puerperal psychosis is inversely related to their severity:
   - Postnatal blues develops after one in two childbirths.
   - Postnatal depression develops after one in eight childbirths.
   - Puerperal psychosis develops after about one in 500 childbirths.

8. **Psychiatric medication in context**

1. **J – Fluoxetine**. SSRIs, e.g. fluoxetine, are first choice antidepressants for patients with cardiac disease due to their relative paucity of cardiac side-effects. Tricyclic antidepressants are associated with arrhythmias and postural hypotension. MAOIs and the RIMA, moclobemide, are associated with hypertension. Note that during the first 6 months post-infarction, patients who develop depression have a fivefold increase in mortality.

2. **C – Lorazepam**. The pharmacological treatment of alcohol withdrawal delirium (delirium tremens) is with large doses of benzodiazepines, preferably chlordiazepoxide. However, when patients refuse, or are unable, to take oral medication, parenteral administration becomes necessary, usually with diazepam or lorazepam (chlordiazepoxide only available in oral preparations). While both lorazepam and diazepam may be given intravenously, only lorazepam has predictable absorption when given intramuscularly.

3. **G – Clozapine**. According to the National Institute for Clinical Excellence (NICE), treatment-resistant schizophrenia is defined as a lack of satisfactory clinical improvement despite the sequential use of at least two antipsychotics for 6–8 weeks, one of which should be an atypical. In these instances, patients should be started on clozapine at the earliest opportunity.

4. **D – Lithium**. Strategies used in managing treatment-resistant depression include augmenting the current

antidepressant with lithium or another antidepressant. Pindolol (a beta-blocker), tri-iodothyronine ($T_3$) and L-tryptophan are also used as augmenting agents.

5. **I – Procyclidine**. Common side-effects with conventional antipsychotics such as flupentixol are parkinsonian motor symptoms. These include muscular rigidity, bradykinesia (lack of, or slowing, of movement) and resting tremor. Anticholinergics, e.g. procyclidine, are the treatment of choice. Also, one should consider reducing the dose of the antipsychotic or switching to an atypical antipsychotic.

### 9. Side-effects of psychiatric medication

1. **F – Agranulocytosis**. The atypical antipsychotic, clozapine, is a very effective antipsychotic, which is used in treatment-resistant schizophrenia. However, it is associated with the life-threatening risk of bone marrow suppression with agranulocytosis in about 1% of patients. Typical symptoms include fever, chills, myalgia, headache, abdominal pain and a sore throat. Patients should be registered with a clozapine monitoring service and have a full blood count (FBC) with differential before starting treatment. This is followed by regular FBCs in an out-patient clinic.

2. **H – Hypertensive crisis**. Phenelzine is an MAOI. Its inhibition of monoamine oxidase A results in the accumulation of amine neurotransmitters and impairs the metabolism of some amines found in certain drugs (e.g. decongestants) and foodstuffs (e.g. tyramine). Because MAOIs bind *irreversibly* to monoamine oxidase A, amines may accumulate to dangerously high levels, which may precipitate a life-threatening hypertensive crisis. An early warning sign is a throbbing headache.

3. **E – Acute dystonia**. Acute dystonia, which is more common in young men, usually develops within the first 5 days of treatment with conventional antipsychotics. It is characterized by involuntary sustained muscular contractions or spasms, e.g. neck (spasmodic torticollis), clenched jaw (trismus), protruding tongue, and eyes rolled upwards and to the side (oculogyric crisis).

4. **I – Prolongation of QT-interval**. Tricyclic antidepressants and certain antipsychotics (e.g. phenothiazines, butyrophenones, pimozide, zotepine) can cause a dose-related prolongation of the QT interval. Therefore, patients who take these drugs in combination or in high doses should be screened for cardiac disease with at least an ECG. A corrected QT-interval (QTc) of above 450 ms is concerning; a QTc above 500 ms may lead to torsade de pointes, which may be fatal.

5. **A – Tardive dyskinesia**. Tardive dyskinesia develops in up to 20% of patients who receive long-term treatment with conventional antipsychotics. It is characterized by rhythmic, involuntary movements of the head, limbs and trunk, e.g. chewing, grimacing of the mouth and protruding, darting movements of the tongue.

### 10. Mental state examination

1. **E – Panic attack**. Panic attacks are discrete episodes of short-lived (usually less than 1 hour), intense anxiety. They have an abrupt onset and rapidly build up to a peak level of anxiety. They are accompanied by strong autonomic symptoms, which may lead patients to believe that they are dying, having a heart attack or going mad.

2. **B – Second person auditory hallucinations**. Second person auditory hallucinations occur when patients hear a voice or voices talking directly to them. They can be persecutory, highly critical, or complimentary. They may issue commands to the patient (command hallucinations). Second person hallucinations are often associated with mood disorders with psychotic features and so will be critical or persecutory in a depressed patient, or complimentary in a manic patient, i.e. mood-congruent hallucinations.

3. **D – Persecutory delusions**. A persecutory delusion is a false belief that one is being harmed, threatened, cheated, harassed or is a victim of a conspiracy.

4. **F – Delusions of control**. A delusion of control, also called passivity or 'made' experience, is a false belief that one's thoughts, feelings, actions or impulses are controlled or 'made' by an external agency, e.g. believing that one was made to break a window by demons. This is a first-rank symptom of schizophrenia.

5. **H – Delusions of reference**. A delusion of reference is a false belief that certain objects, people or events have intense personal significance and refer specifically to oneself, e.g. believing that a television newsreader is talking directly about one.

6. **A – Flight of ideas**. A manic patient may subjectively experience their thoughts or ideas racing even faster than they can articulate them. When thoughts are rapidly associating in this way, in a stream of connected concepts, it is termed *flight of ideas*. When patients have an irrepressible need to express these thoughts verbally, making them difficult to interrupt, it is termed *pressure of speech*.

1. (a) Anhedonia means an inability to derive pleasure or excitement from any activities.
   (b) Further biological or somatic symptoms of depression include:
      - Reduced emotional reactivity.
      - Early morning awakening.
      - Depression worse in the morning.
      - Psychomotor retardation or agitation.
      - Marked loss of appetite.
      - Weight loss.
      - Loss of libido.

2. (a) *Deliberate self-harm* is the blanket term used to mean any intentional act done in the knowledge that it was potentially harmful and includes self-poisoning (overdosing), self-injury (cutting, slashing, burning) and any other form of self-harm. *Suicide* is the act of intentionally and successfully ending one's own life, while, *parasuicide* is the term used to denote an unsuccessful suicide attempt. Suicide and parasuicide are both subsets of deliberate self-harm.
   (b) Strong suicide intent is suggested by the following:
      - The attempt was planned in advance.
      - Precautions were taken to avoid discovery or rescue.
      - A dangerous method was used.
      - No help was sought after the act.

3. (a) Delusions of control (also called passivity or 'made' experiences) is the term used to describe the false belief that one's thoughts, feelings, actions or impulses are controlled or 'made' by an external agency, e.g. believing that God is in control of all of one's choices.
   (b) According to Kurt Schneider, the presence of one or more first-rank symptoms in the absence of organic disease suggests the diagnosis of schizophrenia. First-rank symptoms are described in Fig. 4.6, p. 000.

4. (a) Generalized (free-floating) anxiety does not occur in discrete episodes and tends to last for hours, days or even longer and is of mild to moderate severity. It is not associated with a specific external threat or situation (i.e. free-floating) but is rather excessive worry or apprehension about many normal life events (e.g. job security, relationships and responsibilities). The anxiety experienced in panic attacks has an abrupt onset, occurs in discrete, short-lived episodes and is severe with strong autonomic symptoms.
   (b) The following conditions frequently feature panic attacks:
      - Panic disorder.
      - Phobic disorders, e.g. agoraphobia, social phobia, specific phobia.
      - Post-traumatic stress disorder.

5. (a) Obsessions are involuntary *thoughts*, *images* or *impulses* that:
      - Are recurrent and intrusive and experienced by patients as unpleasant or distressing.
      - Enter the mind against conscious resistance.
      - Are recognized by patients as being the product of their own mind.

   Compulsions are repetitive *mental operations* (counting, praying or repeating a mantra silently) or *physical acts* (checking, seeking reassurance, handwashing, strict rituals) that:

      - Patients feel compelled to perform in response to their own obsessions or irrationally defined 'rules'.
      - Are performed to reduce anxiety through the belief that they will prevent a 'dreaded event' from occurring, even though they are not realistically connected to the event.
      - Are experienced as unpleasant and are, therefore, resisted.
   (b) The following questions may be useful in eliciting obsessions and compulsions:
      - Do you worry about contamination with dirt even when you have already washed?
      - Do you have awful thoughts entering your mind despite you trying hard to keep them out?
      - Do you repeatedly have to check things that you have already done (stoves, lights, taps, etc.)?
      - Do you find that you have to arrange, touch or count things many times over?

6. (a) In the somatoform disorders, the physical symptoms are not under voluntary control, that is, they occur *unintentionally*, as opposed to the *intentional* feigning or production of symptoms that occur in both factitious disorder and malingering. Factitious disorder and malingering are differentiated by the patient's *motivation* for simulating symptoms. In factitious disorder (Munchausen's syndrome), patients are focused on the *primary internal gain* of assuming the sick role, that is, their only aim is to be treated like a patient and to be hospitalized. In malingering, patients are focused on a *secondary external gain*; they seek the secondary consequence of being diagnosed with an illness, e.g. avoidance of military service or evading criminal prosecution.
   (b) Somatization disorder and hypochondriacal disorder are the most common of the somatoform disorders. In somatization disorder, patients express concern about numerous physical symptoms, whereas in hypochondriacal disorder, patients misinterpret normal bodily sensations, which lead them to believe that they have a serious and progressive physical disease.

**7.** (a) It is useful to describe patients presenting with an impairment of cognition in terms of one of three commonly occurring syndromes: dementia, delirium and the amnesic syndrome. A delirium is characterized by an acute impairment of consciousness with cognitive deficits. A dementia is characterized by multiple cognitive deficits, including memory, without an impairment of consciousness. An amnesic syndrome is characterized by memory impairment in the absence of other significant cognitive deficits. See Fig. 9.7 for further factors differentiating delirium from dementia.

(b) See Fig. 7.1, p. 000 for the management of delirium tremens.

**8.** The alcohol dependence syndrome describes a repeated cluster of symptoms and signs that occur in regular heavy drinkers. It was first described by Edwards and Gross (1976) and includes:
- Narrowing of repertoire.
- Increased salience of drinking.
- Increased tolerance to alcohol.
- Withdrawal symptoms.
- Relief or avoidance of withdrawal symptoms by further drinking.
- Subjective awareness of the compulsion to drink.
- Rapid reinstatement after abstinence.

See Fig. 10.4 for a detailed description of each characteristic.

**9.** (a) A personality disorder is said to exist when an individual has personality traits that are persistently inflexible and maladaptive, stable over time and which cause significant personal distress or functional impairment. Personality traits are enduring patterns of perceiving, thinking about and relating to the environment and oneself that are exhibited in a wide range of social and personal contexts.

(b) The DSM-IV has designated three personality clusters based on general similarities. Cluster B, which includes borderline, antisocial (dissocial), histrionic and narcissistic personality disorders, describes individuals who appear dramatic, emotional or erratic. Cluster A includes paranoid, schizoid and schizotypal personality disorders, and describes individuals who appear odd or eccentric. Cluster C includes avoidant, dependent and obsessive-compulsive (anankastic) personality disorders, and describes individuals who appear anxious or fearful.

**10.** (a) A diagnosis of anorexia nervosa requires ***all*** of the following:
- Low body weight (BMI ≤17.5 kg/m$^2$).
- Self-induced weight loss (poor caloric intake, vomiting, exercise, etc.).
- Overvalued idea: dread of fatness; low target weight.
- Endocrine disturbance (amenorrhoea, raised cortisol, growth hormone, etc.).

(b) Electrolyte abnormalities from repeated vomiting include:
- Hypokalaemia.
- Hypochloraemia.
- Alkalosis.
- Hyponatraemia.
- Hypomagnesaemia.

**11.** (a) Cyclothymia is a chronic condition characterized by an instability of mood resulting in alternating periods of mild elation and mild depression, none of which are sufficiently severe or long enough to meet the criteria for either a hypomanic or a depressive episode.

(b) Elderly patients have an increased sensitivity to central nervous system drugs. Therefore, the common side-effects of tricyclic antidepressants will be amplified. These include:
- Anticholinergic effects: dry mouth, constipation, urinary retention, blurred vision.
- $\alpha$-Adrenergic receptor blockade: postural hypotension (dizziness, syncope).
- Histaminergic receptor blockade: weight gain, sedation.
- Cardiotoxic effects: QT interval prolongation, arrhythmias.

**12.** (a) The term 'psychomotor' is used to describe a patient's motor activity as a consequence of their concurrent mental processes. Examples of psychomotor agitation include:
- Being unable to sit still.
- Fidgeting or hand-wringing.
- Frequently standing up and pacing around the room.
- Gesticulating expansively.
- Aggressive or threatening behaviour.

(b) Common causes of acute agitation include: schizophrenia, drug-induced psychosis, mania, alcohol and substance intoxication or withdrawal, dementia, delirium (due to any physical causes), mental retardation (learning disability) and personality disorder.

**13.** (a) The atypical antipsychotics were initially so called because they failed to induce catalepsy (an extra-pyramidal syndrome) when given to animals, as the typical antipsychotics were known to do. 'Atypicals' thus became antipsychotics that were mostly devoid of extra-pyramidal motor effects; the first of these was clozapine. Today, the term atypical has additional meanings. It can also refer to the action of alleviating both negative and positive symptoms, as well as to the capacity to block serotonin 2A (5-HT2$_A$) receptors – a property of most of the atypical agents introduced to date.

(b) See Fig. 27.10: Antipsychotic-induced extra-pyramidal side-effects and treatment.

(c) See Fig. 27.10: Antipsychotic-induced extra-pyramidal side-effects and treatment.

**14.** (a) Postnatal blues, postnatal depression and puerperal psychosis.

(b) • Postnatal blues develops after one in two childbirths.
  • Postnatal depression develops after one in eight childbirths.
  • Puerperal psychosis develops after about one in 500 childbirths.
(c) Puerperal psychotic episodes characteristically have a rapid onset, usually between day 4 to 3 weeks post-delivery and almost always within 8 weeks. They often begin with insomnia, restlessness and perplexity, later progressing to suspiciousness and marked confusion with psychotic symptoms. These symptoms often fluctuate dramatically in their nature and intensity over a short space of time. In 80% of cases, the clinical presentation resembles a mood disorder (depression or mania) with delusions and hallucinations.

15. (a) The ICD-10 groups the psychiatric disorders in children and adolescents into four broad categories:
  • Mental retardation (learning disability).
  • Developmental disorders (specific and pervasive).
  • Acquired disorders with onset usually in childhood or adolescence.
  • Acquired 'adult' disorders with onset in childhood or adolescence.

Fig. 23.1, p. 000, provides an overview of the conceptual framework for other disorders of childhood and adolescence.

(b) The three main characteristics of autism are:
  • Impairment in social interaction.
  • Impairment in communication.
  • Restricted, stereotyped interests and behaviours.
(c) School refusal is the refusal to go to school because of anxiety in spite of parental pressure. It may be caused by separation anxiety (younger children) or be a symptom of another mental illness such as depression, adjustment disorder (change from junior to secondary school) or social phobia. Truancy, on the other hand, is an absence from school by choice and is associated with conduct disorder, poor academic performance, family history of antisocial behaviour and large family size.

16. (a) *Mood* refers to a patient's sustained, subjectively experienced emotional state over a period of time. In the context of the mental state examination *affect* means the observed, external expression of emotion – as perceived by another person; affect is sometimes called the 'objective' assessment of mood.
(b) There are two components to consider when assessing affect:
  • The appropriateness or congruity of the observed affect to the patient's subjectively reported mood, e.g. a schizophrenic woman

with a smiling face who reports feeling suicidal would be described as having as *incongruous* affect.
  • The range of affect. In this sense affect may be:
   i) Within the normal range
   ii) *Blunted*: a noticeable reduction in the normal intensity of emotional expression as evidenced by a monotonous voice and minimal facial expression
   iii) *Flat*: very little or no emotional expression.
(c) A *labile* mood refers to a fluctuating mood state that alternates between extremes, e.g. a young man with a mixed affective episode alternates between feeling overjoyed with pressure of speech and miserable with suicidal ideation.

17. (a) ECT is considered for the following forms of depression:
  • With life-threatening poor fluid intake.
  • With strong suicide intent.
  • With psychotic features or stupor.
  • When antidepressants are ineffective or not tolerated.
(b) The mortality from ECT is the same as that for any minor surgical procedure under general anaesthesia. Loss of memory is a common complaint, particularly for events surrounding the ECT. However, some patients may have impairment of some autobiographical memory. Memory impairment might be reduced by unilateral electrode placement (as opposed to bilateral). Minor complaints such as confusion, headache, nausea and muscle pains are experienced by 80% of patients. Anaesthetic complications (e.g. arrhythmias, aspiration) can be reduced by good preoperative assessment. Prolonged seizures may occur, especially in patients who are on drugs that lower the seizure threshold, e.g. antidepressants and antipsychotics.
(c) Although ECT is an effective treatment for established mania, it may precipitate a manic episode in patients with bipolar affective disorder.

18. (a) Lithium is used in the treatment of:
  • Acute mania.
  • Prophylaxis of bipolar of affective disorder (prevention of relapse).
  • Treatment-resistant depression (lithium augmentation).
  • Schizoaffective disorder and schizophrenia (as an adjunct to standard treatment).
  • Aggression/impulsivity.
(b) Common side-effects include:
  • Thirst, polydipsia, polyuria.
  • Weight gain, oedema.
  • Tremor.
  • Precipitates or worsens skin problems.
  • Concentration and memory problems.
  • Hypothyroidism.
  • Impaired renal function.
  • Teratogenicity.

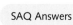

(c) The following investigations are needed prior to initiating lithium therapy:
- Full blood count.
- Renal function and electrolytes.
- Thyroid function.
- Pregnancy test.
- ECG.

(d) Blood levels are monitored weekly after starting treatment until a therapeutic level has been stable for 4 weeks. Lithium blood levels should then be monitored every 3 months; renal function every 6 months; and thyroid functions every 12 months.

**19.** (a) *Primary insomnia* is diagnosed when patients present with insomnia for at least a month not attributable to a medical condition, psychiatric disorder, use of a substance or other dyssomnia or parasomnia.

(b) The assessment of insomnia involves excluding a medical, psychiatric or substance-related cause of insomnia. Many cases of primary insomnia are related to poor sleep hygiene. Therefore it is essential to enquire about sleeping times, daytime sleeping, drinking of coffee, erratic sleeping hours, etc. It is also useful to obtain collateral information from the patient's sleeping partner regarding sleeping patterns, snoring and movements during the night. The most important aspect of management is providing education about correct sleep hygiene. Sleep hygiene, which is described in Fig. 21.3, includes a number of non-specific, non-pharmacological measures that should lead to an improvement in sleep.

There is a limited role for medication in the treatment of primary insomnia. Hypnotics may help with sleep in the short-term, but the development of tolerance to their effects (usually within 2 weeks), possible dependence, and their propensity to cause rebound insomnia limit their use. Therefore, they should only be prescribed on a time-limited basis, ideally for use on alternate or occasional nights rather than every night. Short-acting benzodiazepines (e.g. temazepam) are preferred, as they do not leave patients feeling drowsy the next day and do not accumulate with repeated doses. The related short-acting compounds: zopiclone, zolpidem and zaleplon, which act on receptors similar to the benzodiazepines, are also very effective in the short term.

**20.** (a) Both Sections 2 and 3 are civil Sections that make provision for compulsory admission to hospital.

Patients are admitted under Section 2 for *assessment*. It is used when the diagnosis is uncertain and the response to treatment unknown. It has a duration of 28 days and may be converted to a Section 3 if a longer admission is needed. Medication may be given as part of the assessment process. The application for this Section is made by the nearest relative or an approved social worker (ASW). It also requires the recommendation of two doctors, one of whom should be Section 12 approved. It is recommended that one of the doctors has had previous acquaintance with the patient (this is usually the patient's general practitioner).

Patients are admitted under Section 3 for *treatment*. It is used when the diagnosis and treatment response have already been established. It has a duration of 6 months, but may be extended at 6-monthly intervals if necessary. The application and recommendation requirements are the same as for Section 2.

(b) Section 5(2) is a doctor's holding power that enables the detention of a hospital in-patient receiving any form of treatment in order to allow time for a Section 2 or 3 to be completed. It lasts for 72 hours and is enacted by the doctor responsible for patient's care (RMO) or another doctor nominated by the RMO.

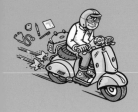

# Index